INSIDER SECRETS

THEY DON'T WANT YOU TO KNOW!

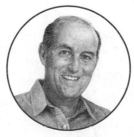

www.jerrybaker.com

Other Jerry Baker Books:

Jerry Baker's Homespun Magic
Grandma Putt's Old-Time Vinegar, Garlic, Baking Soda,
  and 101 More Problem Solvers
Jerry Baker's Supermarket Super Products!
Jerry Baker's It Pays to Be Cheap!

Grandma Putt's Home Health Remedies
Nature's Best Miracle Medicines
Jerry Baker's Supermarket Super Remedies
Jerry Baker's The New Healing Foods
Jerry Baker's Cut Your Health Care Bills in Half!
Jerry Baker's Amazing Antidotes
Jerry Baker's Anti-Pain Plan
Jerry Baker's Oddball Ointments, Powerful Potions,
  and Fabulous Folk Remedies
Jerry Baker's Giant Book of Kitchen Counter Cures

Jerry Baker's Supermarket Super Gardens
Jerry Baker's Dear God...Please Help It Grow!
Secrets from the Jerry Baker Test Gardens
Jerry Baker's All-American Lawns
Jerry Baker's Bug Off!
Jerry Baker's Terrific Garden Tonics!
Jerry Baker's Giant Book of Garden Solutions
Jerry Baker's Backyard Problem Solver
Jerry Baker's Green Grass Magic
Jerry Baker's Great Green Book of Garden Secrets
Jerry Baker's Old-Time Gardening Wisdom

Jerry Baker's Backyard Birdscaping Bonanza
Jerry Baker's Backyard Bird Feeding Bonanza
Jerry Baker's Year-Round Bloomers
Jerry Baker's Flower Garden Problem Solver
Jerry Baker's Perfect Perennials!

To order any of the above, or for more information on Jerry Baker's
amazing home, health, and garden tips, tricks, and tonics, please write to:

Jerry Baker, P.O. Box 805
New Hudson, MI 48165

Or, visit Jerry Baker online at:
www.jerrybaker.com

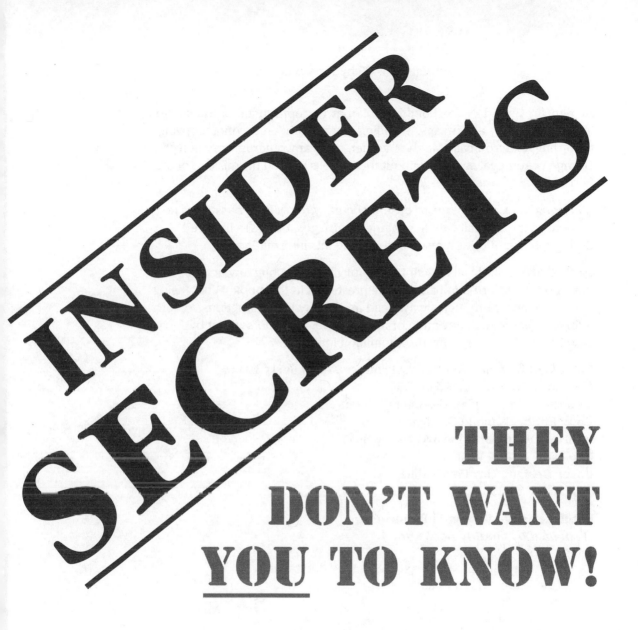

INSIDER SECRETS

THEY DON'T WANT YOU TO KNOW!

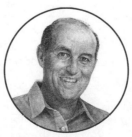

by Jerry Baker

Published by American Master Products, Inc.

Published by American Master Products, Inc. / Jerry Baker
Executive Editor: Kim Adam Gasior
Managing Editor: Cheryl Winters-Tetreau
Copy Editor: Nanette Bendyna
Interior Design and Layout: Nancy Biltcliff
Illustrator: Craig Wilson
Cover Design: Kitty Pierce Mace
Indexer: Nan Badgett

Publisher's Cataloging-in-Publication
(Provided by Quality Books, Inc.)
Baker, Jerry.
     Jerry Baker's insider secrets : they don't want you
to know! / [Jerry Baker].
    p. cm.
    Includes index.
    ISBN-13: 978-0-922433-90-2
    ISBN-10: 0-922433-90-9

    1. Home economics. 2. Health. 3. Gardening.
I. Title. II. Title: Insider secrets : they don't want you
to know!

TX158.B298 2008   640
               QBI08-600145

Printed in the United States of America
2 4 6 8 10 9 7 5 3 1 hardcover

CONTENTS

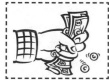 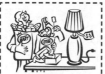 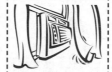 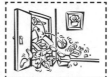 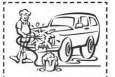

PART ONE
HOME, PROBLEM-FREE HOME

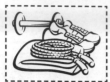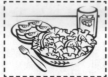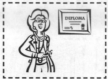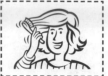

PART TWO
HEALTHY YOU

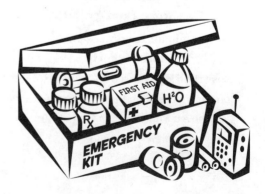

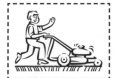 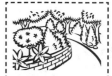 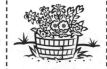 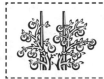 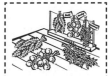

PART THREE
THE JOY OF GARDENING

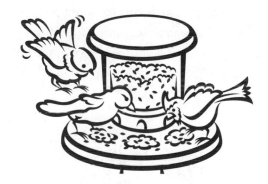

Introduction

Remember when you were a kid and your biggest problem was that imaginary monster lurking in your closet? All you had to do was turn on the light and—poof!—no more monster! Talk about a quick fix…wouldn't it be nice if it was still that easy to solve your problems today?

As a matter of fact, it is that easy! Did you know that you could slash your sky-high heating bills with an old tie and dry rice? Or fast-track weight loss with a fat-burning meal topper? Or get rid of those darn deer with a whiff of a dandy Deer Buster Eggnog? It's all true—and it's just the start of the fast, fun, and easy solutions that follow.

This book is filled to the brim with thousands of tried-and-true tips, tricks, and tonics that have made my life (and the lives of folks all across the country) a whole lot easier. This book really gets down to the nitty-gritty, helping you turn life's major mountains into manageable molehills.

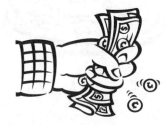

Part One delves into personal finances. What with all the spending and saving options folks have these days, financial planning has come a long way since I stashed my first few pennies in a piggy bank. But no matter how financial strategies have changed, these fundamental money-saving principles still work as well today as they did way back then.

We'll start by dealing with debt, budgeting your expenses, learning the ins and outs of savvy investing, and setting a good example for the kids! (After all, they'll learn smart—or not-so-smart—spending habits by watching you.) Then we'll head on over to the bargain boutique to discover how to get dynamite deals on groceries, clothing, furniture, and even appliances!

Of course, financial planning wouldn't be complete without slicing and dicing expensive energy bills. From drivin' around town to lighting your home to heating and cooling—we'll cut, cut, and cut some more to save you big bucks. In the process, you'll also learn how to be a little kinder to Mother Earth, too.

From there, we'll roam around the house, clearing out the clutter and organizing every room to a "T." Once your living space is picture-perfect, it's time to get behind the wheel of your beloved automobile. Even if you don't know a grease gun from a cap gun, my tips on repairing, maintaining, buying, and selling an automobile are guaranteed to put you in the driver's seat.

Finally, we'll leave your worries behind with some well-deserved R & R. You'll learn how to get the best steals, deals, and meals along the way with terrific tips on efficient packing, low-cost flights and cruises, cheap car rentals, and finding the highest-quality lodgings for the lowest prices.

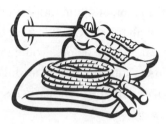

Part Two leads you down the road to good health with super solutions to help you get fit, eat right, and look great. We'll start by tackling problems like smoking, yo-yo dieting, and just plain being out of shape. Don't worry—it's easy to trade in your current lifestyle for a happier, healthier, and more active one!

We'll also explore the healing powers of 10 amazing "superfoods" that you should eat every day. Each one goes above and beyond the call of duty to deliver a potent dose of disease protection. You'll find dozens of remarkable recipes using these foods to help fight major ailments like arthritis, heart disease, and cancer and minor complaints like allergies, dry skin, and "senior moments."

And speaking of senior moments, we might not be able to stop the clock, but we can certainly fight the signs of aging. Get ready to boost your brainpower, prevent hearing loss, keep your vision sharp, combat hair loss, and save your smile—using common, ordinary items you already have in your home!

Of course, eating right and getting fit are only part of the picture. Other problems can sneak up and make you plumb miserable, including stress, headaches, insomnia, and blue moods to name just a few. So I've included dozens of home remedies for a whole host of ailments to keep you feelin' as right as rain.

But it's no fun feeling good if you don't look good, too. Don't worry—we've got you covered in that department. Did you know that there's a four-star spa waiting for you…in your kitchen? That's right you'll discover recipes for an amazing banana-honey moisturizer, a gelatin facial mask, an avocado hair revitalizer, and dozens more beauty treatments that'll make you look like a million bucks for just pennies on the dollar. And you can't beat that!

In addition to helping you feel and look good, we want to help you stay safe, too. Our tips will prepare you for most any kind of emergency that may come along.

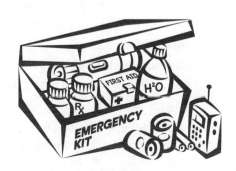

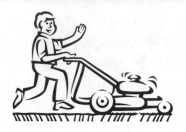

Part Three begins and ends in my favorite place—the great outdoors. After 50-plus years of helping folks all across America, I've learned a thing or three about growing great grass, terrific trees, fabulous flowers, and much, much more. Whether you want the most toe-ticklin' turf in town, the bloomingest beds on the block, or the yummiest vegetables this side of paradise, I've got the tips to get you growin' strong.

Starting with sod, you'll learn all about feeding, weeding, mowing, controlling pests, and solving just about any and all problems that may plague your turf. Whether you're a seasoned sodmaster, or new to the green scene, I'll show you how to give your lawn the TLC it needs to turn into a regular field of dreams.

But what's a lawn without beautiful beds and borders framing it? Not much, in my book. That's why I'm sharing my secrets to growin' the most fabulous trees, shrubs, and flowers in town without having to hire all those high-priced experts. With my help, you'll be growing like a pro in no time at all, and love every minute of it.

Then it's on to the veggie patch. My terrific tips, tricks, and tonics make it easy to harvest big bushels of mouthwatering vegetables with a minimum of time, effort, and expense. You won't believe how fast, fun, and easy it is—yum, yum!

And for a real culinary treat this year, try growing your own cook's garden of herbal delights. Basil, thyme, oregano, and more… all fresh, pungent, and bursting with flavor. Just think of all the delicious dishes, herbal remedies, and handy helpers you can whip up (from the recipes scattered throughout this book), and all the money you'll save when you do!

Finally, since no garden-friendly book would be complete without a nod to my fine-feathered friends, I've included a bunch of bird-errific bits to help you transform your boring backyard into a lively bird sanctuary. I can see it all now, swinging in a hammock on a warm summer's day, sipping a fresh mint julep, and all while being serenaded by a bevy of beautiful songbirds. I tell you, it doesn't get any better than that!

As you can see by now, I've thrown just about everything but the kitchen sink into this book, and for a very good reason. I want to give you the biggest bang for your book-buying buck—and I think I've done that. My goal is for you to use these problem solvers to make your home, sweet home even sweeter, get healthy and stay that way, and grow your own piece of paradise here on God's green earth the fast, fun, and easy way!

CHAPTER 1

Money Matters

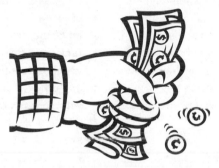

When I was a boy, smart money management was simple: You spent less than you earned and stashed the leftover cash in the bank. That's still the basis of sound financial planning. The difference is that today there are so many more ways to spend *and* save money that the choices are mind-boggling. But they don't have to be overwhelming. Here's some commonsense advice for getting and keeping your financial house in order.

TAKE CONTROL

Money trouble rarely strikes out of the blue. Generally, it comes on over time and for a reason. Make that multiple reasons like frivolous spending habits, poor (or nonexistent) record keeping, overuse of credit cards, or simply taking on too much debt. But take heart: Even if your family finances are headed down a slippery slope, it's never too late to regain the helm and put your financial future on an even keel.

Dare to Dream

If your major financial goal is to pay this month's mortgage, it's time to sit down and do some pondering. Consider what you want life to bring you—*and* what you know it's *going* to bring you—1, 5, or even 20 years from now. For instance, are you itchin' to take a Caribbean cruise to celebrate your 30th wedding anniversary a few years from now? Have you always dreamed of retiring to a beachside cottage? Is the old jalopy beginning to show its age? Or are college tuition bills looming somewhere in the future?

Note: If you have a spouse, you should go through this exercise together, and make sure your wish lists jibe. Having shared goals will help prevent money bickering, which, according to the folks who study such things, is the No. 1 spoiler of wedded bliss. Plus, success will come faster when you work together as a team.

Write All About It

Once you've pinned down your upcoming expenditures, both hoped-for and merely accepted, record them on paper, along with approximate dollar amounts and target dates, or at least time frames. For instance, if your car is running on its last wheel, or you know your roof will need replacing soon, socking away the money for a new one needs to be a short-term goal. Building retirement and college funds are definitely long-term goals.

Build a Budget

The mere mention of the word *budget* makes a lot of folks cringe. But it's simply a tool with which you make your income equal your outgo. (And "outgo" includes saving for the pleasures and necessities we discussed above.) I admit that the process of creating a budget can be unpleasant, to say the least, because it forces you to take a good, hard look at your spending habits. But take my word for it: Once you've started to actually control your cash, you'll feel like a million bucks—even if that isn't *quite* the amount that shows on your bank statement!

Quick Fix

Who says you can't get something for nothing? Why, almost every day, you get a mailbox full of free home-office supplies. Just open the envelopes carefully and set them aside. Then, on shopping day, instead of using tablet paper, grab a business-size envelope, write your list on the back, and tuck your coupons inside. Use the bigger versions to hold receipts, bank statements, and other papers that you need to store with your tax returns. (After all, why pay good money for file folders, when they'll stay in a closed box for umpteen years?)

The Construction Process

You can find all kinds of budget plans on the Internet, or even at your local bank, but you don't really need them. Just grab a pencil and paper, or crank up your computer, and proceed as follows:

Step 1. Gather up all the records you have of your expenditures over the past year, such as your checkbook register, cash and credit card receipts, and bank statements.

Step 2. Divide the expenses into categories— for instance, housing, transportation, loan and credit card debt, insurance, children, pets, and entertainment—and list them on the left side of your paper or your computer document. And remember that one "size" does not fit all, so tailor your list to suit your circumstances. Also, leave plenty of space between these headings. (If you're doing this project by hand, you might want to use a separate sheet of paper for each category.)

Step 3. Write down each expenditure under the appropriate heading. For example, your mortgage or rent payment goes under "Housing," movie tickets under "Entertainment," and so on. Then, for each category, figure out the average amount of money you spend each month, and write that figure on the right side of the paper. Then add up the numbers.

Step 4. Total your average monthly income, including extras like bonuses, interest, or rental payments, as well as your regular salary.

Step 5. Subtract the money you spent from the money you made—or maybe (gasp!) vice versa.

If you have money left over, congratulations! Every month, put that surplus in a savings or investment account earmarked for your financial goals. On the other hand, if you're spending more than you are bringing in, it's time to rethink your habits. But don't lose heart: Read on for a passel of painless ways to cut back on spending, increase your income—and make your financial dreams come true!

DEAL WITH DEBT

Notice that I did not say "eliminate debt." That's because not all debt is bad. In fact, some types are downright good for your economic well-being. For example, taking out a loan to buy a home, pay for school costs, or open a business is a wise move because over time, you'll most likely create capital. What's more, the interest is usually tax deductible. Bad debt is the kind you get when you let credit card spending spiral out of control, charging things that have no lasting value like clothes, restaurant meals, and DVD players. If you've already learned that lesson the hard way, believe me: You *can* tame the credit card monster and reclaim your financial future.

Cut Those Cards!

In this day and age, it's all but impossible to get along without at least one major credit card. For instance, you need to show one when you rent a car or check into a hotel, even if you wind up paying the bill in cash. But if you're like most folks, you probably have more plastic in your wallet than you'll need in a lifetime. Here are my best tips for clearing out the clutter:

Say "no" to annual fees. Even if you pay your balance in full every month, whenever you have a credit card with a yearly fee, you're throwing good money right out the window. If you're carrying a balance and you can't pay it in full right now, you can still close the account—with no ding against your credit rating and no further fees—and continue to make your regular payments until the balance is paid in full. Or, better yet, transfer the balance to a no-fee card that has a lower interest rate. Just make sure you request the closing by certified letter, *not* by phone or e-mail, so that if questions arise, you can prove that *you* canceled the account, not the credit card company.

Take an interest in interest. If you're carrying balances on two or more cards, focus on the one with the highest interest rate. Send in the largest payment you can afford each month, and pay the minimum amount due on your other accounts. Once you've paid off the number one offender, shift your efforts to the card with the next highest rates.

Open a new account. If your credit rating is still in good shape, chances are you get frequent mailings offering you the chance to transfer high-interest balances to a new card with a very low interest rate—and sometimes no interest at all—for a limited period of time (usually six months, but sometimes up to a year or more). Your mission: Apply for a card, and transfer as much as you know you can pay off within the time limit. And make those payments a top priority!

Check out the checks. Some credit card companies send out promotional checks that you can write against your account, with your choice of 0 percent interest for a limited period of time, or a low fixed rate for the life of the loan. This gives you a simple, ultra-low-cost way to transfer high balances from other cards. Obviously, you'll want to opt for 0 percent interest if the time frame suits your budget, but even the fixed rates are much lower than what you're probably paying now.

Be a Savvy Credit Shopper

As you've no doubt noticed, there are a whole lot of banks and other lending institutions that are mighty eager to get credit cards into your hands. That's good news for you, because it means there are some good deals to be had. But to make sure you get the one that's best for you, keep these shopping tips in mind:

- Look for a card that offers something in return, like air miles, train miles, product discounts, or cash rewards. Just make sure that any discounts are for products you plan on buying anyway. And bear in mind that if the card has an annual fee, or if you routinely carry a balance, you may not be getting a bargain at all.

- Read the fine print carefully. In particular, beware of a very low "introductory rate." It may be good for only a few months before it escalates to a much higher number. Also, make sure you understand the fees for cash advances, late payments, and over-the-limit balances.

Don't Be Tardy!

Whether you pay your full credit card bill every month, or you're paying down a balance, make sure you get that money to the "church" on time. If you miss your due date by even a single day, you'll be slapped with a penalty, which is usually somewhere between $35 and $40. What's more, if you've taken advantage of a low-interest balance-transfer offer, a late payment will cancel it instantly and send your rate soaring again. The

---

HOME REMEDY

Don't throw out those promotional credit cards that you periodically get in the mail. Save 'em and use 'em as scrapers around the house. They'll remove ugly wax drippings from furniture or sticky price tags from anything under the sun without scratching the surface. And they also do a pretty good job scraping away ice—either in the freezer or on your car's windshield.

simple solution: If you have the slightest inkling that your check may arrive late, make your payment by phone or over the Internet. Many companies charge a fee for these options, but generally, it's less than a late fee—and a whole *lot* less than higher monthly interest charges.

Pay as You Go

It's easier than ever to use a credit card to pay for everyday expenses like dry cleaning, fast food, and even utility bills. And it's especially tempting if you have a card that offers perks, like air miles, for every dollar you spend. Well, take my advice: Unless you're absolutely sure you can—and will—ante up the full balance due each month, use good old-fashioned cash for your day-to-day purchases. This simple change in habits will boost your bottom line in two ways:

1. It'll stop the financial drain of monthly interest charges.

2. It'll make you more aware of your spending habits. For instance, having to fork out cold, hard currency just may make you think twice about buying that fancy French foot cream.

The Best of Both Worlds

If you're not carrying a debit card that carries the imprint of a major credit card company, you're missing out on one of the best financial deals to come along in decades—at least in my humble opinion. Here's why I never leave home without my debit card:

- You can use it exactly as you would a credit card, and at all the same places. But because the payments come right out of your checking account, there are no bills to pay later.

- It's much safer than carrying large amounts of cash. In most cases, you receive the same

protection against unauthorized purchases that you'd get with a credit card. (Of course, you still need to report the loss within a certain time frame; details vary from one card issuer to another, so read the fine print in your account agreement.)

- For those times when you do need cash and the closest ATM is not affiliated with your bank, you can dodge the out-of-system withdrawal fee with this clever trick: Just use your debit card to buy an item you need, and when the salesclerk says, "Any cash back?" say, "Yes, please." Or if you're using an automated debit machine, just hit the "Cash Back" key.

Escape Trouble in Paradise

Behind almost every personal bankruptcy is overextended credit card debt. If you've maxed out your cards and your bank accounts are drying up, then you could be headed for a riptide of financial woe. You can steer yourself toward calmer waters, but you need to act fast. The longer you wait, the harder it'll be to maintain (or recover) your credit standing and your good name. Here's what you need to do:

Contact your creditors. Most companies can redesign a more comfortable payment plan with lower rates, and deadline extensions (see "Pick Up the Phone" below for the lowdown on working with creditors).

Don't use your credit cards. After all, isn't that what got you into this fix in the first place?

Pick Up the Phone

If you're in financial trouble, contact your creditors as soon as possible, and give them a frank assessment of your situation. They may readjust your payment plan, reduce your interest rate, or even forgive your late fees. Why would they be so accommodating? Because it's much cheaper for them to give financial breaks to their honest customers than it is to pay for the services of collection agencies. Plus, creditors have learned the hard way that although collection agencies usually find their man (or woman), they don't always find their money.

Talk It Out

If self-help hasn't stopped that downward debt spiral, a credit counseling agency could be the way out. A trained counselor will help you create a workable budget based on your income and your expenses, and may recommend a debt management plan (not to be confused with a debt consolidation loan, which I'll explain later). Your counselor will work with your creditors to redesign the fees and terms of your payment schedule. You must make monthly installments to the agency, which will parcel out the money to your various lenders. Sounds fairly straightforward, right? Well, be aware that not all credit agencies are created equal. Here are the details that spell the difference between an outfit that will give you a leg up—and one that just wants to kick you when you're down:

Fees. You won't find an agency that doesn't charge a fee. (After all, they have bills to pay, too.) But if you're asked to pay more than $50 a month, keep looking.

Time. Counseling clients, working with creditors, and arranging payment plans is a complex process, and when it's done properly, it takes time. If a counselor tells you he can design a program for you in half an hour, then he probably isn't being as thorough as he could or should be.

Plan preparation. If a counselor wants to enroll you in a debt management plan without first offering general budgeting advice, or requests money for the plan before she's contacted your creditors, look elsewhere.

Accreditation. A reputable agency will be accredited by the Council on Accreditation and Internal Standards Organization. Make sure this credential is up-to-date.

So where do you find a first-rate agency? The best place to start is with a friend or relative who's used such a service. Your bank or credit union manager or tax accountant should also be able to steer you in the right direction. If at all possible, use a local agency, because face-to-face counseling is a lot more effective than working over the phone or the Internet.

Put It All Together...

maybe. The lenders who offer debt consolidation loans make them sound like the be-all and end-all of fiscal first aid. Could this be your best route to a sound financial future? Well, maybe yes, and maybe no. On the plus side, your payments will be merged into one comfortable monthly bill, and you won't be inundated with overdue statements or calls from rude collectors. On the downside, these loans don't erase your debt; they just stretch it out over a longer period of time. Your monthly payments will be lower, but over the long haul, you could wind up shelling out a lot more cash for fees and interest charges.

Still, a consolidation loan could be your ticket out of debt if you fit one of these descriptions:

● You have a clean credit history. If it's tarnished, you may not qualify for an interest rate that's low enough to make debt consolidation worth your while.

- You have the discipline to swear off new debt.

- You can find a personal loan that has minimal fees and other up-front costs. Nearly all of them have such charges, so read the fine print carefully, and don't be afraid to ask questions.

- You can pay off the loan faster than you would be able to pay off your current debts.

Play It Safe

If you opt for a debt consolidation loan, make sure you steer clear of any that will use your home as collateral. If your payments are delinquent, the lender can send your house into foreclosure, leaving you not only drowning in debt, but homeless, to boot!

FAST FORMULA

Debt-to-Income Ratio

Before you apply for a loan of any kind, find out if you'll meet the lender's financial requirements. Most companies use this straightforward formula to calculate your debt-to-income ratio. Here's what you'll need:

A list of your monthly debt payments
Your monthly gross income

Add up your debt payments and divide the total by your income. This figure is your debt-to-income ratio. Lenders generally view a ratio of 36 percent or lower as a healthy number. If your ratio is between 36 and 40 percent, you may still qualify for a loan, but making your monthly payments could be a hardship. A ratio higher than 40 percent most likely will put you out of the running.

Good Debt Comes Home

Isn't it amazing how may people want to give you money? These generous souls are everywhere, pleading with you from your TV screen, sending you letters and e-mail messages, urging you to *please, please* take their money! Who could blame you for accepting? Home equity loans and lines of credit are two of the most tempting loans around, and for good reason: The rates are generally low, and the interest is usually tax deductible. On the downside, both types of loans tap into the value of what is probably your most precious possession—the roof over your head. I would urge you *never* to use them to pay off credit card bills or to splurge on things like vacations and fancy cars. But if—and I repeat *if*—you use them for the kind of good debt we talked about at the beginning of this section, they can be valuable financial tools. Here's how they work:

Home equity loan. You'll receive one lump sum of cash to use as you see fit. This kind of loan is best for one-time expenses, like home improvements or the purchase of a second property. Your interest is locked in so you'll know what your payments will be from month to month, and your money goes toward both principal and interest.

Home equity line of credit. This is a revolving loan, so you can borrow money as you need it up to a set limit. It works well for ongoing expenses, like college tuition. Your rate will fluctuate depending on the market, so your payments will drop and rise over time. Most lines of credit are "interest-only" arrangements, so your monthly payments don't ever touch the principal. You need to make sure to pay more than the minimum amount each month, or your principal will follow you like a shadow for the rest of your days!

Do Your Homework

Before you take out a home equity loan to make repairs or renovations to your home, there are two factors you need to consider:

1. Some improvements add more resale value than others. And your return on investment will vary (often greatly), depending on the region of the country, the character of your neighborhood, the current housing market, and the latest hot trends. In general, though, according to the National Association of Realtors, two of the most profitable changes you can make are adding a full bathroom or a first- or second-floor laundry room. (A laundry area in the basement can reduce the selling value of your house.)

2. If you plan to sell your home in the next year or two, the best thing you can do to your property just might be nothing at all. It is true that totally renovating your home's interior could increase the potential selling price of your house—but probably not by enough to offset the cash you'd have to shell out on the project (not to mention the time and hassle you'll spend on something you won't even get to enjoy). Before you even start investigating loans, consult with a reputable real estate agent who knows your neighborhood and the current market. He or she can help you decide which improvements will be likely to increase your bottom line, and which ones will be like throwing your money right down the drain. For example, painting a small room in a light color will make it look larger and more impressive to potential buyers. *Note:* Make sure you do this research *before* you put your house on the market, because many banks will not give a home equity loan on listed property.

For more guidance on what to do to your house and when (or when *not*) to do it, visit www.realtor.org.

Get a Line on College

Or rather, *for* college. The interest on a home equity line of credit may be lower than the rate on a student loan. But before you put your home, sweet home at risk, compare the terms of any loans that your would-be scholar qualifies for. If a home equity line makes the grade, estimate projected costs carefully, and borrow just a little more than you think you'll need (thereby covering yourself for unexpected expenses). Then, dole out the cash with care, and only when you have to. (For tips on cutting college costs, see pages 10–11.)

Cast a Safety Net

If you have little or no money set aside for emergencies, but you do have regular income, my advice is to apply for a home equity line of credit *now*. If trouble strikes, it could spell the difference between a challenging time and financial disaster. Some banks charge an up-front fee, but after that, you pay nothing until you actually start using the funds. If, for instance, you lose your job, you can dip into your fund to pay your bills until you're gainfully reemployed. Or, let's say a big storm sends a tree crashing through your roof. You can have it repaired pronto, then just sit there, cozy and warm, while you wait for your insurance company to ante up. Whatever reason you tap into this rainy-day fund for, the interest on your payments will be a lot less than it would be on a credit card. *Note:* Arranging for a line of credit is an especially smart move if you're planning to retire soon, because once you lose that steady income, qualifying for the loan will be a lot tougher.

BE A GOOD EXAMPLE

We all know that children learn their first life lessons by observing their parents—and that includes watching the way you spend money. Even before the tiny tykes know what a dollar is, whatever example you (and Santa Claus) set sinks deep into their little psyches. (Is that a sobering thought, or what?) Here are some tips for launching the youngsters in your life onto the road to riches—or at least financial security.

Plan with the Clan

Many parents make the mistake of treating money as a taboo topic. Don't do it! While children don't need to know the intimate details of your finances, they should understand the importance of living within their means. As soon as the kids are old enough, involve them in your budget-planning sessions. When they see that you need to balance income and outgo, they'll quickly learn that money doesn't grow on trees. Believe me, they'll thank you for that lesson in years to come. (I know quite a few 40-year-old "kids" who wish they'd learned it a whole lot earlier in life!)

Do as I Do

There's a big difference between Scrooge-like stinginess and smart spending. If you routinely pinch pennies till they bleed (even if you don't really have to), your kids might well react by growing up to be compulsive shoppers or "chargeaholics." On the other hand, if you show them by example that it *is* possible to conserve cash and still enjoy the best of what life has to offer, then they're much more likely to hit the high road to financial success.

Frugality Can Be Fun

One way to instill sound fiscal values in your youngsters, and help cut the high cost of child rearing at the same time, is to remember that not everything you buy has to be brand-spanking new. And I'm not simply talking about the classic wisdom of opting for a late-model used car over a new one. In thrift shops, consignment stores, and "junktique" stores, you can find everything from fine furniture to Christmas tree ornaments for a tiny fraction of what you'd pay in a regular retail establishment. Plus, poking around in these places can be a whole lot of fun—and it's absolutely free! In fact, you might even stumble across a nifty nugget that you can turn around and sell for many times what it cost you.

HOME REMEDY

You never know what treasures you might come across in a thrift shop or secondhand store, or on an Internet auction site. Rather than pay full price for new items, I'm always on the lookout for good deals on:

- **Books**
- **CDs and DVDs**
- **Clothing**
- **Sports equipment**
- **Tools**
- **Toys and games**

Money Is Power

As soon as you feel your children are old enough, give them some buying power. Hand over a set amount of money every week, or every month, and make it clear that it has to cover certain expenses. For instance, you might want to give a third-grader cash for a week's worth of candy, baseball cards, and other sundries. As time goes by, you can increase the money and the responsibility to cover things like clothes, entertainment, and sports equipment. You can bet that it won't take the young consumers long to learn some savvy shopping habits!

Once your youngsters reach their teens, they should be mature enough to earn their own spending money by holding down a summer job. Even preteens can dip their toes into the world of capitalism by shoveling snow, pulling weeds, or walking the neighbors' dogs.

It's Their Money, But...

that doesn't mean you can't offer a little guidance on how to spend it. Gently encourage your young workers to put part of their earnings into a savings account, and to donate another portion to a charity of their choice—even if it's only tossing a few coins into the Salvation Army Christmas kettle. (Of course, your suggestions will carry a lot more weight if you're practicing what you preach!)

The Old College Try

These days, a year in college can cost more than the down payment on a modest house did just a decade or so ago. But don't fret. There are plenty of ways to ease the burden on your bank account. Before you put the family homestead into hock, here are a few places to look for help:

Your employer. Some companies (especially the larger ones) offer scholarships, low-interest loans, or other education assistance to their employees' children. Ask the folks in the human resources department at your office about the company's policies.

Your community. In every town, there are service organizations, ranging from the Rotary Club to the American Association of University Women, that give scholarships to deserving youngsters. Your kids' high-school guidance counselor should be able to tell you about the opportunities available in your area and what it takes to apply. You may also find application notices in your local newspaper.

The military. Every branch of the armed services offers scholarships to qualified students. Of course, your child will need to repay Uncle Sam by serving for a few years as a military officer. But that leadership experience will provide a great launching pad into any civilian career. To learn all the details, log on to **www.TodaysMilitary.com**, or call your closest Army, Navy, Marine, Air Force, or Coast Guard recruiting office.

A Is for Articulation

And that word can translate into *big* savings on the cost of a college education. How so? Because all over the country, many community colleges and public universities have formed partnerships called articulation agreements. They enable a student to earn a two-year associate's degree at a community college, then transfer the credits to a pricier, four-year school, with acceptance guaranteed in advance. The result: Your son or daughter lands a valuable bachelor's degree, while you save as much as 40 percent on tuition bills! To find out what your best options are, contact the community colleges in your area, and ask which schools they're teamed up with. You should also be able to find partnership details on the Web sites of your state's public universities.

C Is for Commute

Having your child live at home and commute to classes could save you big bucks in college costs. I say "could" because the price of this daily back-and-forth jaunt can vary greatly, depending on the distance between your home and the campus, and whether your young commuter can use public transportation. Once you factor in the price of gasoline, wear and tear on the car, and increased insurance premiums (see "Drive Down Kid Costs" on page 19), you might be better off paying for dorm fees and finding other ways to cut corners.

Quick Fix

If your young scholar can shoulder a part-time job, one obvious benefit will be less money flowing out of your pocket. But the advantages of student employment don't stop there. If a position is curriculum-related, time spent on the job may transfer into course credit. At the very least, paid work experience will be a big plus when the time comes to write that first resume. Most colleges have student employment offices, where your student can find listings for jobs on- and off-campus. Have him or her also check with the financial aid office to learn about government- and school-sponsored work-study programs, where a student works in exchange for education expenses.

Charge!

It's the first day of college orientation, and there they are: reps from credit card companies, lined up, grinning from ear to ear, and all but pushing their charge cards into students' hands. How can any youngster resist a little piece of plastic that pays for school books, pizza, clothes, concert tickets—you name it? So what if the bills pile up? After graduation, there'll be a big, fat salary check to pay them off. We all know where *that* kind of faulty reasoning can lead. And more and more students are learning it the hard way, as they struggle to earn money for mounting interest payments at the expense of precious study time. The result: ever-growing numbers of debt-ridden dropouts and graduates with hefty debt payments. Here are a few tips to help you keep the apple of your eye from joining their ranks:

Choose one. Limit your child to one card. The fewer options he or she has, the less tempted they'll be to blow their budget.

Pay in advance. Get your offspring a prepaid credit card that's tied to one of your accounts. This way, you can transfer a set amount of money onto the card and set guidelines for when and how it should be used—and you'll know if your advice is being heeded because your statements will show the transactions. Fees and other details vary; to find the best deal for you, search the Internet for "prepaid credit cards."

Keep the limit low. If you'd rather have your budding consumer open an account in her own name—thereby starting to build a credit history—encourage her to keep the spending limit low. She'll be more likely to stick to necessities, and if she does go a little overboard, you can probably come to the rescue before any permanent damage is done.

Deal with a debit. Carrying a debit card makes just as much sense for your favorite student as it does for you (see "The Best of Both Worlds" on page 5). Of course, it won't help your youngster establish credit, but it *will* keep him out of debt, because the charges incurred will come right out of his (or your) checking account.

DAY BY DAY

No matter how budget-conscious we are, we all spend thousands of dollars a year on stuff that's here today and gone tomorrow—or in some cases, here one minute and gone the next. Some of these nondurable goods (as the financial big shots call them) are necessities, such as gasoline and prescription medicines. Others, like restaurant meals, movie tickets, and giant double lattes, are, shall we say, somewhat less essential in the overall scheme of things. In the space we have here, I can't possibly tell you how to save money on *all* your everyday expenses. But here's a roundup of painless ways to cut some of the most draining out-of-pocket costs.

What the Doctor Ordered

If you're taking long-term, prescription medications and the price is beyond your means, put this book down right now and call the manufacturer. Most of the major pharmaceutical companies have patient-assistance plans, and if you qualify, you could get your life-saving meds for free, or close to it. There are also federal and state government programs that may help you pay for prescription drugs. To learn about those, contact the U.S. Department of Health and Human Services. In the meantime, here are a couple of timely tips to help trim drug costs:

Talk to your doctor. I've found that most docs automatically prescribe generic versions of drugs whenever possible, but it always pays to request that option—don't simply assume that it'll happen. And be sure to ask if the office has free samples it can give you. The drug companies send out loads of them, but the doctor may need a gentle reminder to check the supply closet. (Bear in mind that these freebies won't flow forever, but even a few doses will save you some bucks.)

Shop around. As with any other product, the price of prescription drugs can vary from one retail outlet to another. So call the pharmacies in your area and ask what they charge for your medication, how much your insurance company will cover, and what your co-payment will be. And don't forget to check with the pharmacies at local grocery stores, too.

HOME REMEDY

If you're taking medication for a chronic condition, there's a good chance that some simple alterations to your daily routine could improve your health considerably. Ask your doctor whether exercise or dietary changes might translate into a lower dose—and therefore, a lower price tag. If you're *really* lucky, maybe you can even kiss those pills good-bye!

Don't Be Fuelish

If you live where you can walk or take public transportation to work or play, and you're still getting behind the wheel of the old jalopy every morning, I have only two words to say to you: Stop it! You'll save hundreds or even thousands of dollars a year on gasoline—and get some valuable exercise, to boot. (You'll also save on car maintenance and maybe on your insurance premiums; see "All Because of You" on page 18.) On the other hand, if driving is your only way of getting from point A to point B, here are a few simple ways to save on fuel, whether you have a conventional gas-guzzler or a fancy new hybrid:

Lighten the load. When you carry cargo on the roof of your car, the added weight forces your engine to work harder, so it drinks fuel faster. Granted, there may be times when you need to transport, let's say, a couple of bicycles or a canoe on top of your vehicle, but don't *store* them there!

Take it easy. The faster your car goes, the more fuel it consumes. Your auto also takes a big gulp of gas when you hit the brakes suddenly. Your mission: Drive at a reasonable speed, try to maintain a steady pace, keep plenty of distance between you and the car ahead of you, and monitor the traffic flow up ahead. You'll save gasoline *and* decrease your chance of getting in an accident.

Plan ahead. Instead of making a lot of separate trips to and from the grocery store, the dry cleaner, and the hardware store, try to consolidate your errands. The reason: Fuel consumption increases not only with the number of miles you drive, but also with the number of trips you take. That's because a car burns more gas (and also spews out more pollutants) in its first few minutes of operation, before the innards have warmed up. *Note:* This does *not* mean that you should let your car idle in the driveway before you start out— that's a complete waste of gas, because even a cold car is giving you *some* miles per gallon!

Be a Beauty School Drop-In

Whether you're in the market for your periodic haircut or a special treat like a facial, manicure, or massage, you can find a big-time bargain at a hairdressing, cosmetology, or massage school. They all offer hands-on experience to their students, and they welcome customers with open arms. The students who are permitted to work on customers usually have completed most of their courses and are close to graduation. Granted, you probably won't get *quite* the results you'd be assured from an experienced professional, but you'll pay a fraction of the price. And you needn't worry about a true cosmetic catastrophe because a competent instructor is always standing by to make things right.

Dollars for Dining

It's no secret that even a modestly priced restaurant meal will set you back a lot more than your own home cookin'. But that's no reason to deny yourself the pleasure of dining out. Here are some delicious ideas for trimming the fat from those eating-out food costs:

Early does it. These days, many restaurants offer "early bird" dinner specials in the late afternoon, but if you simply want to enjoy good food and good company in a leisurely setting, go out for lunch, or even breakfast, instead. The earlier a meal is, the less it's likely to cost you.

Drink the water. In any restaurant, liquor and even soft drinks add a hefty amount to the check. You'll reap big dividends if you skip those liquid refreshments and just ask for a glass of water (not a bottle, which will be pricey).

Just desserts. Just as drinks (especially fancy cocktails) at a restaurant can set you back a pretty penny, so can the fancy confections intended to top off your meal. If you crave dessert after lunch or dinner, bypass the dessert menu and drop into an ice cream parlor or pastry shop on your way home. Their sweet treats are just as yummy, and a lot less expensive.

Eat Outside the Box

When you're hankerin' to let somebody else do the cooking, your choices are not limited to restaurants or take-out food. Consider these tasty options:

- If you live near a culinary school or a university that has a food-service program, hightail it over there. The budding chefs usually serve up first-class gourmet chow at coffee-shop prices.

- Set yourself down at a church supper (they're usually listed in your newspaper's calendar section). You can get great down-home cookin' for next to nothing. You may even make some new friends.

Go Back to School

If you live in or near a town that has a university in it, you can have yourself a grand old time for almost no money at all. Even in the summer, there's usually plenty going on that's open to the general public. Here are some of the free or almost-free treats I look for:

- Museums, art galleries, and special exhibits

- Concerts and recitals, by either student musicians or visiting performers

- Seasonal festivals of all kinds

- Historic buildings on campus

- Talks and lectures (often by famous visitors)

- Botanical gardens

- Student sports events

PAMPER YOUR PETS FOR LESS

Nowadays, it seems as though every time I turn on the news, there's some fancy new study showing that folks who have pets are happier and healthier than folks who don't. Well, you dog and cat "parents" don't need a study to tell you that! But I'll bet you could use this collection of tail-waggin' tricks for beating the high cost of tender-lovin' critter care.

HOME REMEDY

If you live near a veterinary school, you may be able to get free or very low-cost medical care for your pet—especially if you're a senior. What's more, if your four-footed pal has a serious problem that new, high-tech surgery might cure, a vet school's teaching docs will sometimes operate for next to nothing in the interest of research. So before you give up hope, pick up the phone and give them a call.

Your Best Pal's Best Pal

Sooner or later, almost every pet has a serious medical problem of some kind. When that time comes (if you're anything like me), you want to be darn sure you have a first-class vet on the job. And—for the sake of your pet's health, your peace of mind, *and* your bank account—the time to find that Superguy or Supergal is long before big-time trouble strikes. Why? For a couple of reasons:

1. When your veterinarian has treated your animal for routine matters, knows his overall health picture—and can pull a nice, fat file from the records—it's likely to be much easier for the doc to diagnose and treat a serious problem. And that could translate into big savings for you.

2. When you've had a good, ongoing relationship with the clinic, the financial folks will probably bend over backwards to help you finance the cost of surgery or another major treatment.

Weighty Matters

Of course, you take your dog or cat to the vet for routine checkups and annual vaccinations. Nail trims make good, low-cost visits, too. But here's another, free way to get your pet acquainted with the clinic staff: Stop by every so often to have him weighed. It's an especially good way to introduce a new puppy or kitten, or an older, rescued animal who's a tad nervous about this doctorin' business. Always call first, though, to make sure the clinic isn't overbooked or dealing with an emergency.

Gotcha Covered!

Have you ever wondered why there isn't health insurance for pets? Well, there is: For a tiny fraction of the cost of human policies, a number of veterinary insurance companies will cover your dog, cat, or other pet for X-rays, surgery, hospital stays, lab fees—you name it. In some cases, for a small additional premium, you can get coverage for routine care, including an annual physical checkup, vaccinations, flea-control and heart-worm medications, spay/neuter surgery, and teeth cleaning. Thanks to underwriting by several drug companies, this package will save you *big* bucks on the care that your best friend needs to

stay healthy. To find out all the details, check with your veterinarian or search the Internet for "veterinary health insurance."

Bargain Hunters, Beware!

If you think that one commercial pet food is as good as another, think again. The legal quality standards for pet foods are much lower than they are for human food—and you practically need a Ph.D. in chemistry to understand the fine print on those bags and cans! At best, when you fork over your cash for a low-priced brand, you'll be paying for a lot of filler that isn't worth beans. At worst, your cat or dog could be chowing down on mysterious "by-products" that could (and often do) cause serious and expensive problems.

His Allergies Are Killin' Me!

If your dog or cat is scratchin' up a storm, before you fork out more money on vet visits or allergy meds, take a listen: The answer to Fido's or Fluffy's problem could be right in his food bowl. A lot of dogs and cats are allergic to many of the dyes, preservatives, and other ingredients commonly used in grocery store pet foods—and even in some of the expensive brands that vets sell.

More and more pet foods are coming on the market minus the common itch causers. Just ask the folks at a pet-supply store or well-stocked kennel shop to recommend a high-quality, natural food that'll suit your pet's age, breed, and activity level. And let them know that you don't want to spend an arm and a leg. The nifty newfangled foods with old-fashioned ingredients come in all price ranges. If the store doesn't carry a brand that fits your budget, ask for a recommendation to a store that does.

Change the Menu

Corn, soy, and wheat are all big-time allergy causers in dogs—and they're some of the most widely used ingredients in dog food. Before you start playing expensive games of brand roulette, try any high-quality food that contains none of that trio. It just might solve your problem lickety-split!

COVER YOUR BASES

One expense no one can afford to live without is insurance. The good news is that you don't have to pay high premiums to protect your life, health, home, and belongings from the costs of calamities. I'll show you how to find the coverage you need at prices you can live with.

To Your Good Health!

When you're shopping for health insurance, remember the old adage, "Don't be penny wise and pound foolish." In other words, don't simply jump at the plan that has the lowest premiums. The best bargain is the policy that pays the most for the services you're likely to need, even if the premiums are a tad higher. In particular, look for one that has excellent major-medical coverage, even if you have to opt for a higher deductible to get it. Remember, you can always find a way to come up with a few hundred dollars for a minor incident, but if the company won't fork out the big bucks necessary for things like heart surgery or cancer treatment, you could find yourself in debt for the rest of your life.

Into the Pool

If you have a preexisting medical problem that might (or already has) put you out of the running for health insurance, don't panic. Each state in the Union maintains a high-risk insurance pool for just such cases. As you might expect, the premiums are usually higher than you'd pay for a normal policy, but they're capped by law to keep them within reasonable bounds. Details vary from one state to another, so to get the full lowdown, call your state insurance commission, or type "high-risk insurance pools" into your favorite Internet search engine.

Matters of Life and Death

The concept of life insurance couldn't be simpler: You take out a policy so that in the event of your death, your dependents can continue to live in the style to which they've become accustomed. Here are a few more things you should know about insuring your earthly body without losing your shirt:

Come to terms. There are two types of life insurance: term and whole life. With a term life policy, your premiums, which are usually very low, go toward paying death benefits to the named beneficiary—period. On the other hand, a whole life policy is also an investment account, with a portion of your monthly premium going into stocks, bonds, or other funds. The policy builds cash value that you can borrow against. That may sound enticing, but this investment component, along with high fees and commissions, makes whole life policies very expensive. Besides, there are much more profitable ways to invest your money.

Act fast. The younger you are, the lower your premiums will be. In fact, up to about age 50, if you're in good health, you can get a term policy for practically peanuts. But once you reach 50, rates begin to soar. In fact, many companies won't even sell term insurance to anyone over 65. If you want coverage at all, you may be forced to ante up for whole life.

Take stock. How much life insurance you need depends on your circumstances. And, as we all know, those change as Mother Nature's clock ticks on. For instance, if you have children, you'll want enough coverage to support them until they're old enough to pay their own way in the world. Once your kids have flown the coop, chances are you can do just fine with less coverage—and therefore, lower premiums. Make it a point to reevaluate your coverage periodically to make sure your policy reflects the here and now.

⧗ *Quick Fix*

Of all the important decisions in life, choosing the right insurance can be one of the most confusing. There's so much at stake, and the fine print on the paperwork seems endless—and it's often all but impossible for a layperson to understand. The solution: Find an experienced, independent insurance broker who deals with several companies. Explain the kind of coverage you're looking for, and let him or her find the best deal for you. Believe me, this can be a _real_ time-, money-, and sanity-saving tactic, especially if you've moved to a new state and one or more of your current insurers don't operate there.

Home, Insured Home

Many folks pay a lot more than they need to for homeowner's insurance because they overlook one crucial fact: Premiums can vary enormously from one company to another. For example, a friend of mine recently bought a house that was more than a century old, but in tip-top shape, with brand-new plumbing and wiring from top to bottom. One firm quoted her its standard, astronomical rate for "historic property" and didn't even want to hear about its condition. She said, "No thanks," and found an agency that gave her better coverage at less than half the price. The moral: Comparison shopping pays off.

But before you sign on anybody's bottom line, get rate quotes from at least three reputable companies. Some state insurance commissions provide price comparisons of major insurers, so check with them before you start making random phone calls.

Carry Some Weight

One simple way to cut your homeowner's premiums is to increase your deductible. Of course, this will mean shouldering a greater share of the responsibility for any losses, but you can cover that by putting an amount equal to your deductible into an interest-bearing savings account.

Gimme a Break!

When you take out a new homeowner's policy or renew your current one, find out what discounts you may qualify for. For instance, many companies give price breaks to senior citizens and nonsmokers, as well as houses with features such as these:

- Security systems
- Disaster-resistant features, like storm shutters and shatterproof glass
- Updated plumbing and electrical wiring
- Brick exterior

Hide in Plain Sight

Even if your worldly goods are insured to the hilt, chances are you've got some small treasures that no amount of money could replace. So tuck them away where no burglar is likely to find them—in a literary safe. To make one, you'll need one hardcover book, 3 to 4 inches thick; a pencil or pen; a straightedge or ruler; a craft knife; and some glue.

Open the book to page 5, and draw a rectangle in the center of the page, with a 1- to 2-inch border all around. Working with a few pages at a time, use the craft knife to cut around the rectangle, removing the cutouts as you go, and using a previous page as a template. Continue cutting until you reach the back cover. Glue the back cover closed. Then, for added stability, glue the pages together in ¼-inch layers. Put cash or other small valuables in the center compartment, and set your new safe on a shelf with other books. To make it blend into the scenery, tuck it among volumes of roughly the same subject matter, or the same place in the alphabet.

Deals on Wheels

There's no getting around it: If you own a car, you have to carry car insurance. But you *don't* have to carry the burden of sky-high premiums. And the best place to start trimming those rates just might be right in your house—or, rather, in the company that insures it. If that firm also offers auto insurance, using it for both policies could save you anywhere from 5 to 20 percent on your premiums.

Make and Model Matter

If you have your heart set on a sleek and sassy sports car, by all means go for it—but remember that your premiums will be higher than they would be for a sedate sedan. Insurance companies view sporty cars, and other high-horsepower vehicles, as liability risks. And who can blame them? After all, when was the last

time you saw a Ferrari going 25 miles an hour? Likewise, some kinds of automobiles are proven magnets for car thieves, and if you opt for one of these tempters, you can expect to pay more to insure it. (The roster varies from one part of the country to another, so before you buy a new car, ask your state insurance commission to send you a list of its high-risk targets.)

Feature Attractions

Regardless of what kind of car you drive, certain safety features could translate into big discounts. These four are all but guaranteed to save you money:

- Air bags
- Antilock brakes
- Antitheft devices
- Daytime running lights

All Because of You

Besides your car's equipment, there's another safety feature that insurance companies take into account—and that's *you*. Here are some factors that often result in lower premiums:

Your age. That's because the more driving experience you have, the less accident-prone you are. If you are a senior citizen, you may be able to save up to 45 percent on your rates. Furthermore, some insurers offer seniors low-cost programs that guarantee against cancellation as long as the premiums are paid on time and there are no traffic violations.

Your record. Most insurers offer substantial discounts to drivers who've managed to avoid both moving violations and accidents. Conversely, of course, the more run-ins you've had with either the law or other cars (or even telephone poles), the higher your premiums will be.

Your career. Believe it or not, statistics show that folks in certain professions just naturally tend to be safe drivers. In some states, for instance, artists, biologists, members of the clergy, mail carriers, and teachers automatically qualify for low-risk discounts (except, of course, those individuals who've deviated from the norm).

Your hours behind the wheel. The fewer miles you travel, the less likely you are to have an accident. For that reason, most insurance companies will shave money off your bill if you meet their low-mileage criteria. (Chalk up yet another reason to take the bus, trolley, subway, or good old shoe-leather express!)

HOME REMEDY

I don't know how it happens, but I always seem to end up with extra checkbook registers. For a while I just scrapped them. Then one day, that lightbulb above my head flickered on. Now I use them when I comparison shop for insurance rates. The pages are like mini spreadsheets, and the size is perfect for carrying one with me and fitting it into stuffed files. Now I can't get enough of them—I even ask for extras when I go to the bank!

Pardon Me

Nobody's perfect, and the insurance companies know it. That's why many of them have "accident forgiveness" plans, which guarantee that even if you cause a crash, your premiums won't go up. Some insurers charge you a pretty penny for this option. Others will excuse your first blunder at no extra cost if you've been a good, longtime customer and have few, if any, moving violations. So before you shell out more money for peace of mind, check your policy to see if pardons are already built into your basic coverage.

Drive Down Kid Costs

If you have a teen driver in the family, you've already seen your insurance premiums take off at 90 miles an hour. But if that, um, adventure still lies ahead of you, here's what you can expect: When your daughter takes the wheel, you'll be shelling out up to 50 percent more than you are now. Consider yourself lucky, because a son will drive up those premiums by as much as 100 percent. The good news is that you can cushion the blow. Here's how:

- Insist that your child take (and pass) a driver's education course. This simple measure nearly always ensures lower premiums. Some companies also give discounts for good grades and volunteer work.

- Add your child to your existing policy. It's generally less expensive than taking out a separate one.

- If your child goes to a college that's at least 100 miles away from your home, don't let her (or especially him) take a car along. Most insurers give discounts when they know there's a safe distance between your auto and your offspring.

Don't Drive on Autopilot

When your policy comes up for renewal, don't automatically send off the check. Instead, do some comparison shopping. Rates and discount provisions change frequently, so a little checking could result in big savings. Either log on to company Web sites, contact your state insurance commission, or call a broker and say, "Please find me the best deal!" Whichever route you choose, if you go with a new insurer, make sure you officially cancel your old coverage. Otherwise, the company will renew your old policy and send you a bill for your premium.

The Ties That Bind...

can save you dough! Your old school ties or your current work affiliations could cut the cost of your insurance coverage. That's because some alumni and professional organizations offer auto insurance at group rates, which are almost always less expensive than individual policies. All it takes is a few simple phone calls to find out whether your connections will get you a break.

CAPITAL IDEAS

We've all read stories about 10-year-olds who started buying shares of stock with their paper-route money and wound up retiring as millionaires in their forties. Well, if you're reading this book, it's probably way too late for you to follow *that* example! But it's never too late to make some sound investments that will grow steadily into a nice, tidy nest egg. I'm not going to tell you how to invest your cash—for that kind of advice, you should turn to a professional financial planner. But what I will do is give you some simple tips on solving a very common problem: coming up with money that you can put to work for you.

Can You Afford It?

Lots of people think they can't afford to make any long-term investments until they've paid off every dime of debt and saved enough money to cover any possible emergency. If you're one of those folks, think again. As long as you have savings set aside to cover basic living expenses for three months or so, and your debt is under control, you not only can, but *should* be investing at least a small amount of money each month.

Gain with No Pain

Still think you don't have cash to spare? Then consider this fact: If you invest just $20 a week in a mutual fund with a 9 percent annual return, it'll be worth $250,000 in 30 years. Yep: a cool quarter of a million bucks. What's more, those will be 20 *pretax* dollars if you put them into a 401(k) or SEP retirement account.

Where do you get the $20? Just think about some of the things you buy every day without

HOME REMEDY

If you're like most folks, chances are you've got a fair amount of future cash that's just clogging up closets or gathering dust in the attic. So don't just sit there: Haul that stuff out and hold a garage sale, take it to a consignment shop, or sell it over the Internet. Just one note of caution: Before you sell anything that might have real value, have it appraised by a pro, who can also direct you to potential buyers. To find a good appraiser, contact an antiques dealer, art gallery, or fine-jewelry store.

giving them a second thought. For instance, if you routinely grab coffee and a doughnut on your way to work—or maybe a large double latte—you're probably dropping close to $20 a week right there. Or what about those fast food lunches and take-out dinners you indulge in? They're economical, sure, but the cost of these "cheap" meals really adds up fast!

Fun Money

When you're trying to come up with investment funds, don't think of it as an exercise in self-denial. Instead, make a game of it. First, open a savings account at a bank that's on your daily travel route, or that has branches scattered around town. Make sure you can access the account with an ATM card. Then, every time you come upon extra cash—for instance, some wrinkled bills in the pocket of a coat you haven't worn in a while—tuck it into your interest-bearing "treasure chest." When the balance is large enough (generally around $500), open a money market or mutual funds account.

After that, keep on using your savings account as a sort of holding tank, where you deposit all the stray nickels, dimes, and dollar bills that come your way. When they've grown into whatever minimum deposit your investment plan requires, transfer that amount.

Finders Keepers

Once you discover how valuable tiny bits of money can be, you'll start looking for them everywhere. Here are some absolutely painless ways to find them:

Cash in your coupons. Before you leave the grocery store, note how much you saved by using coupons or buying sale items, and pull that amount out of your wallet.

Change your ways. Take the loose change out of your pocket or purse each evening and toss it into a tin (or even a piggy bank). You'll probably be amazed at how quickly it adds up. *Note:* Your stash will grow even faster if you make it a point to use bills, rather than coins, for cash purchases.

Check your rebates. You can find rebate offers on everything from wine to electric toothbrushes to computers. When you've applied for one and the check arrives in the mail, deposit it pronto.

Deposit your deposits. If you live in a state that mandates a deposit on beverage cans and bottles, count yourself lucky: Every time you return those containers to the store, you'll get a nickel (or even a dime) for each one.

CHAPTER 2

Seize the Deals

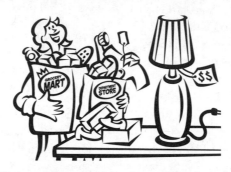

My Grandma Putt never made a fuss about frugality; she just went about life in her commonsense way. But nowadays, it's hard to stay on a budget when prices for the bare necessities are sky-high. Food alone can eat a large hole in your bank account. Then there's the cost of clothing, appliances, furniture, and electronics. You can't do without many of these things, so I'm going to show you how to live well without spending loads of cash!

THE GOODS ON SMART GROCERY SHOPPING

You know me—I'm as frugal and self-sufficient as they come. But even I need to go to the supermarket occasionally. Government statistics say that we spend almost 10 percent of our yearly income at the grocery store! That adds up to a lot of cash. High prices are only part of the story—crafty marketing ploys and so-called bargains drive up the costs of groceries. But you don't have to fall for those come-ons. Here's how you can take a bite out of those bloated grocery bills.

Think First, Shop Later

Saving money at the supermarket starts long before you walk in and grab the cart. You can avoid spending a bundle with just a little bit of planning and organization. I know it's hard to resist the urge to just snatch the keys and go, but I guarantee that you'll save lots of money with just a little prep work if you follow this two-step plan:

Step 1. Gather up all of the coupons you can get your hands on. Check your mail, the Yellow Pages, your newspaper, and your computer. Manufacturers of your favorite foods often have lots of coupons, rebates, and even offers for free samples on their Web sites (the address is usually posted on the side of the package).

Step 2. Make a shopping list. You'll avoid the hazard of buying what the store wants you to buy rather than what you'll need. If that isn't a good enough reason to make a list, then how about this one: Those clever supermarketeers have found a great way to get you to wander all over the store looking for the items you want. How? They move them around the store. (You aren't crazy—that soup really *was* in aisle 7 last week.) Those crafty folks know that your wandering ways will expose you to more products. So avoid overspending by making, taking, and diligently sticking to your grocery list!

Travel Light

You have your coupons and your list, but you're not quite goof-proofed yet! There are a few things you should leave behind if at all possible because they'll only weaken your resolve to make the most of every penny.

Credit cards. That's right—the best way to avoid impulse purchases is to take cash, and cash only. Try to estimate how much cash you'll need before you go, then take an extra $10 (just in case). You might get caught a little short the first time you try this (okay, so leave behind that extra pint of ice cream), but you'll

Quick Fix

Find yourself couponless at the supermarket? No problem! Check out the customer service center. Courtesy counters frequently display the coupons, rebates, and giveaways they receive directly from manufacturers or distributors. And they're all yours for the taking!

get better at hitting your mark every time you shop, and you'll avoid needless purchases.

Kids. Supermarkets can be so cruel! Putting items such as candy in the same aisle as cereal triggers the automatic "I want it, I want it!" response in kids and forces customers to spend more than they planned. If it's not possible to leave the tots behind, keep them occupied with coupons while you shop. Ask them to sort them for you or add up the prices while you go 60 miles per hour past the ice cream freezer.

Your appetite. Never go shopping on an empty stomach! That goes double for your children or grandkids if you take them along. Everything looks much more appealing when your stomach is growling. Make sure you eat before you leave, or take a baggie of popcorn or pretzels to munch on before you go inside.

Test Your Outer Limits

It's time to hit the aisles running! But that doesn't mean racing up each and every one. Have you ever noticed the layout of your grocery store? Chances are that the unprocessed foods (produce, meat, dairy) are on the perimeter of the store, while the higher-priced processed foods (canned, bagged, and boxed goods; junk food; and frozen meals) are in the interior aisles. So if you buy most of your groceries from the perimeter of the store, you'll not only save money, but you'll eat healthier, too!

Head for the Salad Bar

Now, I'm not usually a big fan of prepared foods because they're so darned expensive. But here's an instance when it's okay to break the rules. If your grocery store has a salad bar, a visit there can save you a bundle. The next time you're making soup or stew (or anything else, for that matter) that calls for, say, just a cup of carrots, don't get your veggies from the produce section, where that bag of carrots will set you back $2 or more. Not only will you end up with more than you need for your recipe, but you'll pay more for it, too. That same cup of carrots from the salad bar will cost a whole lot less—and they're already washed, peeled, and sliced, saving you time *and* money!

Shop in Season

Of course, you know that it's a good idea to stock up on your favorite foods when they're on sale, but did you know that many grocery items are at their cheapest when they're in season? Here are a few examples:

Apples. Buy them from October to March, when they are at their peak harvest.

Ham. When Easter rolls around, you're going to find ham on sale, so stock up on it at that time and freeze it for later use.

Sweet potatoes. You'll find great buys on these spuds from October to December. Store them in a cool, dry place, and they'll keep for up to two months.

Turkey. It seems like they're practically giving turkeys away come November! Well, turkey freezes just fine, so buy a couple if you've got the freezer space, and celebrate turkey day well into the new year.

Be Flexible

Now this may sound as though I'm contradicting myself, but as important as a shopping list is, don't use it with blinders on. If you find an item on sale that you normally use, but it's not on your list, then by all means throw it in the cart! It's worth it to buy that item now if you have a few extra dollars on you, instead of waiting

until you really need it when the price is back up again.

Here's a surefire way to keep yourself from going overboard on those kinds of purchases: Set a limit. My personal policy is to limit unscheduled buys to no more than three per trip. You might want to make that number smaller or larger, or even set a dollar limit—but no matter what your limiting method is, stick to it!

Quick Fix

How often have you entered your local grocery store to find an apron-clad employee cheerfully handing out tasty samples of new food products? How often do you stop to try a taste? I used to be mighty suspicious of this "something for nothing" setup until I realized that they were giving away not only free food, but also manufacturers' coupons for the products—and those coupons frequently offered substantial discounts. So now my advice is that if the new product is similar to something you would normally buy, then go ahead and take a sample and a coupon, and give the new product a try.

Give 'Em the Deep Freeze

If you bake or do a lot of cooking around the holidays, you know that supermarkets usually jack up the price of dairy products, such as butter, margarine, and milk, right around that time. If you plan ahead, however, you'll save precious pennies. About a month before you start your holiday baking, buy your butter, margarine, and milk, and freeze them. Then when it's time to make those Christmas cookies, you'll have the provisions on hand without having to hand over a lot of dough (ha-ha!).

Milk can be stored frozen at 0°F for up to three months and will be safe to drink if it is thawed in the refrigerator. Although the flavor and texture may change, it is fine for use in baking. To store butter in the freezer, wrap the unopened carton in moisture- and vapor-proof freezer packaging material or seal in a zip-top plastic freezer bag to keep the butter from absorbing odors from other foods. If properly wrapped and held at 0°F or lower, butter will keep well in the freezer for six to nine months. Then thaw it in the refrigerator. You can freeze margarine for a full 12 months in its original package. Just don't freeze whipped margarine or whipped butter.

Do the Math

Don't get caught by labels that claim you get "10 Percent More Free" in the package. Check the unit price that's listed on the shelf label right below the product. It will tell you the cost per unit (such as ounce, pound, or sheet). If the unit price is missing, use the formula below to easily calculate it yourself. (It's always a good idea to carry a small calculator with you whenever you go grocery shopping.)

Take the price and divide it by the number of units. For example, a 12-ounce bag of pretzels priced at $1.29 costs about 11 cents per ounce. Compare that to a 16-ounce bag that costs $1.40 to see which one is the better buy (the larger bag, in this instance). But don't automatically assume that all larger-size products are cheaper. Sometimes a larger package is much more expensive than the slightly smaller no-name brand, or is actually more expensive than buying two smaller packages of the same brand. So always be sure to calculate the unit cost!

Get the Inside Scoop

I'll bet most of you don't often chat with the folks who work in your supermarket, but it's one of my favorite ways to get the best deals. As I always say, "It pays to be in the know." So shed your shyness and start shopping smart by getting friendly with these folks:

The butcher. Talk to the guy or gal behind the meat counter and ask when your favorite cuts will be reduced or on sale. That way, you can be sure to be first in line and save as much as 50 percent on your next meat bill. Also, don't pass up those family packs, even if you're just shopping for one or two people. Simply ask the butcher to repackage the meat or poultry into smaller portions for you, and they should be glad to oblige.

The department managers. If the store is out of one of your preferred items, or the produce is looking kinda "ripe," talk to the manager in those departments. They can tell you when new shipments are coming in, and you can be at the store bright and early to pick up your favorites. You can also discover when the older produce is going on sale. Remember, wilted veggies are great for making soups and stews!

The store manager. These folks know when promotions and sales are being planned, because they do the planning. So they can let you know in advance, and you can plan your shopping around those big discount days.

Grab Golden Opportunities

If you're a senior—and that often means over the age of 50—you could shave around 10 percent off your total grocery bill! While you're at the customer service counter checking out the coupons and chatting up the store manager, ask if there's a senior discount program. Some stores offer discounts only on certain days of the week or at specific times of the day, so do your homework before you shop.

As a senior, you might also be entitled to free groceries every single week! There are several programs throughout the country— most at a local level—that provide this service. To find out if such a program exists in your town, contact senior citizen centers, community centers, or food banks in your area. They'll also be listed in the Yellow Pages or on the Internet.

Wait for Rain Checks

Missed a sale because the item was sold out? Don't fret—you may have a second chance at saving some money. By law, products advertised as being on sale must be available, or the store has to give you a rain check for that item at the sale price (unless the advertisement clearly states that there are limited quantities). If the item is sold out by the time you get to the store, then ask for a rain check at the customer service counter and use it the next time you go shopping.

Make an End Run

Don't be fooled by those big, fancy displays set up at the ends of aisles. They sure do catch your eye—I mean, they're right there for you to see (and trip over) as you turn the corner into the next aisle. But I'll bet dollars to doughnuts that most times those items are not on sale. Remember, just because an item is singled out *does not* mean that it's specially priced. Look carefully for a sign that states the price; if it's less than usual, great! If not, then walk on by.

Get Down in the Dumps

Wanna save up to 50 percent on selected grocery items? Ask the courtesy desk clerk if

the store has what they refer to as a "dump" section. It might include items in dented cans, items with torn labels, or the last few boxes of a discontinued product. These items are always marked down, usually at a substantial discount. The only catch: Be careful when it comes to dented cans. Inspect them closely to make sure they aren't leaking because a leak might harbor dangerous bacteria that can cause food poisoning.

HOME REMEDY

In spring and summer, the farmer's markets are blooming with cut-rate produce, legumes, and whole grains. But don't let your guard down— specialty items like gifts, homemade breads, and gourmet foods may not be competitively priced, so buy those items wisely. When it comes to farm-fresh food, though, you usually can't find a better deal. And your dollar will stretch even further if you make your purchases at the end of the day, when dealers slash their prices to lighten the load they'll have to haul back home. (Save your egg and corn purchases for the morning, though, since they lose their freshness quickly.) And, if you don't think the prices are low enough, you can always haggle with the dealer—just try to do *that* in a grocery store!

Pass on Disposables

Do you regularly buy disposable items like paper napkins, paper towels, or plastic razors? If you do, then you're throwing your money away as well. You can save big bucks by using things that have more staying power instead. For instance, napkins and paper towels can run you several hundred dollars a year, but cloth napkins and dishrags can be purchased very cheaply and they'll last for years! And if you're buying packs of plastic razors at $6 a pop, you'll have spent about two or three times the price of an electric razor after one year. So think twice before you toss another disposable item into your grocery cart—you'll save more cash when you buy something with a longer life span.

Know Your Generics

Everyone knows that store brands are cheaper than nationally advertised brands, but many people don't like trading quality for economy. The good news is that you don't have to. Many stores now carry more than one variety of house brand, and some have as many as three quality levels. The next time you're wondering how the store brand items stack up against the brightly packaged name brands, keep these in mind:

Generics. The lowest quality products for the cheapest price.

House brands. Equivalent to the better-known "name" brands, but at a price that's about 20 percent less than what the name brands cost.

Premium store brands. Deluxe items that are the equivalent of gourmet products for around 25 percent less than what the gourmet products will run you.

Don't Be Fooled by the Word *New*

Ever wonder what, exactly, it means when one of your favorite products sports a label proclaiming that it's "New and Improved"? Well, it usually means that the product has been *needlessly* improved (New Color! New Scent! New Size!), so the manufacturer has decided

to charge more for it. It's almost as though they were looking for an excuse to raise the price, and so they created one.

Look Up and Down

Most supermarketeers place their most expensive items smack-dab at eye level. Since they're the first items you see and they're easy to get to, you're likely to grab 'em. And manufacturers pay dearly for that exclusive piece of real estate, causing their prices to be even higher. But guess what? Chances are that if you look just a little higher or lower on the shelves, you'll find similar products with kinder prices. Who knew that a simple bend of the knee could be such an economical move?

Another thing to remember is that this eye-level marketing can get pretty sophisticated, especially when it comes to products for kids. The most expensive (and usually least nutritious) children's breakfast cereals are placed at *their* eye level, rather than yours.

Leave the Entertainment Behind

Do your television watching and newspaper reading at home, and you'll save yourself money on groceries. How's that? You see, supermarkets these days do all they can to get you to linger in the store and (they hope) spend more money. Some larger stores even have televisions set up and newspapers available in seated café areas, all with the intention of keeping you in the store a little while longer. So the long and short of it is—don't get comfortable if you want to save money!

Be Counter Intuitive

I usually don't shop in a supermarket with fewer than five regular and two express checkout lanes open during my regular shopping hours, for two reasons. First, remember that time is money: The longer you wait in line, the more money it's costing you. The second reason is that the more overworked the cashier is, the more likely it is that mistakes will be made—and not necessarily in your favor! So if you frequently find yourself in long lines, start shopping when the store isn't as busy, or look for another store that has more lanes open.

Say "No" to Checkout Come-Ons

You may be surprised to know that the most lucrative spot in the entire grocery store is the checkout counter! That's right, that area earns more profit per square foot than any other part of the store. Just think about it—you're held captive in line and you're probably more than a little bored, so it's the perfect place to squeeze more money from you before you leave. But don't give

---

⧖ *Quick Fix*

So you've managed to make room in your home for all of the groceries you just bought, but you may still have one challenge—what to do with all of those plastic grocery bags! Here's a simple solution: Just tuck them inside of an empty tissue box. You can keep the boxes handy in places where you know you'll use the bags, like the kitchen, garage, toolshed, or trunk of your car.

If you <u>don't</u> save your plastic grocery bags, then you may not know how many uses they have—for instance, as trash can liners, pooper-scoopers, and waterproof wraps for packing shoes and cosmetics. There are 1,001 reasons to hold on to your grocery bags, so please tuck those handy helpers into a tissue box for now and put them to good use later on.

---

in! Those lighters, batteries, candy, and other small items may seem reasonably priced, but you can usually find them much cheaper elsewhere. So pass them by and pick up those incidentals on your next trip to the discount store.

Don't Play the Waiting Game

Don't automatically assume that the shortest checkout line will save you time. First, watch the cashiers for a moment or two. Are they paying attention to what they're doing, or do they seem to have their heads in the clouds? Also, be alert for "traffic jams." A line may be short because the cashier is waiting for a price check or some other time-consuming task to be done before he or she can finish up with the person at the head of the line. That makes the line shorter as people get impatient with the wait and move to the other checkout lines. Dash into this kind of short line, and you may be the last one out the door!

Keep It Courteous

It's no fun (and can be downright embarrassing) when you hand the cashier a big wad of coupons, only to discover that some of them have expired, or the store doesn't accept them. So please, toss those expired coupons before you leave for the store, and give the current ones to your cashier *before* she or he starts to ring you up. That way, if the store doesn't accept a particular coupon, you can address it before the item is scanned. Doing it this way will save you money, and spare you time-consuming hassles.

Scan the Scanners

I have to chuckle every time I see a sign in a supermarket that says "We guarantee our scanner price is correct or you get the product free," because I know that the store could be—but isn't—giving away a lot of free groceries.

Why not? Because most shoppers don't pay attention to the screen as the prices get scanned, so they never realize that they're being overcharged.

Errors often occur on the first day of a sale, when the computer system hasn't been thoroughly updated. So how do you avoid this trap? By jotting down the prices of sale items on your grocery list as you put them in the cart, and by paying attention to the cash register screen as those items are being scanned. That way, you'll know right away if a mistake is being made.

Don't Toss Your Receipt

After you've put away all of the groceries and stored your plastic and paper bags (see the Quick Fix at left for tips on putting those bags to good use), don't toss your receipt into the recycling bin! Have you looked at it lately? Many supermarkets print coupons on the backs of or along the bottoms of register receipts. If your store doesn't offer them, switch to one that does—if it's convenient and the prices are competitive. These coupons usually work by tracking your purchases and making offers accordingly. Say, for example, that you buy a few cans of tuna. The cash register will print out a money-saving coupon for the same (or competing) brand of tuna on the receipt. You're almost always guaranteed to get a coupon for a product you want. And by the way, if you're not already scrutinizing your register receipts for mistakes, you're really missing out on a chance to save money!

Consider Clubbing

These days, it seems that just about everyone's joining a buying club—you know, one of those warehouselike super-supermarkets where you can buy everything from groceries to vitamins in bulk quantities. But is it as great a deal as it

seems? Well, as with almost everything else in life, it depends. Here are some questions to ask yourself before you sign on:

- Where's it gonna go? Do you have the closet space for 140 rolls of toilet paper or a 25-pound bag of white rice? And do you have smaller storage containers to break down larger packages if you need to?

- Will you use it quickly enough? Many items spoil or reach their expiration date long before you have a chance to use them, and some things don't store well to begin with. (On the other hand, some items, such as toilet paper, never get old—but that leads us back to the first question.)

- Are you just in it for the thrill? Some folks just can't turn their backs on a bargain—even when it means purchasing quantities of items they will *never* use! How else can you explain the three cases of tomato soup some folks have when they eat soup only about once a month? The bottom line: Don't be lured into buying in bulk just because it's a bargain!

Get Friendly

If you decide to join a buying club and purchase products in bulk, be sensible and split the membership fee with a friend or family member. Think of how much lighter your grocery tab will be. And you won't just be halving your shopping bills, either. You'll be halving your storage space problem, too! Just make sure that you both share the same food preferences and budget ranges. It's also a good idea to shop together when you can, so you can talk about prices. Not only that, but you'll have someone to help you load that 40-pound bag of dog chow into your trunk. Sharing your membership will save you money, and possibly even save your back!

GET DRESSED FOR LESS

When I was growing up, I was one of the best-dressed kids in town. No, my family wasn't rolling in dough—we did, however, wear the best clothes money could buy. Grandma Putt had a keen eye for value, and she could spot quality threads like nobody's business! Whether our outfits were gently used when we bought them at the local secondhand store, or brand-new, Grandma used that same clothing know-how to find the best deals. So if you're breaking the bank to look like a million bucks, heed my advice and try on some new shopping habits, courtesy of Grandma Putt!

HOME REMEDY

Don't overlook bargain clothes just because the sizing is a bit too large. There are some quick "repairs" you can make at home and no one will be the wiser. For example, say you find a shirt you just love, at a great price, but the sleeves are just too darn long. No problem! If the sleeves are cuffed, use a seam ripper to remove the cuffs, cut the sleeves to a shorter length, and reattach the cuffs. Voilà! A perfect fit.

A too-long skirt needs only a simple hem to get it to the length you need. And too-long pants can also be hemmed. If your sewing skills are a bit rusty, bring the clothes to your local dry cleaner or tailor. These alterations are pretty basic, so the charges should be reasonable.

Dress for Shopping Success

First things first: Before you start pounding the pavement, make sure you're wearing your most comfy clothes and shoes. If you plan to try stuff on (and I recommend that you do because it saves you the hassle of having to return ill-fitting clothes), wear clothing that's easily removed. Here's the perfect shopping wear: stretch pants or a skirt with an elastic waistband, a shirt that doesn't need to be tucked in, and slip-on shoes—clogs are great, lace-up boots aren't. With this easy-on/easy-off ensemble, you'll be able to try clothes on quickly. Remember, time is money! And the less time you spend in the store, the less prone you are to making frivolous purchases.

Dodge the Duds

A brand-new $5 shirt (if there were such a thing!) would last about a week before coming apart at the seams—and that's exactly what you'd expect for that price. But if the same thing happens to a $50 shirt, *arrrgh!*—you've been had. High price and high quality don't necessarily go hand in hand. Luckily, you can easily test the durability of a garment once you know where to look:

Stitches. The closer, neater, and stronger the stitching is, the better made and longer-lasting the garment will be. Also, make sure the stitching is straight.

Buttons. Is each button sewn on securely, and is there a button for every buttonhole? If either answer is no, ask for a discount and secure any loose buttons, or sew on new ones at home for less than a penny! And take a look at the buttonholes: Is the trim around them sewn through both sides of the fabric? If the buttonholes aren't solidly trimmed, they'll fray in no time at all, so give that garment a pass.

Seams. Inspect the seams where the parts of a garment are joined together, such as where the arm meets the shoulder. Those seams should be flat, not bunched up. All of the hems should be straight, and you shouldn't see the stitching on the outside of the garment (unless that's the style, of course).

Closures. Be sure that all of the snaps line up and that each one snaps tightly. If there are Velcro® closures, be sure that the "hook" tape and the "loop" tape align properly when pressed closed. Also, check that the zipper is sewn in straight and securely, and that it operates smoothly. If it snags easily or you have to tug at it, put the garment back on the rack!

Pockets. The pockets should be flat and have reinforced corners. If the pockets are supposed to be functional (some are just for show), make sure they are big enough to actually use.

Fabric. The material should look flat and evenly woven or knit with no flaws—unless it's made from a fiber with natural flaws, like wool or raw silk.

Patterns. Plaids, pinstripes, and checks should always match at the seams so the pattern looks unbroken from front to back. On shirts, check under the arms and down the sleeve and side seams. On pants and skirts, check the side and back seams.

Take Your Swatches Shopping

If you're searching for clothing that needs to match something that's already in your closet, take along a swatch or two. It's easy to snip a piece of fabric from your garment without damaging it—just turn the clothing inside out, and cut a small piece of cloth from inside a seam. Then you're good to go.

Don't Get Shortchanged

Say you're buying a new pair of work trousers and you'll need them to last a long time. Here's a clever way to do just that. Buy the pants with the waist size you want, but in a length that's 4 or 5 inches longer than you need. (Of course, they'll cost the same as the shorter pair.) Now take the pants home, hem them yourself, and save the fabric. When it comes time to patch those work pants (and believe you me, that time will come!), you'll have an exact match for the fabric. The extra fabric may be darker if you've washed the pants a lot, but those perfect patches will spare you the cost of having to buy another pair of pants.

Take Credit—Save Money

The next time you're shopping at a clothing store, ask the salesclerk if you'll get automatic savings on today's purchase if you apply for the store's credit card. Sometimes, you can save 30 percent just for applying! I usually do this once or twice a year, then I just cut up the card when it arrives at my house. A word of warning: Don't do this too often, because too many credit applications can negatively affect your credit rating. (For information on controlling that credit card debt, turn to page 3.)

Find a Perfect Price for Imperfections

Has this ever happened to you? You're trying on the perfect shirt or pair of pants, when you notice that it's not so perfect after all. It's missing a button or has a slight stain and, of course, it's the only one in your size. Are you out of luck? No way! Just ask the manager for a discount. Believe you me, he or she is authorized to give it and would probably love to get rid of the merchandise. Ten percent is reasonable. Just make sure it's an imperfection that you can either live with or fix cheaply at home.

Go Halves

You can really rack up the savings on a two-for-the-price-of-one sale. But what if you only need one? Ask a friend or family member if they could use the other one, and then the two of you can split the cost. Now you've saved even more! What if you unexpectedly stumble across a two-for-one sale and just can't pass it up, but again, you only need one of them? You could do what a friend of mine did who found just such a deal on some slippers. She stopped the first lady she saw and offered to go halves with her on two pairs of slippers. It worked! Do I have some mighty clever friends, or what?

Shop with the Big Boys

Attention all you small-size ladies out there! Are you tired of paying top dollar for items such as T-shirts, casual shirts, and even jeans? Then, depending upon how petite you are, head to the boys' or the men's department. The large-size boys' duds and the small-size men's clothing may be just the ticket—and they'll cost you a whole lot less than the ladies' equivalent!

Quick Fix

Tired of ruining (or losing) one sock and getting stuck with the orphan? If you are, then do what I do: Every time I need a pair of socks, I buy two pairs in each color, so I'll always have a complete pair. Here's how it works. If one sock gets a hole or disappears, I use a sock from the new pair to replace it. When the remaining sock from the old pair gets worn out, then I simply use the other sock from the new pair. This way, I'm getting the most mileage for my money!

Stock Up on Staples

My approach to clothes shopping is the same as my approach to grocery shopping: I stock up on staples when there's a good sale. By staples, I mean the basics, such as socks, T-shirts, underwear, and work jeans. For those items, I head to the discount store, *not* the department store, where they'll cost an arm and a leg.

Turn the Tables

When I'm shopping for a major purchase, like a suit, I never buy accessories at the same time. Ever notice those tables of ties, belts, and socks in expensive menswear stores? The store is counting on you to buy them to match the $400 outfit you just bought. Be smart, and buy accessories separately when they go on sale.

Don't Get Taken to the Cleaners!

There's nothing worse than bringing home a bargain, only to find out that it costs a lot more in the long run than you originally thought. That's the case with most clothing that needs to be dry-cleaned. Heck, you could pay for the same shirt two or three times over if you have to have it dry-cleaned every few weeks! Of course, some items (such as suits and blazers, or special-occasion clothing) must be professionally cleaned. But did you know that some "Dry-Clean-Only" clothes can be safely washed at home? You can be sure by checking the label; if it says "Professional Dry-Clean Only," there's no way around it. But if the label says "Dry-Clean Only," there's hope. Here's how to care for those garments in your own laundry room:

Wash by hand. Most of those "Dry-Clean-Only" clothes can be washed by hand in cold water. Silks, cashmere, angora, chiffon, and even lace can all be hand-washed with care. Use a couple drops of clear dish soap, and gently work the suds through the garment. Don't tug or pull.

Roll 'em dry. After hand-washing clothes, try this trick for getting out excess water: Lay the item flat on a clean white towel and roll it up. Press on the towel, then unroll it and let the garment lay flat until it's dry.

Outwit the Outlets

Just because that blouse is for sale in an outlet store doesn't mean it's cheap (or even cheaper than in a department store). Outlets can offer good buys, but finding them takes some shopping savvy. Your best bet for outlet savings is to combine a really good price with a store credit or gift card. Your next cost-saving move should be to understand what you're buying. But those confusing merchandise labels have to be deciphered first, so you'll know if you're getting a bargain. That's no problem! Just use my guide below, and you'll be cracking those codes in no time:

Irregular. Merchandise marked "irregular" is slightly imperfect. The stitching may be a bit off on the hem, or one sleeve might be just a tad longer than the other. Inspect the garment carefully to make sure its imperfections aren't obvious.

Seconds. Anything marked a "second" is flawed—and probably noticeably so. When I go outlet shopping, I head for the seconds whenever I'm buying socks, underwear, casual clothing, towels, and linens, or anything else that I'm not too fussy about.

Samples. This tag means the garment style is something the manufacturer was trying out, or the merchandise was on display. These items can be real oddballs—shoes in size 5 only, or clothing in a variety of strange colors and sizes.

Past-season. Last year's styles are this year's best buys. Don't hesitate to grab a good deal. As long as it's still in good shape, past-season merchandise can be some of the best clothing bargains around.

Discontinued. This merchandise is stuff the manufacturer has stopped making—maybe the style or color is outdated. The items may be top quality, but sometimes, the choice of sizes is limited.

Overstocks. What happens when a manufacturer makes 50,000 pairs of mauve slippers, but only 25,000 people buy them? You guessed it—the leftovers become overstocks. Those items are generally first quality and a first-rate buy, so check 'em out.

Try Thrift Store Threads

Think your local thrift shop is nothing more than a junk store? Think again—there are hundreds of treasures waiting to be discovered in these types of shops. All it takes is a little know-how. Don't miss these clues that separate the rags from the riches:

Worn elbows. If they're on a woman's blouse or a man's shirt, pass it up. But if they're on a blazer or sport coat, you can go the preppy route and sew on store-bought leather or fabric patches for next to nothing.

Too short. There's an easy way to lengthen kids' jeans. Just cut them off at the knee, sew on a band of colorful fabric, and reattach the bottom denim portion; or just add the fabric to the bottom of the pant leg. Unless you're shopping for "kickin' around the yard" clothing, pass on adult-size trousers that are too short.

Missing buttons. That's a no-brainer—it's easy to replace buttons. But torn or misshapen buttonholes are another matter completely. Steer clear of any garment with buttonholes that are in bad shape.

Ragged or frayed hem. As long as you can rehem a garment to make it shorter (and you don't mind the work), a ragged hem shouldn't make much difference on a skirt, dress, or pair of pants. Fixing a ragged hem on a coat can be tricky to do yourself, but any good seamstress should be able to do the job fairly inexpensively.

Catch the Early Bird Deals

You'll find the best thrift store bargains on Monday and Tuesday. Why? Well, most folks clear out their closets (and take clothes to thrift shops) on the weekends—and that means they'll be ready for sale early in the week.

Find Garden-Variety Duds

As you may know, I spend a lot of time in my yard and garden. How do I keep from destroying my everyday clothes? Simply by slipping on my thrift store duds. That way, I know that whatever I'm working in has been broken in and didn't cost me very much to begin with. If you do a lot of gardening or painting or anything else that can get messy, pick up some "play clothes" at the thrift store and spare your casual clothes all of the dirt and stains.

Spend Fewer Fancy Dollars

Got a wedding coming up? Or maybe you're searching for prom attire for your kids or grandkids? Whatever the occasion, you don't have to pony up big bucks to step out in style. Here are several ways to get those special-event outfits for a whole lot less:

- Swap with friends. Most women I know have at least one bridesmaid's dress collecting dust in the back of their closet. Ask your friends and family if you could borrow their finery for an evening (just make sure it's properly

FAST FORMULA

Sweaty Stain Solution

Don't let a few perspiration stains come between you and a perfectly good dress shirt. Before you buy a replacement, tackle those yellow stains with this do-it-yourself recipe that combines lemon and sunshine, nature's best bleach. So far, nothing the detergent industry has come up with can top it!

$1/2$ cup of lemon juice, or 2 lemons
Hot water
1 additional lemon
Plenty of sunshine

Pour lemon juice or squeeze two lemons into a half-full washing machine tub of water. (If you're doing a full load, add twice as much lemon.) Soak your clothes for an hour or overnight, and then put them through the wash cycle. Add the juice of one more lemon to the rinse cycle, and hang your clothes up to dry in the sun.

cleaned before you return it). Even better, start a dress-lending library with your friends. When one member needs a fancy dress, she'll have several to choose from to find just the right one for the special occasion.

- Rent, don't buy. Tuxes aren't the only formalwear you can rent. Check out the usual rental stores as well as costume shops! They may have a low-mileage, stunning outfit that was worn on stage at the local community theater.

- Shop with a friend. If you have a pal who needs some posh apparel too, take her along. If you're about the same size and aren't going to the same event, why not buy one dress and split the bill?

A Magical Transformation

You don't need a fairy godmother, or a king's ransom, to be the belle of the ball. You can transform a dime-store bargain into an elegant treasure fit for the fanciest of occasions simply by attaching small accessories to it with a few sewing stitches or some fabric glue (available at craft stores). Those long-forgotten pumps will come alive with the addition of some well-placed spangles. And a few pearls will really liven up the neckline and hem of that old gown. Heck, even your old rubber flip-flops will look marvelous with the addition of a few fancy flowers!

If the Shoe Fits, Buy It!

The next time you're shopping for shoes, look at the heel and notice how it's attached to the body of the shoe. If the shoes are new, do the heels look sturdy? If the shoes have been previously owned, are the heels so worn that you'll need to have them replaced? If so, then that will boost the price, and may not make them such a great deal.

Make Sure All's Welt

Before buying shoes, check out the welt, which is the seam where the upper part attaches to the sole. Give it a tug to see if it's well attached. Is it stitched, or is it just glued? As you may have guessed, stitched is better.

Get the Inside Scoop

Place your hand inside the shoe: You shouldn't find any holes or deeply worn grooves. Of course, if the shoe is used, there might be slight signs of wear, but avoid shoes that look worn out or abused, because they're nothing but trouble.

Uncover a Cover-Up

Many women's pumps have heels that are covered in the same material as the upper part. Make sure that this material is in good shape and is not fraying around the bottom on the heel or at the inside seam. If it is, walk on by! That material is usually impossible to repair.

Take a Walk

Isn't it funny how shoes often seem more comfortable in the shoe store than at home? It's no accident. Most stores have carpeting that's so thick and cushy, you'll feel like you're walking in slippers. So the next time you're shopping for shoes, make sure to walk on a hard surface in or outside of the store (if they'll let you) before you buy anything.

Rescue and Recover

I'm always shocked when I see people throwing away perfectly good shoes. I mean, don't they know they could *double* the life of their shoes just by visiting the neighborhood shoe repair shop? Of course, not all shoes are salvageable. Those $10 sneakers with a hole in the sole belong at the dump, but "hard" shoes, such as loafers, pumps, and bucks, can all be repaired. Keep that in mind when you're visiting the local thrift shop and you walk past the shoe aisle. Those once-proud pumps you're eyeing can regain their former glory for just a few dollars!

Check the Lost and Found

Speaking of shoe repair, stop by your local shoe repair shop to see if they have any shoes for sale. That's right—most shoe repair shops will hold repaired shoes for only a limited time (usually 30 days). Once that time is up, they may be willing to unload those freshly repaired shoes for a song. After all, they're in the business of repairing shoes, not warehousing them!

Night Moves

Has this ever happened to you? You buy what you thought were the most comfortable shoes in the world, only to find out later on that they pinch like the dickens! If so, then you probably bought them during the day. You see, your feet actually swell as the day progresses, and by nighttime, your dogs are at their largest. The simple solution is to hold off on your shoe shopping until the late afternoon or early evening, so you can find the best fit. Your tootsies will thank you!

APPLIANCES AND ELECTRONICS ON THE CHEAP

For lots of folks—me included—appliances and electronics are the two things we're most intimidated about buying. First, there are all those complicated doodads, and who knows if you really need them? Even the models without the doodads cost a small fortune! You could save money and buy used appliances and electronics, but how much life do they have left in them before you are back to needing a new one? Then there's the issue of utility bills. Appliances and electronics are hungry beasts that eat up your energy month after month after month, and older ones eat up more than new ones. Confused? Don't be. Here are some of my best ideas for saving money on big-ticket purchases, whether you are in the market for a brand-new dishwasher or a used stereo system.

Mind the Season

Most of us think of shopping in season as something we do only for fresh fruit and clothes. But there are shopping seasons for appliances and electronics, too. You'll usually find these items offered during two kinds of sales: clearance sales (because no one is buying them) and competitive sales (because everyone wants one). I always wait for the clearance sales because, in my experience, they save you more money. Of course, that may not always be practical—especially if your washing machine has just spun its last cycle! But if you aren't in an emergency situation, try to plan your purchases during times of the year when the pickings are ripe. Here's a rundown of when to look for what:

January and February. This is traditionally a dry period for retailers, so there are usually plenty of good sales to be found. Look for clearances on last year's models. They may not be the flavor of the month, but they are top-of-the-line, fully warrantied versions of last year's flavors.

May and June. Spring-cleaning sales offer low prices on vacuum cleaners. Discounts on air conditioners and refrigerators kick in just before Memorial Day and last well into June.

July. If you can hold out until July for your new air conditioner, prices will start heading toward clearance levels by midmonth.

November. Heating appliances go on sale, spurred on by lots of competition.

December. "Gift" appliances and electronics, such as vacuum cleaners, microwaves, televisions, and computers, are usually on sale. The best bargains, however, are after Christmas, when the stores want to clear out holiday returns and outdated models to make room for the latest and greatest.

Do a Little Digging

Most of the time we spend shopping for a new, big-ticket item would be better spent doing a little research. The biggest problem shoppers face is being overwhelmed with too many choices (all of which add to the purchase price, of course). If you want to make a smart purchase, tap these resources before you buy:

- Ask an expert. Is there a service person who's been coming to your house for years, someone you count on? Ask for his or her opinion on which brand to choose before you head to the stores. (Just be sure you talk to someone who services *all* brands.)

- Get the scoop from Uncle Sam. To find out if the product you're considering buying has any recalls or blemishes on its safety record, call the Consumer Products Safety Commission hotline at (800) 638-2772 or (800) 638-8270 (for the hearing impaired), or check out its Web site at **www.cpsc.gov**. Records go all the way back to 1972, so this is also a great source of information if you're thinking of purchasing a used item.

- Read all about it. Take a quick trip to the library to read about the models and brands you have in mind. Now I know that time is money, but in this case, it's well worth the effort. The last thing you need is a washer or dryer with a record of not washing or drying! Check out a copy of the *Consumer Reports*® annual buying guide, or log on to the *Consumer Reports* Web site at **www.consumerReports.org** to find out how various models rate on quality and performance.

- Scan the ads. If you're in the market for any major appliance or electronic equipment,

browse through the ads in the Sunday newspaper for three or four weekends in a row before making a final decision. Once you've got all the info, make a beeline for the store that offers the best deal.

Keep It Simple

I try to look at it this way—every button and function on an appliance or electronic gadget

---

FAST FORMULA

The Wall Wipe-Up

You've just purchased a new dryer. Now you need to remove the old one—and it's been in the same spot since 1966! You could probably knit a sweater with all of the lint underneath it. Dirt and dust can be easily swept away, but stains on the walls behind old appliances (especially ranges) are more of a challenge. Use this simple solution to wash away grease, grime, or any dirt smudges from your walls.

2 oz. of borax
1 tsp. of ammonia
1 bucket of water

Dissolve the borax with the ammonia in the water. Scrub down the wall, starting at the top. Then dry the wall with a clean, soft cloth or paper towel immediately. *A word of warning:* If you live in a recently built home that was painted by the builder, chances are that only a very thin layer of paint was sprayed on. If this may be the case, wash only a small section of the wall as a test; otherwise, you could end up looking at patches of drywall!

is a potential malfunction. Does the usefulness of that switch outweigh the risk of its breaking and needing repair? (In other words, do you really need 16 different cycle settings to clean your dishes?) If the answer is no, then I'd look for a more streamlined (that's pronounced "less expensive") model. A good friend once told me that the secret to good appliance and electronics buying is sticking with KISS. "It stands for 'Keep It Simple, Sweetie'," she said. That's one of the best bits of advice I've heard yet!

Don't Cry Over Scratches and Dents

You'll find fantastic open-box deals on new appliances and electronics right after Christmas. You can't help but be jolly about those savings…unless you're the type of person who's uncomfortable about scratches and dents. If a few blemishes make you cringe, think about whether the imperfection will even show. If your new refrigerator will be butting up against a counter or cabinet, no one will ever see that dent on the side.

Most stores have a scratch-and-dent corner, but some warehouse and outlet stores specialize in carrying marred models. Just be sure the item comes with the complete manufacturer's warranty on its performance. An appliance without a warranty is never a true bargain!

Find the Best Been-Used Deals

I'm just as certain that there are some fantastic deals sitting in the classified section of your local newspaper as I am that there are a few lemons there as well. If you're going to buy used appliances or electronics, here are the questions you should ask:

If it's so great, why do they want to sell it? Generally speaking, appliances are used until they fail. Ask the owner why it's on the market. The answers you'd like to hear? "We're moving

and the new house already has one," or "My mother just moved in and she doesn't need it anymore." Make sure the reason it's being sold is due to circumstances, not the appliance itself.

Does it work? You'd be surprised at the number of folks who don't bother to find this out before they buy an appliance. Always plug it in and try it out before you reach for your wallet. If the sellers have nothing to hide, they'll be more than happy to demonstrate how well the item works.

How does it compare? If you have a talent for appliance or electronics repair, you risk much less when buying a used item. But if you don't have the skills to make at least minor repairs, don't buy from a private seller until you check to see if a used-appliance dealer has a similar item. Dealers can offer you a warranty that includes parts and labor—something you'll never get from a private seller.

How high-tech is it? While used appliances can often work just as well as newer ones, be wary of buying high-tech products—especially computers and "digital" anything—that are more than two years old. Technology is developing at lightning speed, so even recent models won't hold up to the standards of the future. Last year's TV or dishwasher, warranties and all, can be a fantastic buy for a smart shopper, but an older computer or digital camera may not be compatible with today's technology, let alone the programs and upgrades of tomorrow.

Wheel and Deal

When it comes to making big purchases, you've got to act like a gambler, knowing when to hold 'em and when to fold 'em. In other words, when to push for a better deal and when to make tracks out of the store. The rules are a bit different depending on where you shop, so follow this guide to play your best hand:

Retail stores. Most retailers won't deal on price, but many will throw in something extra, like free delivery or no sales tax, to sweeten the pot if they think you are going to walk away. If you'll be transporting it home yourself, ask to have an accessory thrown in (some places even sell the power cord separately!). The only exception to this rule is on scratch-and-dent or open-box items, since they are already deeply discounted.

Wholesale and discount centers. These centers expect you to handle your own delivery, so transportation won't be a bargaining chip. But you can probably deal on price here, so offer 20 percent less than the asking price, and work down from there.

Dealing one-on-one. Private sellers know they're going to have to negotiate, and most take that into account when they set their asking price. So the rule here is—deal your heart out!

Be Wise to Warranties

There are two kinds of warranties you'll have to consider for any major appliance: the manufacturer's warranty that comes with your

---

⏳ *Quick Fix*

Need to load that heavy appliance into a pickup truck or van? Don't risk injuring your back! Make a loading ramp by leaning a ladder against the back of the vehicle, and covering the ladder with a strong board or two. Then set your cargo on the ramp, and slide it right in.

---

purchase, and the extended warranty that the salesperson will pitch to you. You should always get the most complete, extensive warranty possible, but never pay a single penny for an extra one. Why? Because if the item does break down past the manufacturer's warranty period, the cost to repair it is usually about the same, if not less, than the price of an extended warranty. And here's another reason to just say no—some credit card companies will lengthen the term of the manufacturer's coverage, so be sure to check your card agreement. The only time that an extended warranty might be a good idea is if the manufacturer guarantees repair and labor costs for a very short period of time. But if that's the case, you might want to think about purchasing an item with a more solid guarantee instead.

Freeze High Fridge Prices

If your refrigerator is more than 10 years old, I guarantee that you are losing money each and every month! In fact, two of today's models use about the same amount of electricity as one older, less efficient model. Your savings, of course, will depend on the style you choose. Refrigerators with a freezer on the bottom will save you the most energy, and models with freezers on top come in second. Side-by-side models are the costliest to run. The most efficient styles usually have a higher price tag, but the extra money may be worth it, especially when it comes to refrigerators. They'll eat up more energy than any other household appliance, so you'll probably recoup most of that money during the first year of use.

You'll save even more money (and electricity) if you skip those water and ice dispensers on the front door. Personally, I can do without this convenience. I can just as easily fill my glass with tap water from the kitchen sink, and since I've been making ice myself for 50-plus years,

I don't see any compelling reason to stop now. The fact is that fridge-produced water and ice drain your wallet in three ways:

1. These built-in conveniences always inflate the purchase price.

2. A plumber will need to run a water line from the refrigerator to your water pipes. Average cost: about $150.

3. Water dispensers will increase your electric bills by as much as 20 percent each month.

Used Refrigerators, Cool Prices

As I mentioned earlier, if your refrigerator is over 10 years old, you would probably save more money in electric bills by buying a recent model. But I know that there are times when a new refrigerator just isn't in the budget. If a used fridge has to do the job, here's how to make sure you get a good one:

Go for youth. The newer the model, the less you'll pay in utility bills.

Take its temperature. Make sure the refrigerator cools to between 38 and 40°F and the freezer is between 0 and 10°F. The refrigerator should be plugged in for at least 24 hours before you can get an accurate thermometer reading.

Give it the paper test. Close the door on a sheet of paper or dollar bill. If the paper falls or slips, the door hinges or the seal will have to be repaired and/or replaced.

Don't forget the yardstick. Measure your refrigerator space to make sure your new appliance will fit nicely in the current opening.

See the rear view. Are the coils clean? If they aren't, but the fridge works great, clean them the minute you get home. Vacuum the coils and then wipe them down with a damp cloth, rinsing it out often.

Clean it later, alligator. Don't let crumbs and stains stand between you and a great deal.

HOME REMEDY

Baking soda has thousands of uses around the home, from sunburn relief to flea removal. But when it comes to pure scouring power, it's truly a shining star. So don't let stains or odors stop you from buying an otherwise great used appliance—just seal the deal and let your baking soda do the dirty work. Here's how:

- Remove grease from stovetops and refrigerators using a sponge dampened with hot water and sprinkled with baking soda. Scrub lightly, then rinse.

- Kill mold and mildew with a no-rinse, all-purpose spray formula using 1 cup of clear ammonia, $1/2$ cup of distilled white vinegar, $1/4$ cup of baking soda, and 1 gallon of water. Mix the ingredients in a bucket, pour the solution into a spray bottle, and aim for the stains. No need to rinse!

- Tackle tough appliance stains with a scouring powder made up of 1 cup of baking soda, 1 cup of borax, and 1 cup of salt. Combine the ingredients in a container, and scrub away. The powder lasts a long time, so store it as you would any other powdered cleaner.

If the refrigerator seems sound, make your best offer, and then give the shelves a good scrubbing once you get home with my baking-soda-and-borax formula, at left.

The Do's and Don'ts of Dishwashers

Most new dishwashers are equally capable of washing a load of dirty dishes. And isn't that what we really want from a dishwasher? Unfortunately, it's all the fancy options that take a bite out of your wallet. Here are some features that can either save you some cash or empty your pockets:

Temperature controls. The ideal water temperature for getting dishes germ-free is about 140°F. But it would be wasteful, not to mention dangerous, to set your water heater this high. If you buy a dishwasher with a temperature-boosting feature, you can keep your water heater at an economical (and safer) temperature.

Stainless steel cases. Think about passing up any dishwasher with a stainless steel case, which is the decor option of the moment. The steel helps the washer hold in heat a little better, but not enough to make up for the extra cash you'll spend for that fashionable finish.

Adaptive cycles. You can buy a dishwasher with six or seven cycles and settings that adjust for pots and pans, china, crystal, dishes with baked-on food, and so on. But if you never use anything other than the "normal" cycle (who does?), then don't waste your money on features you don't need.

Dirt sensors. A sensor measures the purity of the water used to wash the dishes. Why the heck would we need that? Of course the water gets dirty because the dishes are dirty—that's why we're washing them!

Sound barriers. Have you seen the dishwashers that are whisper-silent? You'll pay almost double the price for one that doesn't *swish-bang*. I know that silence is golden, but let's not get ridiculous!

Avoid Loaded "Deals"

Washing machines and clothes dryers have huge appetites when it comes to energy. Front-loading washers are the most energy efficient, but they cost hundreds of dollars more than the top loaders. It will take you several years to make up the difference you'll pay for a front-loading machine. On the other hand, gas dryers, which are about $100 to $200 more than electric, are energy efficient enough to make up that cost difference quickly. Here are a few more considerations to mull over when you're in the market:

Moisture sensors. What a great idea! A sensor will reduce your electric bill by automatically shutting down the dryer when your clothes are dry. No more paying extra each month for burning your clothes to a crisp. This nifty feature is good for your wallet *and* for your wardrobe.

Pricey extras. If you want to save big bucks, don't buy models with lots of different cycles and/or special fabric settings. Basic cycles and settings are quite capable of cleaning and drying most types of materials and load sizes.

Get the Dirt on Used Washers and Dryers

Fortunately, washers and dryers pose the least risk when you buy them used. Why? Because although there have been recent advances in convenience and efficiency, the basic machines have largely remained similar to the ones made 5, 10, and even 15 years ago. While used washing machines and dryers aren't as likely to break down as other used appliances, there are still two common pitfalls you should avoid:

1. If you find rust in the washer tub, it will have to be replaced. But keep in mind that rust might not be limited to just the tub. Other parts you can't see could be rusted, which means that the whole machine could have to be replaced in the not-too-distant future.

2. When shopping for used dryers, make sure the air gets hot. The heating element is usually the first thing to go on a dryer, and it can be quite costly to replace.

Save Big on Small Appliances

Microwaves, vacuums, air conditioners, and other small appliances can all eat a hole through your wallet if you're not careful. But if you take this advice, you'll learn how to shop smart and save a bundle of money, to boot:

Microwaves. Does the oven fit your cooking style? If all you really want to do is bake a potato, you don't need a huge turntable and a lot of fancy cooking options. Keep in mind that you can find some great deals at moving and garage sales, since more new homes are coming equipped with built-in microwaves. To make sure the oven works, heat a cup of water for two minutes. If the water comes out close to boiling, it's time to make a deal!

Air conditioners. Believe it or not, a too-large-capacity air conditioner won't cool your room any better than one that's too small. Your biggest cost-saving move is to measure the room area you want to cool *before* you start shopping for an air conditioner.

Vacuum cleaners. Of all appliances, vacuums may have the biggest price range for the least difference in performance. A vacuum with a $1,000 price tag might clean just as well as a $200 model. My advice is to go with the companies and models that you've had success with in the past.

Scout the Repair Shop

If you have an appliance repair shop in your neighborhood, count yourself lucky! It could be housing a treasure trove of hugely discounted, working appliances. Most repair shops will hold a repaired item for a fairly short time, because storage space is limited. So appliances that aren't claimed within that holding period are usually priced to sell quickly to make room for other items. Trek on over to see what freshly repaired appliances are sitting there, just waiting for a good home—maybe yours!

Stay Tuned for TV Technology

There's good news for bargain shoppers like me: high-definition (HD) technology means fantastic deals on standard televisions (those "prehistoric" sets that don't have fancy LCD or plasma screens). The TVs of yesteryear are being phased out and all programming is slated to go digital by 2009, so TVs without HD capability are now fairly cheap. If you're considering buying a TV this year, keep in mind that if it isn't made to show HDTV channels, you won't be getting the breathtaking pictures your neighbors will see on their HDTVs in the future. Before you purchase that TV, consider these factors:

High-definition. Although there are several types of HDTV technologies, plasma (which gobbles up the most electricity) and LCD (which has the highest price tag) sets are the ones that hog the spotlight. Their sleek, flat panels easily mount to the wall and take up minimal counter or tabletop space. The higher the number of pixels, the more brilliant resolution you'll have. But if you want to cut your costs by settling for fewer pixels, you'll save even more by choosing another HDTV technology called direct-view, or CRT. This type of HDTV uses picture tubes, so they're bulkier than their slim-jim cousins, but the image quality is great. Plus, they don't need special maintenance, and they have a long life span, which gives you the best of both worlds.

Size. You may have the wall space and ceiling height for a big-screen TV, but is it suited to your viewing area? If you'll be sitting less than 10 feet away from your TV, a 27- or 32-inch screen is ideal. Anything larger would literally be a pain in the neck!

Settings. The images should be equal in brightness, color, and contrast. Remember that televisions on the showroom floor are usually set at the brightest picture setting possible, so it's difficult to judge the overall quality. When in doubt, ask the salesperson to readjust the picture controls for a more normal, homelike setting.

Price ranges. Just seven years ago, an HDTV would have cost you well over $5,000. But today, you can find them for as little as $500! Just be sure you know what the price includes before you buy; sometimes, you have to pay extra for speakers, cords, controls, and the like. Check your Sunday newspapers and the Internet for great deals.

Compute the Savings

If you have children at home, then you've undoubtedly been introduced to the wonderful world of A drives, C drives, e-mail, and online everything. You might have found some terrific deals on the Internet, or maybe you're thinking

of checking out local retailers. No matter where you may get your gear, the good news is that as technology for these machines gets better, in a strange but pleasant twist of fate, the prices continue to come down. A word to the wise, though: No matter what kind of system you buy, look for a deal that includes free technical support. Otherwise, if your system develops kinks, you may be stuck paying $50 an hour to have it diagnosed. Here are some other smart shopping tips:

- If you buy your hard drive, monitor, and printer together, you'll probably get a good discount. Sometimes, you'll even get hundreds of dollars' worth of software—free! Check your local newspaper and the Internet for the best prices.

- Compare the fees to what other providers are charging before you take the plunge on an offer for a "free" computer. The offer will come with the stipulation that you commit to

---

HOME REMEDY

If your favorite TV show starts looking a little snowy (and it's not being taped in Siberia or some other chilly locale), it's time to fine-tune your TV set with the help of your owner's manual. But if you can't recall where your manual is, then you have another problem to fine-tune—unorganized paperwork. Fortunately, keeping owner's manuals, warranties, and receipts tidy and in one place is easy. Just store your appliance, furniture, and electronic paperwork in a recycled three-ring binder. That way, all of your records are together, and easy to find when a problem crops up.

a specific online access provider for a specific amount of time, usually three years. But the cost of 36 months of service fees may be just as much as the cost of a new computer, so be sure to compare!

- Make sure you are getting technical support with your purchase because there's a good chance you'll need it. Also, find out if the support number is toll-free or if there is a per- hour, per-phone-call rate, because tech support has a way of keeping you on the telephone for hours.

- Consider reconditioned models—and no, I don't mean ones with dented, beat-up metal boxes. "Reconditioned" usually means that somebody sent it back or canceled an order, and the maker can't sell it as "new" anymore. If you're thinking of buying a reconditioned computer, stick with a major manufacturer you know and trust. They usually sell their refurbished models direct to consumers, or through retailers at huge discounts. Also, be sure to get a good one- to three-year warranty with convenient technical support. Finally, pass it up if it doesn't come with a return clause. In general, refurbished computers are in great shape, but you want the option to return it if you end up with a lemon.

GREAT FURNITURE FINDS

Furniture: You can't live well without it, but how come it costs so dad-burned much money? The standard markup on new furniture is somewhere in the neighborhood of 300 percent, and those lovely pieces in a high-end store can be marked up 400 percent or more!

Price doesn't always reflect the quality of the furniture, either. You can find real gems at outlets and garage sales, and real rubbish in expensive showrooms. And some manufacturers are masters at hiding flaws with fabric, finishes, and fancy detailing. Luckily, there are lots of clues that'll tell you whether the piece is solidly crafted or shoddily made. I'm going to show you how to find top-of-the-line wood and upholstered furniture without the inflated price tags. They say a man's home is his castle, and here's how you can decorate yours without paying a royal fortune.

Get the Goods on Wood

Before you buy a piece of wood furniture, you need to know what kind of wood it's made of. There are various grades and types of wood, and they all have qualities that can make the difference between a bargain and a rip-off. As a master gardener, I have more than a little knowledge to share with you about trees and wood, starting here:

Hardwoods. These types of woods are rock-solid, so they're tough to scratch or dent and they resist warping. Hardwoods include oak, cherry, maple, walnut, and mahogany. Furniture made from hardwood is top-quality, enduring, and fairly expensive.

Softwoods. Pine, cedar, and poplar are softwoods, and their flexibility makes for some really beautiful furniture. They do wear and show their age sooner than hardwoods, but they are less expensive. So if you're looking for furniture that won't have to stand up to heavy use, softwoods can be a real bargain.

FAST FORMULA

Perfect Polish for Wood

Here's a great furniture polish that's easy to make and can be used on any type of wood.

$1/2$ cup of linseed oil
$1/4$ cup of malt vinegar
1 tsp. of lemon or lavender oil

Put the linseed oil and vinegar in a clear jar with a tight lid, and shake the jar vigorously. Stir in the lemon or lavender oil. Apply the polish to your furniture with a clean, soft cotton cloth, and buff with a second, clean cloth. In hot, humid weather, reverse the proportions and use $1/4$ cup of linseed oil and $1/2$ cup of vinegar. Why? Because damp heat tends to make oil, well, oilier.

Veneer. Pieces made with veneering can be very strong and durable. A veneer is composed of either thin sheets of wood that are glued together to form a "sandwich," or one sheet attached to a solid wood core. Veneer gets a bad rap for being cheap and flimsy, but if the veneer and the material under it are both hardwoods, then you've got yourself a quality piece of furniture. If the veneer is attached to particleboard, the construction won't last long, so search for something sturdier.

Plan Ahead

Now that you know what type of wood you want, you have to decide what you are willing to pay for it. Otherwise, you'll be vulnerable to sky-high prices and furniture that is more like kindling than it is kingly! You can save a lot of time and trouble if you plan ahead, so before

you hit the stores, give some thought to these important details:

- Check your seasons. How's the weather? If it's either brutally cold or scorching hot, then your timing is just right. The best times to look for furniture are in January, February, July, and August because that's when the new furniture lines arrive in stores. Last year's trends are deeply discounted, so stores can move them out quickly and make room for the latest and greatest.

- Don't buy just one. If you'll be needing more than one piece of furniture, then you have some bargaining power. You'd be surprised how low salespeople can and will go if they see a multi-item sales ticket at the end of the tunnel.

- Get in line with credit. Plan to shop in stores that offer same-as-cash credit lines. This allows you to make payments without interest charges, and every dime goes toward your purchase price. As long as you pay it off before the deadline, it's like a layaway you can take home today!

- Make a deal. Just remember that prices are almost always negotiable. You may even be able to work in free delivery and setup. So decide ahead of time what your budget will allow, put on that poker face, and get going!

Drawer Your Own Conclusions

When buying furniture, the quality of the drawers says a lot! A drawer has all of the critical elements in one small piece that's easy to inspect thoroughly. Here's how:

Step 1. Roll it out. Well-made drawers slide easily in and out on guides or rollers. They also have built-in stops, so you won't pull them out too far and drop them on your toes—*ouch!*

Step 2. Test the hardware. Drawer pulls on new furniture should be snugly attached and evenly placed. If you are looking at used furniture, the drawer pulls aren't as critical. They can be repaired and replaced in a matter of minutes once you get the piece home.

Step 3. Check the joints. Dovetail drawers and drawers joined by wooden dowels are well made. If they are joined with glue or nails, the craftsmanship isn't good quality. And if they are joined by staples, the furniture is shoddily built.

Step 4. Look for a dust panel. If the piece has panels between each level of drawers, it's a sign of quality. If you pull one drawer out and see the drawer underneath it, then the manufacturer hasn't bothered with this very inexpensive, yet very practical, feature.

Avoid Funny Finish Business

When inspecting furniture, make sure the entire piece is finished, not just the front and top. This will tell you how much effort has been put into making it. Does the finish feel rough and gritty, instead of smooth? Can you find any bubbles, blisters, cracks, or flaws? If the answers are "yes," ask for a discount or keep on searching until you find something without these flaws.

Another important thing to check is the label. If it says the piece has an "oak finish," that means it is the *color* of oak, not that it's *made* of oak.

A Lesson in Labels

You have to read furniture labels carefully, or you may find yourself paying more for the piece than you need to. Here is a list of commonly used terms and what their translations *really* mean (I've used walnut as an example):

"Walnut veneer." A layer of walnut has been used on the outside or top. If the label doesn't specify another type of wood, then the inside should be made of walnut as well. If another wood is mentioned, then it's not 100 percent walnut.

"Solid wood." All of the exposed surfaces are made of wood.

"Walnut finish." The product is the color of walnut wood. It may not be made of walnut or, for that matter, may not even be made of wood!

No label at all. Heads up—there's nothing worse than not being able to find a label. Any retailer that removes labels is probably hiding something about its wares. By all means, take your business elsewhere as fast as you can.

Check the Cushions

Getting to know upholstered goods is a little like solving a mystery because most of the features that indicate how well it's made are buried beneath layers of fabric and padding. Fortunately, cushions hold the best clues about the quality of upholstered furniture. If they're well made, then the rest of the sofa or chair is, too. Find out how durable the cushions are with these three easy steps:

Step 1. Sit on it. Now stand up and turn around to look at the cushion. If there's still an indentation, then the stuffing isn't up to snuff. That tiny depression in the fabric will eventually get bigger.

Step 2. Read the tag. Do the cushions have springs wrapped in layers of padding? If that's the case, then you can be sure it's made with quality materials.

Step 3. Zip it up. While not all cushions with zippers are good quality, most cushions without zippers are poor quality. Look for zippers with material plackets (that's the fabric lip that hides the zipper). If the manufacturer has gone to the effort of protecting the zippers, chances are the company is conscientious about construction as well.

Take the Fabric Test

The condition of the fabric used to make upholstered furniture can speak volumes—it can tell you if you're looking at high-quality craftsmanship or cheap knockoffs. See if the upholstery makes the grade with these simple tests:

Scratch and sniff. Gently scratch the upholstery on new furniture with your fingernail to make sure it doesn't have a tendency to pull apart. If it's used, give it a good sniff. If it has an odor now, you'll probably never get rid of it.

Read the label. Check the fabric-care label to find out how the upholstery should be cleaned. Some fabrics, like linen, don't respond well to spot cleaning. If the furniture is used and the label is missing, ask the owner what type of fabric the upholstery is made of. (For the lowdown on fabric washability, see the Home Remedy box at right.)

Color coordinate. Don't laugh, because you'll thank me later. Try to color coordinate your upholstery and your pets! I'm not suggesting that you shouldn't clean your furniture. I just know that if your white couch is really owned by your black cat, you'll spend a lot of time trying to de-fur your furniture.

Perfect prints. A good print can hide a multitude of sins, which means that stains and tears won't be so obvious. The longer a piece of furniture looks good, the more likely you'll keep it. But buying printed upholstery is tricky for the exact same reason. It's hard to detect flaws, so it deserves close inspection. Make sure the pattern matches up throughout the piece and the fabric is sturdy and unblemished.

Love leather. Leather is one of the toughest fabrics around. The simple style of most leather furniture means you can dress it up or down with pillows and throws to keep up with fashion trends. That's a good thing, since it's likely to last a lifetime. Just one word of warning: If you own a pet, those claws and nails can cause nasty rips!

HOME REMEDY

It's simply a matter of time before you'll be cleaning up splatters and drips from your upholstered furniture, so if you're looking for washability (and I suggest you do for furniture that will be heavily used), look for furniture made from these materials:

- **Nylon.** This material holds up well against stains and stain removal, and it's fairly durable.

- **Cotton.** Heavy cotton blends, such as canvas and denim, are long lasting and respond kindly to cleaning solutions.

- **Acrylic.** Coverings made from acrylic blends are usually machine washable and shrink resistant.

- **Polyester.** This fabric maintains its shape well and is easy to wipe down.

Don't Forget the Frame!

Take a moment to squeeze the armrests of upholstered chairs and sofas. If you can feel the frame underneath, then sooner or later, it will wear through the fabric. Also, if you can easily lift one side of a sofa, then it's probably not strong enough to support a furniture-bouncing child or a crash-landing adult.

Find Fine Furniture Discounts

Every store accumulates returned, damaged, and just-one-left items, even those fancy fine furniture stores. So ask the salesperson where the clearance room is and you may discover a wealth of bargains. Also find out when the floor samples go on sale, and make it a point to check them out when they do.

Shop the Outlets

High Point, North Carolina, is the mecca of American furniture outlets, but there are a few regional and national retailers that have outlets sprinkled here and there around the rest of the country. Search the Internet and check in the Yellow Pages under "Furniture" to see if any are located near you.

Other outlet prospects are big catalog operations like JCPenney, Sears, and Spiegel. They can't reship returned items as new merchandise, so they often end up with lots of flawless pieces of furniture for sale. If there's a department store in your area that sells its wares through a catalog, call to find out if it has an outlet near you.

Buyer Beware

The No. 1 rule of outlet furniture shopping is to know what the furniture is worth when you see it. Don't be fooled by those tags that tell you the manufacturer's suggested retail price (MSRP) is thousands of dollars more than the sale price.

Retailers rarely charge the MSRP. In fact, you can easily find discounts of at least 35 percent off of the MSRP, even in the fanciest furniture stores. So if that "rock bottom" outlet price isn't more than 35 percent less than the MSRP, you're not getting a special deal after all.

Phone It In

Here's a little-known way to save a lot of money when buying furniture. Write down the exact name and a detailed description of the pieces you want, then call the manufacturer to see if it can put you in touch with its own outlet or preferred discounters. You'll have to pay for shipping, but depending on your state, you may *not* have to pay sales tax. You will also have to wait a few weeks for delivery, but the savings could be worth the wait.

Hitch a Ride on the Freight

Most of the time, furniture shipments arrive at the showroom safe and sound. When a shipment *does* get lost, misdirected, or separated from its bill of lading, the trucking company ends up with loads of product and no place to put it. Freight liquidation sales don't usually have a large selection of furniture, but you can find some fantastic deals. Call around to local trucking companies and ask if they have liquidation sales—there's a good chance that you'll save a bundle!

Buy from the Builder

You can get a great deal on furniture if you buy it directly from the craftsmen. I've seen plenty of mighty fine tables, chairs, and other goods for sale at a fraction of their furniture store value in the workshops of Amish and Mennonite craftsmen and even folks who make furniture as a side business. You'll take away a handcrafted, one-of-a-kind work of art at a modest price.

Used Is Good

Sometimes, the best deals aren't found at a furniture store. For the price of a few brand-new lamps, you just might find a full dining room set at a good garage or estate sale. And if you shop with cash and a truck, you have it made! Most sellers would sooner give you a big discount if you pay cash; if you can cart it away yourself, you'll be absolutely irresistible to someone who wants it gone immediately. So leave the checkbook and the hatchback at home! You'll find bargains by the boatload in these locations:

Flea markets. These are the true treasure troves for furniture shoppers. First, there are the standard flea market staples: furnishings that need a little TLC. But sometimes, you'll also find furniture craftsmen who don't have their own stores to showcase their wares. They stand to make the most money by selling directly to consumers, and you stand to get a great deal on handmade pieces.

Yard sales. This is where being the early bird really pays off! Any decent piece of furniture will be picked up before most of us sit down to breakfast, so make sure you're the first one there. If the items are overpriced and the seller won't budge, walk away and hope that no suckers come along. Then return later in the day to see if the furniture you had your eye on is still there. If it is, then the sellers may be anxious to get rid of it, so repeat your original offer, and see if they'll bite. Also, check out the sales in upscale, pricey neighborhoods where folks often sell barely used furniture simply because they've changed the decor of their rooms. Beverly Hills 90210, here I come!

Rental shops. I'm not suggesting that you rent your furniture. But I am suggesting that you look at buying rental furniture. Plenty of rental shops sell previously rented items at deep discounts, so give the stores in your area a call to find out if they do sell their merchandise and when their sales will be.

Thrift stores. Clothes and small household goods are not the only charitable donations that people make; they often donate furniture, too. So check out your nearby Salvation Army and Goodwill stores—you may be surprised to find some decent used furniture in among all the other stuff they have for sale.

⏳ Quick Fix

Moving new furniture into a room, or rearranging your old furniture is exciting—unless you're the one doing the moving. Then it can be excruciating, especially if you have a bad back! Fortunately, you can shuffle furniture around with a lot less risk to your back using one simple tool (and I'm willing to bet that you already have it)—a soft, thick sock! Just slip a sock over each leg of that heavy piece of furniture and it'll glide right into place. You'll not only save your back, but you'll also save your hardwood floors from nasty scratches! For moving heavy pieces over carpeting, invest in a pack of those plastic gliders—they really do the trick.

CHAPTER 3

Cut Your Energy Bills

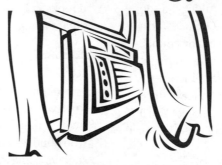

It's easy to use more energy than we need to—it's behind
every switch, dial, and faucet handle, just waiting to do our
bidding. And if your utility bills have grown out of reach, then
all of that easy access to power may have gone to your head!
The good news is that it's never too late to begin controlling
your energy costs. And there's no time like the present to
get a leg up on high utility bills. Let me show you how.

AUDIT FOR ENERGY LOSS

Do you have a closet that could
double as a walk-in freezer? How
about an attic that feels like a
sauna? If the room temperatures in your
home seem to have a mind of their own,
then your house is either underinsulated
or leaking air—not to mention cold, hard
cash! While lots of just-built houses are
equipped with energy-efficient features
that make them tight as a drum, you don't
have to build a brand-new house to save
big. In fact, even if your house is as old as
the hills, my tips will help you kick those
high utility bills to the curb!

Hunt for Leaks

I hate leaky faucets! Those steady *plip-plops*
not only keep me up at night, they also send
good money down the drain. Air leaks in your
home are even more wasteful when the air that
you pay so dearly to heat and cool is escaping
through cracks in your home. Luckily, sealing
those cracks can be fairly easy to do—it's
finding them that can be a challenge. Unlike a
drippy faucet, you can't hear or see air leaks, but
there are a few places where they are most likely
to occur. The usual suspects? Areas around
doors, windows, chimneys, and fireplaces.
Here's how to check these areas for leaks:

Shake things up. It's easy to test the soundness
of your doors and windows—just give the

frames a little rattle. If they move, then they're not tightly installed, and air is escaping around them.

Shed some light. If you can see light shining around the perimeter of your doors and windows, then they're letting the outside air in, and the inside air out.

Read the paper. Close your windows and doors on a piece of paper. If you can pull the paper out without tearing it, then the seals aren't sealin' too well.

Use a little H$_2$O. Dampen your hands and hold them around the places you suspect are leaky. If your hands feel cool, you've found a leak.

Grab the incense. Pass an incense stick around your door frames, window frames, and fireplace damper. If the smoke forms a horizontal line, then you have a draft.

Go Beyond the Obvious

As I mentioned earlier, the designated openings in your home are where you're most likely to find air leaks. But there are less obvious places that can seep air, too. So when you're hunting for leaks, test these spots as well to make sure they're properly sealed against the elements:

Inside: Attic hatches, vents, crawl spaces, mounted air conditioners, mail slots, baseboards, electrical outlets, pipes, and wires.

Outside: Vents, mounted air conditioners, electrical outlets, exterior corners, faucets, pipes, wires, and anyplace where two different materials meet, such as between vinyl siding and brick.

Fill in the Gaps

You can plug up most leaks with just a little bit of time, money, and effort. Many cracks and gaps can be patched easily with caulk, weather stripping, or shrink-wrap.

Use caulk to plug holes and cracks around outlet covers, pipes, and door and window frames. Caulk can also be used to form a seal between two different materials, such as between vinyl and brick. It works best when applied on days that aren't humid, and the temperature is above 50°F. There are several types of caulk, so read the labels carefully to be sure you choose the right compound for the job. You can use caulk to seal small gaps and holes on the top of interior walls, but expanding foam and strips of board insulation are best for larger

HOME REMEDY

Don't put pressure on yourself to plug up every last air leak in your home. First, it's nearly impossible to seal all of the leaks, and second, making your home completely airtight is dangerous! You need a healthy exchange of air in your home to filter out toxic fumes and odors, keep moisture levels balanced, and allow fresh air to circulate around fuel-burning appliances.

So before you seal up those cracks, make sure that outdoor vents aren't blocked, exhaust fans are in fine working order, and appliances fueled by wood, natural gas, propane, or oil are properly vented. And, if you use these appliances, it's a good idea to invest in one or more carbon monoxide detectors. Fuel-burning appliances can release dangerous levels of carbon monoxide if they malfunction, or if they're poorly vented. One final note: Have all systems cleaned and maintained on a regular schedule.

holes. Those types of insulation, however, are best left to the professionals.

Use weather stripping to stop air leaks under your doors and at the base of your windows. Make sure the weather stripping you buy is designed to withstand the friction, temperature, and wear and tear associated with the area you'll need it for.

Use shrink-to-fit plastic wrap around your windows to form another barrier against outdoor air. A roll of shrink-wrap is inexpensive, and it's an easy do-it-yourself job.

Bring in the Pros

You can have every nook and cranny in your house tested for air leaks by a professional, if you'd rather not do it yourself. And it may not be as expensive as it sounds. Just call your home utility company to find out if it offers energy audits for free or for discounted prices. If your local utility doesn't offer this service, request a referral to an energy auditor. Auditors have special equipment that can detect thermal defects and measure how airtight your home is. Plus, they'll suggest how to plug up the leaks.

Keep It Under Wraps

Heating bills that are through the roof are sometimes caused by a very large "hole" *under* the roof—your attic. If your home was built in the "old" days (that would be before 1980), then you may need another layer of insulation over your head. Some experts say that only 20 percent of the homes built before 1980 have the proper amount of insulation. If you have an unfinished attic, here's a quick way to tell if it has enough padding: Take a look at the level of insulation on the floor. If it is at or below the floor joists, you could probably use some more insulation. If you have a finished attic, look at the insulation in an exposed attic wall

---

FAST FORMULA

Crafty Draft Dodger

If you have an old necktie that's seen better days, then turn it into a stylish draft blocker for under your door! All you need are some odds and ends, and one drafty door.

1 old or unwanted tie
Thread or fabric glue
Stuffing, such as batting, newspaper, rags, or old pantyhose
Dry beans or dry rice

Fold the tie in half lengthwise, and either sew or glue the side and bottom edges together to form a tube shape. Insert your stuffing, and then add dry beans or rice to give it some weight so your blocker will stay in place. Stitch or glue the top part closed, and voilà—you've saved yourself a bundle of money!

(it's usually adjacent to unheated rooms, such as garages and basements). If the insulation is less than 12 inches thick, then you should add another layer. And while you're up there eyeballing it, look for any dirty or discolored insulation. Those marks could mean that air is moving through the insulation and you have a leak.

Adding attic insulation is fairly easy. In most cases, the best types of insulation are blanket and loose-fill insulation. Blanket insulation, which comes in batts and rolls, is made of flexible fiber that can be cut to fit your space. Loose-fill insulation contains tiny bits of fiber or foam, and is usually the less expensive of the two. However, when it's installed properly, it will give you better coverage. The amount you need depends on the type of house you live in and the climate conditions in your area. Generally speaking, colder climates require insulation with higher R values (which is a measurement of heat resistance) than warmer climates. Your local utility company or state energy department can tell you what the best-dressed homes in your area should be wearing. One other thing to keep in mind—installing insulation yourself requires skill, some construction knowledge, and sometimes, even special equipment. So if you would rather play it safe (and who could blame you?), call a few contractors and get estimates. You can bet your bottom dollar that the ones recommending a higher R value will give you the highest estimates. Weigh your options carefully and remember, sometimes paying more for solid experience and quality assurance is a bargain in the end!

WATTAGE WISDOM

When I was young, my Grandma Putt often scolded me for leaving the lights on when I left a room. Fortunately, some of us outgrow this habit, but others don't, and they carry their wasteful ways into adulthood. If you're one of them, then I'd like to assure you that Grandma Putt was right—leaving a blazing trail of lights behind you is a waste of your hard-earned money. So, for goodness sakes, "When not in use, turn off the juice!"

Plant Bulbs in the Right Spot

Lightbulbs get no respect! Some folks don't give much thought to the whys and wherefores of choosing the right bulb. The fact is that when you put the right bulbs in their proper place, they'll use electricity more efficiently, and they'll also last a heck of a lot longer. So follow these guidelines, and I guarantee you'll find the perfect home for your bulbs:

Incandescent lights. These are the least expensive bulbs of the bunch, and that makes them very popular. They're also the least efficient, and that makes 'em very expensive in the long run. Incandescent bulbs convert only about 15 percent of the electricity they use to light. The rest generates heat, which is why they're extremely hot to the touch. Why, halogen bulbs (the hottest type of incandescent bulb), can reach temperatures of 1,100°F! Halogen lights, however, do recycle some of the heat they generate, so while they're hot enough to fry an egg on, they're more efficient than the average incandescent bulbs. Just don't put them in rooms that heat up quickly (like small bathrooms), or in fixtures that could be brushed up against. If you use standard incandescent bulbs, avoid putting them in fixtures you use the most, or you'll be changing them often.

Fluorescent lights. This type of lighting costs more than incandescent lighting, but lasts up to 10 times longer, and uses electricity more efficiently. You can now buy compact fluorescent lamps, or CFLs, which are smaller versions of the tube-shaped fluorescent bulbs and have screw-in bases that fit into standard light fixtures. Their average life span is between 6,000 and 10,000 hours, while incandescent bulbs will burn for just 750 to 1,000 hours. And CFLs use only about a third of the electricity that an incandescent bulb does. The downside is that they don't generally work well in dimmers, enclosed fixtures, or rooms that hold a lot of moisture. Since CFLs won't burn out quickly, they're perfect for hard-to-reach spots, both indoors and out, where changing bulbs is a hassle. And because every flick of the switch cuts into their life span, they're more efficient in high-traffic areas where the lights will be on for at least 15 minutes at a time.

Don't Leave the Porch Light On...

especially if your porch fixture uses natural gas! Using eight decorative outdoor gaslight fixtures all year round will burn up enough energy to heat an entire home during the cold winter months. So if your outside lights are powered by gas, replace them with electric fixtures and use CFLs to get more glow for your dough.

That Hits the Spot!

Your entire living room doesn't have to be lit up like a Christmas tree if all you want to do is curl up with a good book. Use lamps, under-cabinet, and recessed or track lights to direct those beams just where you need 'em. To avoid eyestrain, place lamps so that they're over your shoulder or to the side of you when you're reading or doing paperwork. Small, but detailed projects, such as crafts or sewing, are done more comfortably with overhead lighting from under-cabinet, and recessed or track lights. If your home wasn't built with these lighting options, consider contacting an electrician to have them professionally installed. And if you have some electrical experience, pick up a do-it-yourself kit to retrofit your existing fixtures.

Dim the Lights

Dimmers are an inexpensive way to save you lots of money. They're fairly cheap and easy to install. Dimmer switches allow you to make your lights as bright or as soft as you want, so in the process, you control how much electricity you use. They're perfect for those rooms that the family uses the most, such as the kitchen or den. If you make it a habit to dim the lights while dining and when watching TV, you'll see immediate savings on your next electric bill.

Keep 'Em Filled

Never remove a burned-out lightbulb without replacing it right away with a new bulb. Believe it or not, that light fixture is still feeding electricity to the socket, even if it is empty. So keep your family safe by making sure all of your sockets are occupied!

Quick Fix

*Here's an old-time way to remove a broken lightbulb that's still in the socket. **First, make sure the power to the fixture is turned off!** Next, push half a potato, cut side first, against the broken bulb. Turn the 'tater just as you would to unscrew a whole lightbulb. Once it's out of the socket, don't try to remove the bulb from the potato— just throw the whole thing in the trash!*

Welcome the Rays

Even if you're using energy-efficient lighting, there are probably very few rooms in your home that need artificial light during the morning hours. So take full advantage of the natural (and free-of-charge) sunlight that's offered to you every day. Just open up the curtains and blinds on the south-facing side of your house, and let the sun be your guiding light (unless, that is, there are dark-colored upholstery or rugs in the line of fire—ultraviolet rays will cause fabrics to fade and weaken). If you don't want to lose your privacy, try replacing heavy, dark-colored curtains with ones that are loosely woven and lightly colored. The sun's rays will still shine through, and you won't feel as though you're living in a fishbowl.

Clean the Bulbs

Don't let dirt leave you in the dark! Dusty buildup on lightbulbs can reduce light output by as much as 50 percent, even though the bulbs are still operating at full power. To maximize the lighting in your rooms, wipe down your fixtures and lamps every six months or so. If you use incandescent bulbs, make sure you turn them off before you take a damp rag to them. The cool moisture could cause bulbs to blow their tops! And if you really want to brighten things up, clean your walls and windows at the same time. Dirty walls don't reflect light as well as clean walls do, and we all know how dirty windows can make even the sunniest day look dingy gray.

CLOSE THE FLOODGATES ON WATER BILLS

If you're like some folks, you don't give much thought to how much water you use every day. After all, it's odorless, colorless, and tasteless, so it doesn't exactly command attention... unless, that is, your water bills are leaving your pocketbook high and dry! And you not only have to pay for the amount of water you use, but you also have to shell out money to heat the water. *Now* we're talking big bucks! In fact, keeping your water hot is likely to be your biggest heating expense. Luckily, your water expenses are easier to control than any other utility you have. I have lots of simple solutions for pulling the plug on high water and heating bills—and not one of them involves taking an icy cold shower!

Flush Bad Bathroom Habits

No matter how small your bathroom is, it uses up more water than any other room in your house! Just take a look around. You can flush, shower, bathe, shave, brush your teeth, and wash your hands all in one convenient spot. But while there are lots of opportunities to waste gallons of water in your bathroom, there are just as many opportunities to use it wisely. And best of all, conserving water in the loo is very easy to do. Take these simple steps to heart and you can start savin' plenty of water (and money!) right away:

1. Turn off the faucet while you're brushing your teeth and shaving.

2. Keep your showers short, or turn the water off while you're lathering up.

3. Close the drain *before* you start to fill the bathtub. You'll save all of the water you use trying to find just the right temperature.

4. Take a bath with only half the amount of water you usually use.

5. Don't flush your toilet frivolously. If you don't have low-flow toilets (which use 1.6 gallons per flush), every flush sends 5 to 7 gallons of water out to sea. So resist using your toilet as a trash can: Instead of flushing those tissues you use to blow your nose, fix your makeup, or clean up razor nicks, throw them in the wastebasket.

Stop the Drops

Did you know that a drip of water a second will cost you $1 per month? That doesn't sound like much, but put a bucket under that drip, and you'll collect gallons of water in no time at all. That's precious H_2O you could be using to shower, clean your dishes, or wash your hands. So grab that wrench and screwdriver, and put an end to the waste now.

Test the Waters

Which do you think is more wasteful, a shower or a bath? The answer depends on how long you like to stand under the shower, and how deep you like to fill the tub! To find out which one is your most efficient option, plug

---

HOME REMEDY

If your showerhead is old, sputtering, and/or spouting off in 10 different directions, chances are that your water bills are overflowing. It's easy to tell if your showerhead is wasteful. Just turn your shower on at your usual volume, and hold a bucket or pan under the showerhead for 15 seconds. Then calculate how many quarts of water you've collected. That number is equivalent to how many gallons of water you're using per minute. If that number is more than 3, think about replacing your showerhead with one that'll conserve more water. According to the National Resource Defense Council, a slow-flow showerhead can save a family of four up to 20,000 gallons of water a year, and that's enough to fill an average-size swimming pool!

---

up the bathtub drain, and take a shower. After you're done, check the water level. Is it higher than it would be for your typical bath? If so, then you'll probably save more money by taking baths instead of showers. If not, then stick to showers.

Lower the Heat

If you were to lower your water heater temperature by just 10°F, you would reduce your energy costs by 3 to 5 percent. So check the thermostat on your water heater. If you've never adjusted the temperature, it's probably sitting at 140°F, which is where many manufacturers set it. However, the hottest temperature you'll ever really need is 120°F (except if you have a standard dishwasher, which I discuss on page 64). Anything higher than that could cause a nasty scalding. So bring the temperature down to 120°F if it's not already there, and your wallet will thank you. Your water heater will say *gracias*, too—a lower temperature will reduce the amount of mineral deposits that collect in your heater, which means it'll last longer. And whenever you plan to be away from home for three or more days, make sure you turn the thermostat down to the lowest setting.

Cook Kitchen Costs

Whether you're a culinary master or a fan of frozen dinners, you can save lots of dough on your water bills by making a few slight changes to your cooking style. Here are some simple ideas that'll keep those bills from boiling over:

- Plunge your produce into a bowl of water, and give it a good scrub with a stiff brush instead of holding it under a running faucet.

- If you want a nice, cold glass of water, don't run the water until it's cold. Just fill your glass right away, and put it in the fridge. Better yet, fill a pitcher with tap water now and refrigerate it, so you'll always have cold water on hand.

- Steam your veggies. You'll use less water and save more nutrients than if you boil them.

- When you have to boil water, for say eggs or pasta, pour it into a container after you're done. Use it later to water your plants.

Shade Your Swimming Pool

Swimming pools cost you money in several ways—they require electricity for the pump, gas for the heater, a lot of chemicals to keep it clean, and, of course, water. And not only do you have to fill the darn thing, but you also have to replace any water that's lost through evaporation. A simple pool cover will reduce evaporation by a whopping 30 to 50 percent! So don't let your pool go topless, and you'll save a bundle of money.

Low-Water Landscaping

Conserving water doesn't have to leave your lawn and garden parched and dry. Here's how to reap what you sow without using lots of H_2O:

Add a layer. Compost, peat moss, and mulch help your plants retain water.

Weed more. Those dandelions are stealing water away from your prized plants.

Time your water. Do your watering in the morning, not in the afternoon, when the sun will cause much of it to evaporate. And don't water in the evening either. The plants will stay cool and wet overnight, making them prime targets for fungal disease.

Landscape with care. Choose and use native plants in your yard because they're more likely to survive on rainwater alone. Also use less grass (a real water hog!) and more groundcovers, shrubs, and rock gardens.

COOL DOWN THE HIGH PRICE OF HEATING

There are few things that can chill you to the bone like a huge heating bill that's in the triple digits! Most of us have lowered our thermostats and piled on the blankets to lessen the blow of high heating costs. After all, what else can you do? Actually, plenty! Believe you me, you *can* keep those home fires burning without getting raked over the coals. So pull up a chair, make yourself cozy, and settle in for some heart- (and home-) warming advice.

Maintain and Prosper

One of the best ways to put a lid on fuel bills is to keep your heating system properly maintained, so it'll function for many years to come. That means changing your furnace filters every three months, making sure all air ducts are sealed, and draining any trapped air from hot-water radiators. Gas heating systems should have a thorough physical every two years, and oil-fired boilers should be checked every year.

Turn *On* the Fan

Contrary to popular belief, ceiling fans can actually keep you warmer in the winter. Most fans are equipped to run both clockwise and counterclockwise. If you run yours clockwise at a low speed, the fan will circulate heat that's gathered at the ceiling, forcing it down into the room. Once you feel warmer, you can set your thermostat a few degrees lower.

Turn *Off* the Fan

The exhaust fan, that is! It can get rid of an entire house-worth of heat in no time at all. Bathroom exhaust fans will move out up to 20 cubic feet of air per minute, and kitchen fans will suck out up to 25 cubic feet per minute. So don't run them continuously for more than 20 minutes. Otherwise, your furnace will be working overtime to replace all of that warm air.

Dress for Success

When we feel chilly, our first instinct is to put on more clothes. Of course, it makes sense to dress in heavier clothing or add more blankets to the bed. You can make the most of that extra insulation, however, when you take full advantage of your own body heat. So lower the thermostat a few notches, and then try out these red-hot ideas:

Bundle up. Throw on a few layers of clothing. Putting on a second or third garment will insulate your body better than one outfit of heavy clothing will. Try wearing a lightweight shirt, then topping if off with a bulkier shirt or sweater. The same goes for socks. Just make sure they fit loosely, so air can circulate. And the old-fashioned long underwear Grandpa used to wear? It's great for keeping heat close to the body, as are those thick stockings that Grandma wore. Guess our grandparents really *did* know a thing or two about keeping warm!

Start your blood pumping. Take a jog to the bathroom, do some jumping jacks while you're watching TV, or walk up and down the steps while you're reheating leftovers. When you move around, your blood will circulate faster, which naturally warms you up.

Eat for heat. There's nothing like a piping hot bowl of soup or a cup of hot chocolate to warm your insides. But spicy-hot food can warm you up just as well. Mouth-tingling ingredients such as hot mustard and red pepper give your body a sudden burst of heat that can last for an hour or more. So dig into some five-alarm chili, and you'll be sizzlin' in no time!

Join the crowd. Ever notice how even on the most frigid days, you find yourself sweating at parties, in church, and in crowded malls? That's because lots of bodies mean lots of body heat. So invite some friends over, gather your family into one room, or just cuddle up with your favorite snuggle buddy. I guarantee that it's the best way to warm you, body and soul.

Put Out the Fire

There's nothing romantic about a fireplace if it's sending huge amounts of money up in smoke! The No. 1 way to snuff out high heating bills is to close the fireplace damper when it's not in use. When the damper isn't closed, your fireplace acts like one big hole in your house, with all of the heat escaping right up the chimney. Here are other ways to keep the home fires burning without losing your shirt:

- When you use your fireplace, open up the damper or the nearest window about one inch, close off the room from the rest of the house, and then reset your thermostat to between 50 and 55°F. This will minimize your heat loss.

- If you never use your fireplace, then for goodness sakes, consider sealing and plugging up the flue! Eating by candlelight can be just as warm and cozy, and will save you enough money on your heating bills to buy tons of roses and bottles of wine. Now, *that's* what I call romantic!

Don't Hinder the Heat

Most folks lay out their furniture based on convenience, traffic patterns, and visual appeal. But not a lot of folks consider air flow when they're making these decisions, and sometimes, their decor is hindering the heat. Take a good look around your rooms, making sure the floor vents and radiators aren't blocked by furniture, rugs, or curtains. If they are, then it's time to do a makeover so the heat can circulate freely.

Quick Fix

Extra! Extra! Read all about it! What's the most efficient insulation you can buy for under $1? Newspaper! It combines the insulating features of wood and air to stop those chills in their tracks. In fact, it's so effective that manufacturers use it to make cellulose insulation. Here's how a tabloid can help you feel toasty:

- *Does your bed feel like a giant block of ice? Just take a few sheets of newspaper, and put them between your box spring and mattress. All of that precious body heat will be trapped between your blankets and mattress, and you'll be snoozing shiver-free. Sweet dreams!*

- *If your feet tend to get cold, or the soles of your shoes are wearing a little thin, then line your insoles with newspaper before you head out the door. It'll keep your feet from frostin' over so you can take the nippy weather in stride.*

- *Lay a few sheets of newspaper under area rugs and doormats to stop floor chills dead in their tracks.*

*Now, **that's** what I call hot front-page news!*

Cover Your Conditioner

If you have a window air conditioner, either remove it or protect it from the chilly elements with a tightly fitted cover, which is available in home centers and hardware stores. This is also a good time to make sure the seal between the air conditioner and the window is in tip-top shape. If the seal doesn't look up to par, apply duct tape around the inside edges between the unit and window frame. Or, give it a double blast of protection and use shrink-wrap to encase the whole kit and caboodle, window and all!

DEFROST YOUR COOLING COSTS

Once upon a time, air-conditioning was for rich folks only. Back then, beating the heat was actually *fun*, especially for kids! When I was a boy, I swam in the lake, sipped ice-cold lemonade on the porch, or cooled myself with a homemade fan when the temperatures got a little steamy. These "old-fashioned" chillers still work today, but since nearly two-thirds of all American homes have air conditioners, we've become accustomed to simply flippin' on the AC. All told, homeowners spend almost $16 billion a year in energy to keep their homes cool, which is a high price to pay for comfort. But you don't have to join the ranks—whether you have an air conditioner or a few electric fans, I guarantee that you can chill out for a lot less money than you're spending now. Here's how.

Control Your Fans

When it comes to cooling your home, fans don't do a darn thing. But when it comes to cooling your *body,* they're worth their weight in gold! Fans work by lowering your body temperature, rather than the room temperature, and you can probably guess which method will cost you less money. And when you feel cooler, you won't need to rely on the AC as much. So conserve electricity by raising the thermostat setting by about 4 degrees and turning on your fans. Even though the air conditioner will be blowing less cold air, I guarantee your fans will keep you as cool as a cucumber.

Ceiling fans are the most efficient way to cool down because they circulate the air in the entire room. If you're in the market for a new one, keep these guidelines in mind:

1. Ceiling fans work best in rooms that are at least 8 feet tall.

2. The blades should hang between 10 and 12 inches below the ceiling, and 18 inches from the nearest wall.

3. Ceiling fans that are 36 to 44 inches in diameter will cool rooms up to 225 square feet. If your room is larger, you'll need a ceiling fan that has a 52-inch diameter.

If you have a portable fan and you aren't sure which room it will work best in, keep the size of the blades in mind. Portable fans with larger blades make fewer rotations at low speed, so they're ideal for rooms with lots of paper, or other loose items that are easily airborne. Fans with smaller blades rotate more quickly, so use them in rooms with heavier items.

Put On Airs Cheaply

The quickest and easiest way to conserve air-conditioning energy is to raise the temperature on your thermostat. Every 1-degree increase can reduce your cooling costs by 3 to 5 percent. If you have central air-conditioning, try raising the thermostat from your usual setting by 5 to 10 degrees to see if you can still maintain a level of comfort. If you have a room air conditioner, then set it at a warmer temperature, and when you leave the room, either adjust it again or turn it off. And, if you can, install your air conditioner in a shaded part of the house; direct sunlight can cause your unit to run up to 10 percent less efficiently.

Keep It Humming

Make sure your air-conditioning unit is in tip-top shape. If the unit is clogged with debris, it'll struggle to pump out cool air, and use more energy in the process. Help it run more efficiently by replacing or cleaning the filter every month during the hot weather. And if you run your AC a lot, or if you have furry pets, clean or replace that filter more often. Also, keep any shrubbery that's around the outdoor compressor trimmed back, so branches are at least 2 feet away. And clear away any tall grass, piled-up leaves, and other yard debris that is close to the unit.

Find Some Cool Shades

When the temperatures soar, most folks seek out the shade of a tall, leafy tree. Believe it or not, tree shade can reduce air temperatures by as much as 9°F! And the best part is that you don't have to be outdoors to reap the benefits of shade. A few well-placed trees on the south side of your home will shelter it from the heat, and you won't need to rely on those fans and AC units as much. Obviously, a tree takes time to grow, but with a little patience, your energy bills could start dipping significantly by next summer. A 6- to 8-foot-tall deciduous tree can begin shading your windows and walls as early as the first year. After about five years, it'll start to shade the roof. As I mentioned earlier, a shaded air-conditioning unit uses 10 percent less electricity than one that bakes in the sun, so planting trees near your unit (but at least 2 feet away) is especially helpful.

If you prefer to get a faster return on your investment, then install a trellis or lattice board on the south side of your home, and grow some vines like ivy, clematis, or honeysuckle on it. They'll spread quickly in the first year, and the shade from their branches will reduce the warming of your walls.

HOME REMEDY

Has this ever happened to you? You've got every fan you own spinning its little heart out, but your house still feels hotter than Hades! If so, then maybe your fans aren't positioned properly. Table and floor fans that are less than 36 inches in diameter will cool you best in a 4- to 6-foot-diameter area, while larger fans are suitable for areas up to 10 square feet. And if you have a room that is more than 18 feet long, you'll need at least two fans to keep you cool. Since window fans work by bringing outdoor air into your home, they're only effective when the outside temperatures are cooler than your inside temperatures.

The most important thing to remember about all fans, though, is that they cool *you* down, not your house, so don't leave them running when you're not around. Otherwise, your energy dollars will be gone with the wind!

Haul Away the Heat

Check out the location of your thermostat. Are there any heat-generating appliances nearby? If so, then your thermostat will run harder and longer to adjust for the warm air. So if you have a TV, lamp, computer, or any other hot items near the thermostat, relocate them to another area.

Chill Out

Of course, you can take a big bite out of keeping cool by turning down or turning off the AC, but then how do you keep from sweating buckets? With these refreshing ideas, that's how! Try one or more of them out for size:

- Dress in light-colored, loose-fitting clothes, so air can circulate around you.

- Avoid wearing any fabric that doesn't "breathe" (like nylon), and forget the stockings!

- Ice your wrists, wrap a cold towel around your neck, or plant your feet in a bucket filled with cool water.

- Body heat escapes from the top of your head, so pull your hair back, or keep it cut short in hot weather.

- Position a bowl of ice near a fan or two, so the air will hit the cubes and send a cool breeze around the room.

- Cool off on someone else's dime by visiting an air-conditioned building, such as your local library or mall. Just don't spend the energy dollars that you're saving!

Run 'Em at Night

When the temperatures are sizzling hot, don't use your dishwasher or washing machine during the day. Those appliances generate heat, so your air conditioner will have to work harder and longer to keep your house cool. Nighttime is the right time to take care of those dirty clothes and dishes, since that's when air temperatures are cooler. And if you want to find out how to keep your everyday appliances energy-friendly, then keep on reading!

APPLIANCE GUIDANCE

Everyone knows that an ounce of prevention is worth a pound of cure. You brush your teeth so you don't get cavities. You change the oil in your car to keep it running well. But do you wash your towels and your delicate garments separately? Do you clean your refrigerator's condenser coils once a year? Appliances can eat up anywhere from one-third to one-half of your energy costs, depending on how you operate them and how well they're maintained. Luckily, you can tame these hungry beasts with a little tender, loving care that can save you lots of hard-earned cash!

Outwit Your Oven

If you can't stand the heat, *don't* get out of the kitchen—just stop opening the oven door! Every time you take a peek at your food, your oven loses heat, and its internal temperature drops by 25°F. Keep your eye on the clock (or timer) instead, so that the heat will stay inside the oven where it belongs, and your food will cook faster.

Here are some other cooking and baking tips that'll cut your utility bills:

- Match the size of your pan to the size of the burner. Cooking with a 6-inch pan on an 8-

inch burner can waste as much as 40 percent of your stove's heat.

- Use smaller appliances, like your toaster oven or microwave, to cook or reheat smaller meals. They use up to 50 percent less heat and electricity than a full-size oven does!

- Never line the bottom of your oven with aluminum foil—it reduces airflow and can actually increase cooking time, which will increase your energy bills.

- If you have an electric stove, use mostly flat-bottomed pots and pans that make full contact with the burner. Rounded pots and pans tend to waste most of the heat.

- If your food needs to stew awhile, use a slow cooker instead of your stove. A slow cooker uses a lot less energy to simmer food.

FAST FORMULA

Microwave Magic

Microwave ovens are great, but if you don't keep them clean, then you're in for a load of trouble. Here's a super-simple formula for keeping your microwave spotless, fresh smelling, and trouble free.

Microwave-safe bowl
Water
Lemon wedge

Pour some water into the bowl, and add the lemon wedge. Heat the water for about three minutes, then let it sit inside the microwave for five minutes. Remove the bowl from the oven. Any dried-on particles on the oven walls will wipe away in a snap, and the interior will be odor free.

Clean the Cooker

Your kitchen range is probably the hardest appliance in the whole house—much less the kitchen—to keep clean. But clean we must; otherwise, it won't operate at top efficiency. Maintaining a spot-free range is easy if you just clean up the spills as soon as they happen. For routine cleanups, wipe down the burners and range top once a day with a paste made of baking soda and warm water. Use the same paste to tackle nasty oven stains instead of those smelly (and expensive) cleansers.

If your oven stains are *really* stubborn and the paste isn't cutting it, then try this trick. Even the hard, baked-on grease will be gone before you can say, "Vamoose"!

1. Set your oven on warm for about 20 minutes, and then turn it off.

2. Place a small pan of full-strength ammonia on the top rack, and a large pan of boiling water on the bottom rack. Shut the oven door, and let it sit overnight.

3. In the morning, open the oven door, take out the pans, and let the oven air out. (It's a good idea to open the kitchen windows, too.)

4. When all the fumes have flown, wipe down the inside surfaces with soap and water.

Give Your Fridge the Cold Shoulder

I'm the kind of guy who sees the ice cube tray half full, rather than half empty. That's how I keep from worrying about the high costs of running a refrigerator, which is the biggest energy hog around! Those chillin' expenses are just begging to be controlled, and now's your chance to make thriftiness pay off, big time. These tips will help you use your fridge more efficiently:

Fill 'er up. A full refrigerator is far more efficient to run than an empty one, and in case of a power outage, fuller fridges stay cooler longer. Just make sure you leave some space between items, so the cool air can properly circulate under normal running conditions.

Don't linger. Discourage anyone (including yourself) from standing in front of an open refrigerator, looking for inspiration! An open door will let as much as 20 percent of the cold air escape. Place the foods you use the most front and center, so they can be retrieved quickly, and try to make your food choices *before* you open the door.

Block the heat. If your refrigerator is sitting next to your oven or dishwasher, it will work overtime to keep your food cold. If you can't move it, place a piece of plywood between your fridge and your heat-generating appliances to absorb the heat.

Keep it in good standing. Your refrigerator should never lean forward—the door could fail to shut completely, and that means higher electric bills!

Don't shelve it. If you use the top of your refrigerator to store stuff, pile it someplace else. That excess weight makes your fridge burn more energy.

Unplug the spare. If you have a second refrigerator or freezer that you only use on occasion, make sure it's unplugged when it's not in use. You could save up to $15 a month. And don't worry about damaging the compressor; plugging it in from time to time won't harm it one bit.

Clean the Cooler

Giving your refrigerator a vigorous scrubbing will not only help it run more efficiently, but it'll also provide sanitary storage for your food. Here's how to keep your fridge clean, safe, and cool as a cucumber:

- Whisk away stains with a sponge dampened with hot water and a little baking soda. Just scrub lightly, and rinse. To tackle tough mold and mildew, try my all-purpose stain formula in the Home Remedy box on page 40.

- As part of your routine kitchen cleaning, wipe down the door gasket with a mixture of 1 tablespoon of baking soda dissolved in 2 quarts of warm water. It'll remove dust, dirt, and any odors, while keeping the gasket soft and flexible.

- It's a fact: A refrigerator with clean condenser coils runs for shorter periods of time. So clean those coils at least once a year, and more often if you have pets that shed. You can buy a special coil brush, but save your money because a vacuum cleaner will do the job just as well. And while you're at it, remove the dust on the wall behind the fridge, before it ends up on the coils.

Wash Your Dishwasher

You would think that your dishwasher would be the cleanest appliance in the kitchen. After all, it takes more hot showers in one week than most folks do! But mineral deposits from all of that water can clog the insides, and that means the appliance will use more energy to clean dishes. So try these tricks for spotless dishes—and shockless utility bills:

Clean the interior. Stand 1 cup of vinegar in the upper rack, and 1 cup of vinegar in the lower rack, along with a full load of dishes. Then run the dishwasher as usual. The vinegar will be dispersed throughout the machine, removing

any mineral deposits or soap residue. You should give the insides this good all-over shower once or twice a year.

Unclog the heating element. It's easy to clean the element with a paste made of vinegar and baking soda. Just apply the paste generously to the element, rinse with a little full-strength vinegar, and watch those mineral deposits magically disappear.

Give the spray arm a good poke. Pull the spray arm out of the machine, and poke a strand of thin wire through each hole. When you're through, shake the arm gently to make sure nothing else is caught in there. Then scrub those mineral deposits away with a solution of vinegar and hot water. You should clean the arm at least twice a year.

Maintain the racks. Use a steel-wool pad to remove rust from the tips of your dishwasher racks. And, to keep those racks spic-and-span, clean them once a month with a paste made of baking soda and water.

Sponge the strainer. Every couple of months, lift out the strainer, put it into a sink full of hot, soapy water, and scrub it gently with a sponge.

Discipline Your Dishwasher

The convenience of having a dishwasher (no more dishpan hands!) comes at a price—mainly hundreds of dollars' worth of energy expense every year, and most of that is just to heat the water. So make your dishwasher earn its keep by heeding this advice:

- If your dishwashing water temperature isn't between 140 and 150°F, then the soap won't dissolve; it'll just build up until you've got a miniature mountain of soap gunk—and dirty dishes, to boot! If your dishwasher has a temperature-boosting feature, make sure it's set between 140 and 150°F. If it isn't, then run hot water in the kitchen sink for a minute or so *before* you turn on your dishwasher.

- Don't wash small loads. You'll get more for your money by running your dishwasher once you fill the racks. But don't overload it, either, or your dishes won't get the full force of the cleaning cycle.

- Use your automatic "air dry" switch instead of the "heat dry" switch. If your dishwasher doesn't have an air dry feature, then simply turn the control dial to "off" after the final rinse and prop the door open so your dishes will dry faster.

Reduce Washer Wattage

Ninety percent of the money you spend running a washing machine goes toward heating the water. So if you want to save money, simply wash your clothes in warm or cold water, not hot. Just a quick switch of the temperature setting from "hot" to "warm" will reduce your hot water use by almost half! What's that—your whites will look dingy? Not to worry. Warm water will do an admirable job of cleaning those undergarments and towels as long as you throw in a little bleach. The only time you really need to use hot water is to wash diapers or greasy clothes, or to kill dust mites and other parasites.

Size It Up

Try washing full loads of laundry to make the most of your water and electricity use. Just don't be tempted to overdo it. If your load of clothes is higher than the agitator axle, then they won't be cleaned properly. Also, don't pack your clothes down to fit more in—doing this will also strain the motor. And always match the water setting to the size of your load. Using too little water

Quick Fix

Lots of folks limit how much salt they use. I'm not one of them—I use table salt every chance I get, just not at an actual table! I reach for the salt when I want to keep my non-dishwasher-safe kitchenware clean and sanitary. The next time your fragile items need a bath, ask someone to "please pass the salt" and start shakin' it on! Here's how:

Wooden cutting boards. *Cover the surface with a layer of coarse salt, and rub it in thoroughly with the cut side of a lemon half. Then rinse the board with hot water, dry it, and rub on a light coat of vegetable or mineral oil.*

Metal cook- and bakeware. *Combine 1 cup of salt, 1 cup of baking soda, and 1 cup of borax, and use the mix to scrub away grease, just as you would any powdered cleaner. Store leftover cleaner in a closed container in a cool, dry place.*

Glass vases and decanters. *Pour a handful of salt and 2 teaspoons of white vinegar inside the glassware and give it a good swish. Then rinse with clear water.*

to wash a full tub of clothes can damage the agitator and the motor.

Move It or Lose It

If your hot water has to travel only a short distance through the pipes, it'll lose less heat. So, if you can, position your washing machine as close as possible to the hot water tank.

> ### FAST FORMULA
>
> ## Homemade Dryer Sheets
>
> Here's how to make your own dryer sheets and get the same anti-cling power of store-bought kinds for a fraction of the cost.
>
> Liquid fabric softener
> Water
> Bowl
> Washcloth
>
> Mix 1 part fabric softener and 1 part water thoroughly in a bowl. Soak the washcloth in the mixture for a minute or two. Wring it out, and toss it into the dryer with your clothes. You can reuse the washcloth several times before laundering it and having to make a new batch of softener.

Save Your Soap

If your tub bubbleth over, then it's using that much more energy to rinse out all of the excess soap. The bottom line: Don't use more detergent than the package recommends. And here's a neat trick—if you've accidentally added too much soap, just add 2 tablespoons of vinegar to the water to counteract that extra detergent.

Keep It Level

Make sure your washing machine stays on level footing. Otherwise, it may literally start to walk around the room! That'll not only ruin your floor, but it can also wreak havoc on the inner workings of your washing machine. Leveling the machine is easy—to raise the legs, turn them clockwise; to lower them, turn them counterclockwise.

Launder Your Washing Machine

Sounds silly, doesn't it? Your washing machine pretty much cleans itself. But what about those liquid fabric softeners, which are very waxy and can gunk up the innards? Help your washer work more efficiently by filling the washer tub with warm water and about $1/2$ cup of vinegar (but no clothes!). Then run it through a complete cycle and you'll avoid the whole ball of wax.

Don't Tire Your Dryer

Dryers that are in fine working order all use about the same amount of energy. One model isn't that much more or less efficient than the next. It's the dryer *owners* who use these machines in vastly different ways that makes the difference between money-saving efficiency and money-wasting expense.

The most energy-efficient (and no-cost!) way to dry your clothes is to hang them on a clothesline, and let the sun do its thing. Now I know this isn't practical for many folks, so here are some other ways to dry out your duds:

- Don't dry your towels and other weighty cottons with delicate fabrics. If you separate your heavy materials from your delicate ones, both will dry much more quickly.

- If your machine has moisture sensors, use them. Sensors are great money-saving (and clothes-saving) features. They'll cause the dryer to shut down automatically once the clothes are dry, so the machine won't have to run any longer than it needs to—and you'll save on your utility bill!

- Make sure you remove lint from the trap after every drying cycle. That way, the hot air can travel freely and dry your clothes faster. (You'll also be reducing the risk of starting a fire.)

Make the "Moist" of Your Clothes Dryer

It really doesn't take much to help your clothes dryer live a long and prosperous life. These appliances are usually very agreeable, and they don't ask for a whole lot of attention in return—just an occasional bath, a few strokes of the brush, and a new seal of approval every now and again, and they're good to go for a couple of years (how many of us can make *that* claim?). So follow these easy steps, and you won't have to fire your dryer any time soon:

1. Clean the screen. Every month or so, wash the lint screen in warm soapy water, and let it air-dry overnight. Then follow that up every four months by scraping all of the built-up lint out of your outdoor vent with a stiff-bristled brush.

2. Dust out the duct. Remove the exhaust duct from your dryer twice a year, and give it the once-over with a vacuum cleaner.

3. Test the seal. Make sure the seal around your dryer door is as tight as a drum, so heat doesn't escape. To do this, just hold a piece of tissue paper next to the door edge while the dryer is running. If it sucks the tissue in, then you've got an air leak. All you need to do is take a quick trip to a hardware or appliance store, and buy a new seal. They're relatively inexpensive and easy to install.

Give Your Appliances a Vacation

While you're baring your belly in Bermuda, all your appliances are still hard at work if you didn't unplug them! Now that's not always a bad thing; it all depends on what appliances you have and how long you'll be on holiday. Here's how to leave your appliances before you leave town:

Refrigerator. Emptying your fridge and cutting the power before you leave for a week or two is usually not a practical idea—it'll cost you about $7 a month to keep your food from spoiling, but it'll cost you a whole lot more to restock the fridge with fresh food when you return. Your refrigerator will run more efficiently in your absence if you toss out food that spoils quickly, like veggies and milk, and raise the temperature a degree or two, but no higher than 38°F (and no higher than 5°F for the freezer). Then place gallon jugs of water on the shelves to help the fridge maintain a stable temperature while you're gone. If you'll be away for a while, say longer than two weeks, your best bet is to empty out and clean up your refrigerator, turn it off, and leave the door(s) open. This will prevent the insides from developing a not-so-pleasant odor.

Electric water heater. If you're going to be away for more than a few days, turn off your electric heater at the breaker box. When you return, turn it back on, and give your heater a few hours to produce hot water. Since every 10°F reduction will save you between 3 and 5 percent of your monthly energy costs, turning the heater off will save you plenty!

Heat pumps. Think about your goldfish or houseplants before you turn down the heat—if the temperature's too low, you may come back to frosty fins and a frozen ficus. But if you *don't* have anything in your house that thrives on warmth, then take the thermostat down by 10°F, and you'll save a few bucks. *Caution:* If you're leaving town when the temperatures are frigid, don't drop the thermostat below 50°F because your pipes could freeze while you're gone.

Monitor Your Computer

Now, I'm no computer whiz, so I can't tell you how to surf the Web without wiping out. And I certainly can't help you pick up the pieces after your system crashes. But there's one thing I *can* do: give you some high-speed ideas for keeping your computer clean. That may not sound like much, but take my word for it that many computer problems can be traced back to dusty drives, cruddy keyboards, and murky mouse balls. I may not know much about high-tech electronics, but I'm a master when it comes to good old-fashioned dirt! So boot up and sign on for these dirt-busting ideas:

Trap that mouse dust. When your computer mouse quits cold turkey—and the cord is plugged into the right hole in the back of the computer—chances are that the tracking ball on the bottom of it is dirty. Remove it from the mouse housing by either twisting off the cover with your fingers or unscrewing those tiny screws. Then clean the ball with a cotton swab dipped in a bit of warm water. Use your finger to move the rollers in the ball housing, then replace the mouse ball, and secure the cover. Your mouse is now ready to roll!

Wipe down the screen. Computer screens are dust magnets in the first degree. But if you gently rub a fabric softener sheet or some old pantyhose over the surface, those dirt particles will take a flyin' leap, and land right on to the fabric.

Clean the casing. First, make sure the computer is off before you clean the casing. Then make a paste of baking soda and water, and gently wipe down the exterior of your computer until it sparkles like new. Just be careful not to let any liquid seep into the unit.

Turn the key...board, that is. The safest way to clean your computer keyboard is to unplug it, turn it upside down, and gently shake it to get out any crumbs and loose dirt that are stuck between the keys. Then blow on the keys (try not to spit), and clean the tops of them with a cotton swab moistened with rubbing alcohol.

CHAPTER 4

Clear the Clutter

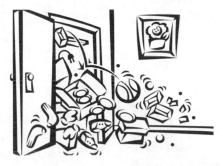

Behind every door and drawer is stuff that's just waiting to tell
a story, and it can be a messy tale indeed. But if you simply try
to close the door (or drawer or lid) on small piles of clutter,
they can quickly outgrow their hideaways and spread all
over the house. So the moral of the story is to tackle the mini
messes *now*, before they turn into mighty big ones later on!

KITCHEN CHAOS

The kitchen is at the heart of every home. It symbolizes nourishment of both body and soul. Unfortunately, all that nourishment tends to clutter up cabinets, pantries, and drawers. Remember the last time you reached for something in the back of your pantry and a big can of "nourishment" fell on top of your toes? Avalanches of food aren't the only disasters waiting to happen. The backs and corners of crowded shelves and drawers are usually filled with long-forgotten food. By the time you discover it, the only thing it should be feedin' is

the trash can! But you can save your money (and your toes!) with just a few organizing tricks that'll stop clutter in its tracks. I'll show you how to quickly turn your cabinets, pantry, and drawers into neat storage spaces so your food will stay fresh longer.

Shelve Cabinet and Pantry Clutter

Here's a dandy project for a rainy afternoon: Clean out your pantry and food cabinets. Now that may be the last thing you want to do, but I bet you're harboring scads of unwanted and/or outdated food that's hogging up valuable shelf space. So just grit your teeth and find some empty trash bags and/or sturdy boxes. Then open a door—any door—and start grabbing things. As you pull out each item, put it into one of the bags/boxes that you've assigned to one of the following categories:

Trash. Bulging cans, stale snacks and bread, leaky jars or those whose warning buttons have popped up, and anything else that's older than its printed sell-by date. Bag these relics, and haul 'em out to the curb on your next garbage pickup day.

Food bank. Anything that's still good, but you *know* you won't use—such as last year's cranberry sauce, or those extra cans of chili you bought at half price. Drop off these goods at your local food bank.

Use soon. Food that is still good and that you routinely use.

Get creative, *now.* Items that you bought on impulse, such as pickled peppers, because you thought they'd be a great new taste treat. Well, they will be, *if* you eat them or work them into a recipe before they migrate to the "food bank" category.

Now that your shelves are bare, take this opportunity to wipe them down so that the leaks and crumbs don't attract any multilegged munchers. Once you've cleaned up the bug (and other thug) chow, it's time to get organized and restock those shelves!

Find Your Cup of Tea

There's no right or wrong way to organize a kitchen cabinet. The best plan for you is the one that puts food where you can easily find it—before it gets old or outdated and turns into wasted cash. The system you choose should fit your space, your time, and your cooking personality. Whether you're a hurried cook with one small cabinet, or a creative cook with a

pantry the size of Texas, one of these plans will work for you:

- For simplicity, you can't beat the good old standby of arranging foods by category. For instance, group all canned fruits and veggies on one shelf, and soups and stews on another. All baking ingredients should be grouped together, as well as all cereals, and so on.

- If you like to put meals on the table pronto, this system is just for you: group together all the foods you use to prepare a meal. For example, put the refried beans, taco sauce, and salsa next to the taco shells, gather all the broth and canned stew veggies into one big huddle, put pasta and sauces together— you get the idea.

- If you have lots of shelves to work with and really want to boil things down to the basics, label each shelf with a color. Then store your food according to its color. For instance, pickles and green beans would go on the "green" shelf, pasta and mayonnaise would go on the "white" shelf, and tomato sauce and chili peppers would go on the "red" shelf.

Once your shelves are arranged, keep them that way. It's easy if you draw up a basic diagram showing where foods are located, so you won't have to dig around for them later. Then attach the diagram to a clipboard, and hang it on the inside of the pantry or cabinet door so everyone in the family knows the new system. By the way, no kitchen should be without a clipboard or two. They're ideal for holding placemats, takeout menus, grocery lists, and even notes reminding you where your seasonal kitchenware is stored.

Embrace Your Junk

You may think that I'm against "junk drawers," but think again because everybody needs at least one. In fact, even Grandma Putt had a junk drawer! She knew it was better to have all of those little knickknacks corralled in one place, particularly in the kitchen, where lots of useful stuff won't fit neatly into a silverware tray. So do what I do and use these things to keep miscellaneous items contained and ready to use:

Small jars. Use baby food or condiment jars to store corncob holders, pastry tips, and twist ties.

Rubber bands. Bundle up skinny things like chopsticks, shish kebab skewers, mixing beaters, fondue forks, and pencils.

Wide masking tape reel. Rubber bands can control clutter, but they can also create their own jumbled mess. A masking tape reel will tame 'em. Just snap the bands around the reel, and they'll stay in place.

Binder clips. Keep coupons, takeout menus, or cooking guides fastened together with a clip, so you can easily find and grab them.

Once your kitchen odds and ends have found their own little homes, be vigilant about keeping things that way. If you put loose items back into their containers after you've used them, then your junk drawer will always look, well, less junky.

Clip Coupon Overload

If you're like me, you're always clipping out money-saving coupons. But once you've clipped 'em, where do you store 'em? I file my coupons in an expanding file folder and keep the file in a kitchen drawer, so I know exactly where it is. If you don't want to get that fancy, simply store coupons in a recycled envelope. When it's time to make up your grocery list, write it on the back of the envelope, and you're ready to go!

HOME REMEDY

Is your kitchen screaming for some breathing room? Well, you could always knock down some walls and rebuild it with huge cabinets and plenty of shelves, or you could free up some space by storing items in a different way. Give any or all of these inexpensive and creative ideas a try:

- **Hang a clean, clear plastic shoe bag in your pantry, or on the back of a large cupboard door. The pockets are perfect for storing dried herbs, spices, nuts, and other small packaged goods.**

- **Install metal cup hooks under your cabinets and dangle your prettiest coffee cups and mugs from them. You'll free up more cabinet space and give your kitchen a fresh, homey look.**

- **Transform an old baby gate (the expandable kind with a crisscross pattern) into a wall rack. Simply attach a 1-inch-thick piece of wood behind each corner, and drive screws through each corner into the kitchen wall. Then add S-hooks and hang up pots, pans, and measuring utensils.**

As you can see, it just takes some imagination and a couple of pieces of hardware to create a whole lot of extra room. So put that sledgehammer away!

Quick Fix

Don't have a spice rack or lots of shelf space for your spices? That's not a problem! Take a space-saving lesson from Grandma Putt: Tack a strip of elastic to each interior side of a drawer and tuck the little jars inside the stretchy bands. They'll stay upright, organized, and easy to reach.

Spice Things Up

A complete set of spices is nice to look at, but do folks use even half of them? I doubt it! So go through all of your spices and throw away the ones you've never used (or never even heard of). As for the spices you always reach for, give them a good sniff. If they've lost their aroma, then they're probably not fresh, so toss them out. But don't throw away those spice jars. Wash them out and fill them up with other essential ingredients you may need just a sprinkle of—like salt, powdered sugar, or cocoa—and put them right back on the rack. Or expand your horizons and use them in other places to store nonculinary items, such as plant seeds, baby powder, or bath salts.

A TIDY BOWL AND BATHROOM

Bathrooms are the *only* rooms that cause family squabbles. After all, no one ever fights to use the laundry room or home office! Bathrooms are used by everyone in the family, multiple times every single day,

and that's an invitation to clutter. You'd think that the most heavily used room in the house would be built with plenty of storage space, but that's rarely the case. If this sounds like your bathroom, don't despair—I guarantee you can transform your cluttered lavatory, no matter how small it is, into an organized oasis.

Counter Your Blessings

Everyone has a stash of pretty gewgaws, but just how many vases, candy dishes, and fruit bowls does one person really need? If you have a surplus of home decor pieces, I have the perfect way to show them off *and* put them to good use at the same time. Take them out of hiding and use them to contain soaps, cotton balls, and lotions on your bathroom countertops or shelves. Here are just a few lovely holders that'll prettify your powder room—and free up some valuable cabinet space:

Kitchen canisters. Tuck cosmetics, cotton balls, bath beads, wrapped guest soaps, and the like inside of them.

Ceramic teapots. Use these as decorative containers for cotton balls, wrapped guest soaps, or trial-size bottles of lotions.

Crystal decanters. No law says that they can only hold liquor. So go ahead and fill them with mouthwash, bath oil, and cosmetic lotions. (Just don't put them in a bathroom that is used by small children.)

Wine racks. They're perfect for holding rolled-up towels and washcloths.

Recovery Room

If opening your medicine cabinet triggers an

avalanche of lotions and potions, then it needs first aid, stat! Follow these three easy steps to making a respectable receptacle, and show the world that you have nothing to hide (at least not in the bathroom):

Step 1. Take an inventory of your pills, ointments, creams, and all other medicines that are currently stuffed into your medicine cabinet. If any have expired, aren't sealed properly, are leaking or damaged, or you simply can't tell what they are, then dispose of them now. It's better to be safe than sorry.

Step 2. Check out your cosmetics because, unlike fine wine, they don't get better with age. Toss out that two-year-old glitter lipstick, not because it's tacky, but because it's unhealthy! Old cosmetics are more likely to become contaminated and cause infections or skin irritations. So throw away any mascara that's more than four months old, foundations and lipsticks that are more than one year old, and eye shadows and powders that are more than two years old. That should free up a lot of space!

Step 3. Finally, gather up all your hygiene and first aid items, such as bandages, cotton balls, and cotton swabs. Consolidate same-type products into one box or container, and toss out the half-filled boxes. If you find that you still have lots of loose items that need to be lassoed in, then by all means, read on!

Round 'Em Up

Those small and/or easily toppled toiletries are destined to spoil your best-laid reorganizing plans. But you can stop the spillage and control the clutter by putting loose items in small containers like these three handy helpers.

Note: You can also use them to store small stuff in vanity drawers.

Lozenge tins. Use them to hold small bandages, bobby pins, and other tiny odds and ends.

Laundry detergent caps. These big, sturdy caps make dandy organizers for your medicine cabinet contents. Fill 'em up with lipstick tubes, tweezers, small makeup brushes, bobby pins, and cotton swabs. Just be sure to rinse the caps thoroughly before you put them to work in your bathroom.

Spice jars. Pop the shaker tops off, wash the jars well, and use them to store small makeup brushes, safety pins, cotton swabs, and makeup pencils. They're perfect!

Stick 'Em Up!

Use the power of attraction to give your medicine cabinet just a smidgen more storage space. Simply add a long magnetic strip to the inside back wall of the cabinet, and then stick lightweight metal items, such as tweezers, bobby pins, and safety pins, right on it. Now you can do a quick strip search the next time you need one of those tiny doodads.

Make Your Tub *Berry* Tidy

Tub time can be playtime, especially for small children. But between their toys and your bathing supplies, the area around your bathtub may be filled to the brim. If that's the case, keep your rubber duckies and other accessories in a row—or at least in a nifty, water-resistant shower caddy. If you don't have one, just hang a plastic berry basket or two on your shower wall with small suction cups. Then tuck in soaps, bath beads, razors, and other personal items—and don't forget the toys!

Give Small Bathrooms the Boot

And a basket, too! There never seems to be enough space in a typical bathroom to hold large, bulky accessories such as blow-dryers, curling irons, and hairbrushes. Here are two novel ways to store your stuff, while giving your bathroom a funky new look:

- Attach a hanging shoe bag to a wall or the back of the bathroom door. It's ideal for holding brushes and blow-dryers, and smaller items, such as cosmetics, toiletries, bath toys, and first aid supplies.

- Hang the loops of a wicker or plastic bicycle basket from a towel bar, or from two hooks that you've screwed into the bathroom wall. Now you can store your extra towels and grooming gear in a receptacle that has a nostalgic touch.

REC ROOM WRECKAGES

The family that plays together, stays together…until, that is, it's time to clean up the mess that's left behind! No matter what room your family gathers in most, whether it's the living room, rec room, great room, or den, it undoubtedly has the word *family* written all over it. This room probably has the biggest hodgepodge of clutter in it, from books and magazines to catalogs and craft supplies. And that's just for starters, because when odds and ends start tussling with each other, there's mighty big trouble brewin'! So follow my advice on how to divide and conquer your rec room clutter.

End Sloppy Hobby Habits

Hobbies are a terrific way for you to express your creativity, but unfortunately, they can leave behind one imaginative mess! To keep your creative juices from flowing all over the carpet (and coffee table and couch), put your supplies in one container, if possible, in one central location. Here are some clever storage ideas for corralling your crafting clutter:

Baby wipe containers. They're tailor-made for storing beads, glue, ribbons, small scissors, and tubes of paint.

Film canisters. Use them to hold pins and needles, tiny buttons, and beads.

Mayonnaise jars. Their tight-fighting, screw-on plastic lids and multiple sizes are ideal for large items, such as markers, knitting needles, scissors, and clay and for smaller pieces such as embroidery floss and embellishments.

Handbags and tote bags. Stuff them with yarn and quilting gear. And, since they're portable, you can craft on the go!

Shoe bags. Use the kind with clear plastic pockets to stash paper, yarn, scrapbooking supplies, glue guns, and the like. Then hang them from a rod in the nearest closet.

Jewelry boxes. Fill the pouches, ring holders, necklace hangers, and drawer compartments with thimbles, beads, ribbon, buttons, and other tiny treasures.

Read All About It…

then get rid of it! If your family room furniture is buried under a mountain of reading material, then it's time to dig yourself out. Old news is not good news for your living space, so don't be a pack rat and save outdated newspapers and magazines. You *know* you're never going to read it all, so turn that paper tiger into a pussycat with these four easy "to dos":

1. Visit your local library to determine what magazines it subscribes to, then cancel any of your subscriptions that duplicate theirs. After all, why pay good money for information you can read for free?

2. It's silly to hang on to 200 pages just because you want to save one or two of them. So clip (or rip) those pages out, put them in a folder, and file it in a cabinet. But be fussy about the articles you keep, or you'll soon have one overstuffed file cabinet! And if you follow this route, be sure to check out my advice on page 79 for weeding out bloated files.

3. As I always say when it comes to reading material, "the fresher, the better." So give yours a "read-by" date, and once that date passes, throw it out whether you've read it or not. And if you haven't read your newspapers and magazines by the time the next issue arrives, then give those expired papers the heave-ho, too!

4. Fire the paperboy and let modern technology deliver the news instead. Nowadays, you can catch up with current events, finances, job opportunities, hobbies, the latest celebrity gossip, and so much more with a few simple clicks of the mouse. And you're already paying for the Internet connection, to boot!

One final bit of advice on this subject: I firmly believe that information is meant to be shared, so be a good neighbor and donate your unwanted magazines to local hospitals, schools, and libraries. Their patrons will appreciate your generosity, and it'll make you feel good!

FAST FORMULA

Soap Box Derby Magazine Holder

The big boxes that dry laundry detergent comes in are just as strong as those upright file boxes that are designed to store catalogs and magazines—and they're free! Here's how to make your very own publication holder.

Large, empty laundry detergent box
Ruler
Pen or pencil
Scissors or utility knife
Fabric, wallpaper, or adhesive plastic
Plain white labels

Cut off the top of the box, and clean out any inside residue. Then lay the box down on its back side and, with a ruler to guide you, draw a diagonal line from the upper right corner to about 8 inches from the bottom of the left corner on the front of the package. Flip the box over, and draw a diagonal line from the upper left corner to about 8 inches from the bottom of the right corner on the back of the package. Using your scissors or knife, slice along the front and back lines that you've drawn. Now slice a horizontal line across the side of the box to connect the cut on the lower left hand to the cut on the lower right hand on the front and back of the box, respectively. (Use a commercial magazine file, or a picture of one, as a guide if you need to.) Then attach your decorative covering of fabric, wallpaper, or plastic to the outside of the box, stick on a label to show the contents, and put those magazines in their new resting place.

THE BEST-DRESSED CLOSETS

Do your linens come tumbling down every time you open the closet door? Is your prom dress from 1968 still hanging in your bedroom closet? Most every room in your home probably has a closet in it, and that's an open invitation to simply shove things inside, slam the door, and forget about them. Sometimes, the tidier the room is, the messier the closet is—after all, it's a very convenient hiding place when unexpected guests drop by. If your closets are about as organized as a child's toy box, then these terrific tips will show you how to neaten things up, double your storage space, and, yes, even help you find exactly what you need in your closets.

Harness Your Clotheshorse

Most of us have gained or lost a few pounds over the years, and we have a history of clothing sizes to prove it! Make a habit of shedding all those outdated, ill-fitting duds as you come across them. Simply tie the handles of a drawstring trash bag to a coat hanger and hang one up in each closet. Then each time you spot a garment that you haven't worn in ages, toss it in the bag. When the sack's filled up, take it to your local thrift shop, Salvation Army, or Purple Heart store.

Access Your Accessories

No doubt your clothes are sharing space with lots of accessories, including scarves, belts, and handbags, and they can be the dickens to keep orderly. You can buy accessory organizers that are specially designed to corral them all, but sometimes, the solution is right inside your four walls. If your accessories are out of control, give these items a try:

Napkin rings. Keep two or three scarves bundled neatly together by threading them through a napkin ring. Then store those beauties on a shelf or in a drawer.

Shower curtain rings. Pop them over the closet rod and use them to hang scarves, belts, and handbags in one place.

Wooden clothes hanger. Screw cup hooks at intervals of 1 inch or so into the base of the hanger. Then put it on the closet rod and hang your belts and handbags from the hooks. (This is also a great way to organize necklaces and bracelets.)

Get Out of Space Debt

If your clothes need some more elbow room, then you can increase your closet space by making some quick and easy (and cheap) improvements. One of my favorite ways to add more storage is to install a simple hook—after all, who doesn't have room for at least one or two in a closet? Screw them into closet walls and use them to hang robes, pajamas, and accessories.

Here's another trick for doubling the storage potential of the shelf above your clothing rod: Just add another shelf above it. Many closets have one shelf with space that extends straight up to the ceiling. Take advantage of all that room and install a second shelf to hold seasonal clothing or special-occasion accessories that you don't need to reach for very often.

With a little bit of tweaking, most closets can accommodate up to twice as many items as they were originally built to hold. Take a tip from the decorating and designing pros—rather than

Hot Rod How-To

Let's face it: Clothes almost always look better when they're stored on a hanger, so clothing rod space is usually at a premium. Fortunately, most closets can easily accommodate a second clothes rod. Just install it underneath the first one to hang shirts, vests, and folded pants. And adding another rod doesn't have to involve a whole lot of handyman know-how (or money, either). Here's a quick and easy way to get the job done.

Broomstick or dowel (cut to fit)
2 small eye hooks
2 chains (The length depends on how low you want to go.)
2 large S-hooks

Take the broomstick or dowel and insert the eye hooks on the top of each end. Attach a length of chain to each hook. Hang the chains from the closet rod above it with the S-hooks. Now that rod is ready for action! This is a great addition to a child's closet. Since the second rod is within little ones' reach, there's no excuse for piles of clothes on the floor. Not only that, but it kind of gives a whole new meaning to "Spare the rod, spoil the child," doesn't it?

focusing on a lack of space, zero in on the space you do have and make the best use of it.

Know Your Linen-tations

Linen is such a tidy little word, but let's look at what it really means: bath towels, bedsheets, quilts, tablecloths, dish towels, and on and on

and on. It's darn near impossible to cram all those things into one tiny linen closet, but we try to anyway! If your linen closet is stuffed to the gills, then the problem might be that you simply have more linens than you (and the next several generations) will ever need. Here's how to draw the line on linen overload:

Bath linens. You do the math! If you take a shower every day and wash your linens three times a week, then you'll need at least two complete sets of towels (7 showers per week ÷ 3 launderings per week = 2.3 towels per person). Use this formula for each household member (some of them may bathe more frequently than others) to figure out how many sets of towels they'll need, and then add up the totals. That'll give you the minimum number of towel sets, including washcloths and hand towels, you should have on hand.

Bed linens. Keep no more than three complete sets for each bed in your home. That way, you've got one set in use, one set to change out with a dirty set, and one set as a spare. It's also a good idea to keep a few extra pillowcases, since they tend to wear out sooner than other bed linens.

Table linens. You should never use a dish towel for more than one day because a damp, dirty dish towel can spread food-borne bacteria from plate to plate to plate, and that's no good for anyone! With this in mind, the number of dish towels you need depends on how often you wash your linens. If, for instance, you do your laundry twice a week, then you'll need about four dish towels so you'll have a clean one ready to use every day.

Once you've gone through your stash and separated the good from the bad from the ugly, don't be tempted to throw the tattered ones away. Old washcloths and dish towels are perfect for dusting and cleaning around the house. They also make great packing material for delicate items. Donate the ones that are in decent condition to an animal shelter or your favorite charity, or take them to a thrift store.

Lay Down Linen Laws

I'm sure all of us at one time or another have opened up the linen closet door and been on the receiving end of a toppling towel or two. Luckily, a falling towel has never knocked anyone senseless. But don't wait for it to happen; use this easy-to-reach arrangement to say good-bye to those fabric fallouts:

Upper shelves. Use these for seldom-used holiday tablecloths or other linens, and any items you don't want children to reach, such as cleaning supplies.

Eye-level shelves. Put your smaller items, such as washcloths, folded pillowcases, and toiletries here, so you can see them easily.

Middle shelves. This is the place for linens you use frequently, including bath and dish towels.

Bottom shelves. Reserve these for big items, such as bedsheets, blankets, comforters, and other large linens.

Banish the Bulk

Sometimes, there's no room in the linen inn for really big bedding—like quilts, comforters, and pillows. If your hefty wares can't bunk with the rest of your linens, then give them a new home by storing them under your beds. Plastic wading pools, plastic sweater boxes, and even old suitcases are perfectly sized for under-the-bed storage, and what's even nicer is that they'll glide right in and out without a struggle!

Get Down in the Trench Coats

Coats draped on the backs of chairs, scarves hanging from railings, hats on end tables— these are all signs that your coat closet is overflowing. After all, it's much easier to toss a coat over a chair than it is to find hanging space in a parka-packed closet. If you've got outerwear everywhere, then your coat closet is crying for help. Relieving that bloat starts with donating some coats (and scarves, hats, mittens, and so on). Those items that no longer fit your body or your taste are desperately needed by charities that minister to folks in need. So take the castoffs you haven't worn in two years to a local charitable organization, such as the Salvation Army or Purple Heart, and give the gift of warmth.

Closet Cleanup

Now that you've pared down the outerwear in your coat closet, it's time to take a fresh look at your closet space. See that overhead shelf? Well, it's the biggest clutter magnet in most

Quick Fix

Most folks have at least one giant-size gift tin that once held popcorn or other snack treats lying around the house. If it's at least 18 inches tall, you can transform it into an umbrella stand. Just cover the outside of the tin with paint, fabric, or Contact® paper, and spray the inside with a waterproof sealer. Then place a plastic saucer in the bottom or line the inside with a plastic bag. Pour in 2 to 3 inches of sand or gravel to absorb wetness and weigh down the stand. Set it by your door, and you have one splashy umbrella stand!

coat closets. By their very shape and size, hats, gloves, and scarves tend to create chaos, so they need their very own space. That's where shelf dividers come in handy. They'll stop the hats and gloves from crossing the line into other territories. Or you can use old shoe boxes and dish tubs to house and separate your scarves, gloves, and mittens. Here are some other nifty ways to put an end to coat closet chaos:

- Help your kittens find their mittens (and gloves) with the old cardboard tubes from gift wrap, paper towels, and toilet paper. Tuck gloves and mittens inside the tubes and write the wearer's name on the outside, so there's no doubt who they belong to. Or hang a clear plastic shoe bag from the closet rod or a hook on the interior wall, and stuff the pairs into the pockets!

- Another great use for cardboard tubes is for corralling wayward scarves. Assign one or two tubes to each family member, and wind their scarves around them. Or drape scarves over the closet rod and thread the ends through a napkin ring to keep the scarves from tangling up or slipping to the floor.

- Keep knitted hats in a clothespin bag and hang it from the closet rod (this also works for scarves, mittens, and gloves).

MAKING THE HOME OFFICE WORK

For the record, not every home needs an official "home office" that's equipped with a computer, fax machine, wall-to-wall bookshelves, and file cabinets galore. For most folks, a space that's big enough for a small desk where they can balance their checkbook or keep important files will suffice. But no matter where you do your paperwork, that area should be organized so you can focus on the task at hand. Record-keeping messes, jam-packed file cabinets, and desktop litter will sabotage your concentration just like fingernails scraping down a blackboard! So if your office area resembles a train wreck, fire your disorganized ways, and hire a clutter-buster professional—me!

Organize the Folder Holder

Record keeping can easily take over your life, especially if you've been hoarding every invoice, contract, tax return, and warranty since 1972! There comes a time when all of those important documents go from safeguards to space hogs. Let's face it—file cabinets are usually made of pretty sturdy material, but the weight of decades' worth of paper is enough to test any cabinet's mettle (*and* metal). If your file cabinet is bursting with papers, then it's probably holding records you don't need. So grab a chair, open that overstuffed drawer (if you can), and use this guide to document life span:

Three years: Banking statements, credit card statements, stocks, bonds, and receipts for deductible income and expenses

Seven years: Tax documents

For as long as you own it: Vehicle titles, licenses, purchase and service receipts, and current warranties

Toss 'em out: Outdated insurance cards, old registrations, grocery store receipts, and receipts for unwarrantied, uninsured, or nontaxable items you no longer own

Once you've discarded all that paper poundage, you can organize everything you've saved into files/folders that are neatly labeled as "tax returns," "insurance policies," "bank statements," "warranties," and so on. Remember that the purpose of a file cabinet is to put important documents right at your fingertips without needing a crowbar to pry open an overstuffed drawer.

Quick Fix

Don't let important notes, reminders, and phone numbers get lost in the desktop shuffle. Help those little scraps of paper rise above it all by attaching them to a bulletin board. If you don't have a spare one, you can make your own with some fabric, some wood or corkboard, and several extra-long rubber bands. Just glue fabric around a 1-foot-square, 1/2-inch-thick piece of wood or corkboard, and stretch the rubber bands around the board in both directions to form a grid pattern. The bands will hold your papers securely—and you won't have to search high and low for thumbtacks or pushpins.

Take Desk-erate Measures

A desk is the heart of all home offices. And, just like the heart, it should be kept clean of any and all debris that could clog it up. A lot of valuable time is wasted looking for "missing" pens, sticky pads, staples, and so on. But as long as you practice some healthy habits, your desk will function the way that it was meant to. Here's how to use common household items to corral not only those little office supplies—like pens, paper clips, and rubber bands—but also larger

items, to help you work smarter, not harder:

Ice cube trays. Put small piles of paper clips, pushpins, stamp rolls, and sticky pads in each little compartment.

Lozenge tins. Store business cards, sticky pads, rubber bands, pushpins, paper clips, and other odds and ends that tend to drift into the far corners of your drawers.

Plastic berry baskets. Fill them up with 3 1/2-inch computer discs, or turn them upside down and fill the grids with pencils, pens, and lightweight letter openers.

Small photo albums. Slip your business cards inside the vinyl pockets.

Cutlery organizers. Keep pens, pencils, markers, staples, and erasers from rolling around, helter-skelter, in your drawers. Or keep one on your desk to hold items you use regularly.

Shoe bags. Hang one on a hook on the back of the office door or on a nearby wall, and stash pens, notepads, ink-jet cartridges, and envelopes inside the see-through pockets.

Plastic plant trays. After you've planted your flats of annuals or groundcovers in the spring, don't throw away the trays. Clean 'em up and save 'em because they're just the right size to hold papers or outgoing mail.

Sweater boxes. Use them to corral papers, folders, envelopes, and pamphlets.

Copy-paper boxes. These sturdy boxes are great for holding folders, record-keeping books, large envelopes, and, of course, plain white paper. You can even dress up the box with a bit of fabric or wrapping paper to match your office decor!

GIVE YOUR GARAGE A LIFT

Contrary to popular belief, garages aren't *just* crash pads for cars. More and more folks are utilizing that extra space for noncar things like workbenches, gardening tools, sports equipment, and backyard toys. The result? A room so jammed with clutter that it's no longer fit for a car! Transforming a garage back into the safe automotive shelter it was meant to be doesn't have to involve a three-day trash fest and a posse of people. Luckily, sorting out your garage can be done in baby steps and in your spare time. The secret is to focus on one area and break it down into little doable parts. Here's what you need to do.

Bench Workbench Litter

The area around a workbench probably attracts more clutter than any other part of a garage, often including paintbrushes, tools, scraps of lumber, and nails—and let me tell you, nails and tires don't mix! Fortunately, there are lots of containers already lying around your house that'll keep tiny bits and pieces from scattering around. Not all of them are sturdy enough to survive a rough-and-tumble environment, but some hardware holders, such as the following, are more than up to the task:

Lozenge tins. Use 'em to separate your nails, screws, nuts, bolts, drill bits, thumbtacks, and small batteries.

Laundry detergent caps. Line up a bunch of them on a shelf, and toss a separate size of screw into each cap.

Film canisters. Tuck screws, tacks, fishhooks, lead weights, and other small hardware inside, and write the contents on the lid with a permanent felt-tip pen.

Baby wipe containers. They're perfect for storing spare electrical parts, screwdrivers, pliers, pens, and pencils.

Toilet paper tubes. Wind up loose cords and stuff them in the tubes. And if the cord is attached to an appliance, wind it up until it's long enough to reach from the tool to the outlet, and then stuff the excess into the tube.

Prune Garden Tool Messes

When garden tools seem to take root in your garage, they'll spread out faster than dandelion seeds on a windy day. No matter where you keep your gardening equipment, whether it's in a spacious shed or a cramped garage, you can stop those tools from tumblin' down around you with these nifty storage ideas:

- Store bags of potting soil and fertilizer in plastic sweater boxes, or make those soil additives mobile by putting them in a wagon.

- Attach binder clips (from your neatly organized office) to gardening gloves and sun hats, and slip the clip handles over any hookable surface.

- A galvanized steel bucket makes a great garden hose hanger. Just drill three holes in a triangular pattern in the bottom of the bucket, and screw it to the wall with the open end facing out. Coil the hose around the bucket, and store extra nozzles and hose-end sprayers inside of it.

- Slide hoes and rakes into an old rolling golf bag, and stuff hand tools, seed packets, and other odds and ends into the pockets. Then your gardening gear can travel with you!

- Hang hand tools from empty thread spools that are screwed into the wall, or corral them inside of a giant-size laundry detergent bottle. Just make a big hole on the side of the bottle that's opposite the handle, and put your tools in the hole. Then you can simply grab the handle and go.

Are We There Yet?

Well, not quite. We *still* haven't addressed your automobile, which is the biggest space hog in any garage. Even if you have room to actually park your car, you may not have room to park all the tools, fluids, rags, and grease monkey duds that you need to maintain it. If that sounds like you, then take these clutter-busting ideas for a test drive:

Car caddy. If you still prefer to drink your beer and soda pop from bottles, then save the six-pack carton. Use it to store windshield-washing fluid, brake fluid, and motor oil. Or make yourself a car-cleaning kit by putting your sprays, sponges, car wax, and scrubbing pads in the cubbies. Now all your supplies are together and neatly stored in one handy place.

Tool hangers. Dangle an old tool belt or shoe bag from a hook on the wall or the edge of a shelf, and slip all of your car repair tools inside the pockets.

Toolboxes. If you've got a plastic sweater box or old plastic cooler lying around, use it to hold jumper cables and hand tools for the car. Just make sure you throw in a few sticks of chalk before you close the box to absorb moisture and keep your tools rust-free.

Now that your garage is free of clutter, your car finally has a place it can truly call home! But what if your auto itself it hiding pockets of litter? If that's the case, then carry on to find out how to give those minor messes the red light.

The Clutter Compartment

Glove compartments have become a convenient catchall for the stuff we use or collect in our travels, such as snacks, receipts, and small toys for the kids. But this little storage cavern is within easy reach of the driver's seat for good reason—it's meant for items that the driver may need to grab quickly. It's no fun fumbling through bags of pretzels and a year's worth of gas receipts to find a pair of sunglasses while you're driving on a blindingly bright day. The only residents of your glove compartment should be the car manual, maps, sunglasses, a pen, a pad of paper with emergency phone numbers written in it, and insurance and registration documents. You should still have some room for small necessities, such as coins for the highway tolls (which I like to keep inside of an empty film canister) and a disposable camera in case you're in an accident and want snapshots for insurance purposes.

Quick Fix

Before you start dismantling anything that has a lot of teeny-tiny parts, lay a length of wide, double-sided tape on your workbench. Then as you remove each little piece, stick it on the tape. The pieces will stay put and you won't have to hunt around for them when you're ready to put the appliance (or whatever) back together again.

For safety's sake, toss out everything else that's taking up precious compartment space. Throw away papers you don't need, and put incidentals like snacks and toys into a tote bag that a passenger can be in charge of. Once your glove compartment has been decluttered, keep it that way by weeding out the trash every few months, or after a long road trip.

De-Junk the Trunk

Car trunks are perfect little dens for stashing weather gear, sports equipment, toys, compact discs—but, wait! Where's the stuff you really need, like a roadside emergency kit? Unfortunately, many items in the trunk of a car are more about lifestyle and less about saving a life. It may take a little work, but you can make room for the things you need *and* the things you want. Read on for my tips on getting a handle on your trunk junk.

Divide and Conquer

Before you can organize your car's trunk, you'll have to clean out the debris. So grab a garbage bag and a sturdy box, and dig right in. Start by putting all the items you don't need or want, like old magazines, expired advertisements, empty cups, and fast-food bags, in the garbage bag, and haul it over to the trash can. Then place the stuff that never made it into the house, like those garage sale books you couldn't pass up, or the canned peas that fell out of the grocery bag last month, into the box and take it inside. Store

those things in their rightful places the next chance you get. What's left should be plenty of wide-open trunk space.

Trunk Tamers

Now that your trunk has been de-junked, it's time to organize all the keepers. The best way to tame car trunk clutter is by placing a few containers in it to hold like items together. You probably already have these inexpensive containers lying around the house. Use them to keep emergency supplies, groceries, toys, pet gear, and such from rolling around and migrating into the four corners of your trunk. Among the best are:

- Coolers
- Laundry baskets
- Milk crates
- Plastic sweater boxes
- Sturdy file boxes

Lose Weight, Save Gas

No, not you—your car! When you have to transport heavy items like luggage, furniture, or sports equipment, don't drive around with them in your trunk any longer than you have to. That extra weight causes your car to guzzle more gas and cuts down on your gas mileage.

And as a final reminder, try to clean out your trunk every few months, so your home away from home is as safe and clutter-free as it can be!

CHAPTER 5

Auto Biographies

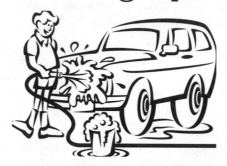

There are two sides to this story: yours and your automobile's. You shell out big bucks to buy, maintain, and repair your car. But loads of money won't solve every car conundrum, and replacing your car with another one can cause even bigger headaches. So how does this story end? Well, that depends on how much time and money you're willing to spend. Here's what you need to know.

REPAIR SHOP POTHOLES

It's inevitable—if you keep a car long enough, then there's a breakdown in your future. It may not be today or tomorrow, but one day, trust me, it'll happen. Every vehicle, whether it's on the assembly line this very second, or standing outside in your driveway, only travels so far until it starts to shake, rattle, and eventually, not roll. And when that happens, you know what that means— pricey repair bills, and sooner or later, a pricier car to replace it. But even though all automobiles need some fixing, you can delay or even prevent some of those costly

repairs with common sense and proper maintenance. Just remember that a bit of timely TLC can help prevent your car from going to pieces.

Use Manual Labor

Remember the owner's manual that came with your car? You know, that thick book that's probably still sitting in its original wrapping in your glove compartment? Well, crack it open and start reading because it's literally a bible of betterment for your vehicle. The manual spells out exactly what each car system does and when it's due for maintenance. And even if your car is running smoothly, don't neglect the checkups because they will almost always prevent costly repairs down the road. You say you don't have a manual, or you can't find it? Then order another one through a local dealer (like the one you bought the car from), or contact the car's manufacturer; every major automobile company has an easy-to-use Web site for handling these types of issues.

Make Pit Stops

There is no "ideal" time to give your vehicle a thorough checkup; it all depends on the make, model, age, accessories, and how and where the vehicle has been driven. Nevertheless, all vehicles will benefit from these monthly checkups done by you, your mechanic, or someone with a bit of mechanical know-how:

Engine oil. First, make sure the auto is on level ground so you can get an accurate reading. Then check the color (the lighter, the better) and feel of the oil (it shouldn't be gritty). And if your car is old or loses oil, check the level of the oil more often.

Finish. Give your car's finish a good scrubbing at least once a month to wash away any and all corrosive road grime. If the water beads are larger than a quarter, then it's time for a wax job, too.

Tire pressure. Check this when the vehicle has been sitting awhile, or has been driven only a short distance. Tires should be inflated to the pressure that's listed on the driver's side door frame, the interior side of the glove compartment door, or the trunk lid. While you're at it, check for signs of leaks, bulges, or other defects. And don't forget the spare tire in the trunk!

Checkin' Things Twice

A year, that is. To keep things whirring and purring, there are certain items in, or areas of, your vehicle that should be serviced every six months or so. Have your mechanic perform these checkups twice a year (I've included tips for checking the less complicated parts in case you're so inclined):

Air filter. Hold the filter up to a bright light. If you can't see the light, then the filter should be replaced. You can save yourself time and money on parts and labor by buying an air filter at an auto parts store and installing it yourself. It's really easy—just take off the filter cover, remove the old one, and drop in a new one. If you take a lot of short trips or drive on dirt roads, then your air filter should be checked more often.

Battery. If your battery has removable caps, check the fluid level every few months. Make sure the terminals and cables are rust- and corrosion free and are attached snugly. If any corrosion has built up, clean the posts and cable connectors with a paste made of 3 parts baking soda to 1 part water. Then dry the cleaned parts with a soft cloth, and coat them lightly with petroleum jelly. *Caution:* Batteries contain sulfuric acid, so ALWAYS wear latex gloves and protective eye gear whenever you're handling them.

Brakes. If you rack up a lot of miles, or if you do a lot of stop-and-go driving, then have your brakes checked at least twice a year. And if you hear any grinding or squeaking, or the brake pedal suddenly feels different, get them checked out ASAP!

Constant velocity (CV) boots. These rubber sleeves protect the CV joints against all manner of road grime. It's easy for a mechanic to check them out while your vehicle is up on a hoist for an oil change.

Oil change. Generally speaking, it should be done every six months or so, but that depends on where you live (dusty climates will gunk up the oil faster) and what kind of driving you do (short, frequent trips eat up more oil than longer ones do).

Radiator. You can wash the outside of the radiator yourself with a garden hose. Sweep away any debris (bits of leaves, paper, and so on) with a soft-bristled brush, wipe down the radiator with liquid detergent, and then hose it off.

Same Time Next Year

Some systems and parts of your car need to be serviced only about once every couple of years. As I mentioned, your owner's manual has the final say when it comes to maintenance schedules, but here are a few things that need to be checked more frequently:

Belts and hoses. They may not show signs of wear and tear, but belts and hoses should still be replaced every two to three years. If one of them suddenly breaks, you're stuck, whether it's in the middle of a rush-hour traffic jam, or a nice drive in the country. Either way, it'll cost you a lot in terms of time, money, and aggravation.

Cooling system. Have it checked every fall, just before the cold weather sets in, to make sure you've got adequate winter protection. The mechanic should also be able to determine when the system needs to be flushed. Since old antifreeze must be safely disposed of, most folks prefer to leave this job to the pros.

Transmission. In many cases, the transmission fluid and filter should be replaced every 36,000 miles, but it depends on the make and model of the vehicle. Check your owner's

manual to determine what the manufacturer recommends, and then follow up on it.

Naturally, as your car starts to age, all of its parts need to be checked and maintained more often. It may seem costly and inconvenient, but as the old saying goes, "An ounce of prevention is worth a pound of cure." Or in this case, an ounce of maintenance is worth a pound of repair.

FAST FORMULA

Concrete Cleanup

Has your do-it-yourself auto tinkering left oil spills on your concrete garage floor? Whatever you do, don't clean up the mess with toxic chemicals. Instead, try my all-natural solution to oily spills and splotches.

Baking soda
Cornmeal

Cover the spills with equal parts of baking soda and cornmeal. Wait until all of the oil has been absorbed, and then sweep up the residue. If any stains remain, wet the floor with clear water, scrub the spots with baking soda on a stiff brush, and rinse well. Then keep that cornmeal handy, because it works wonders absorbing oil on car upholstery, clothes, and even oil-stained hands.

Make Tires Go the Distance

There's a lot riding on your car's tires, but many folks put more thought into choosing the color of their car than they do choosing the right tires. We generally tend to go with whatever tires the service person recommends, but that's a mistake that could cost you several hundreds of dollars! As with everything else, it pays to comparison shop. The very same make and model of tires can have one price tag at, say, an auto shop, and a very different price tag at a department store. So before you make a deal on your wheels, compare prices at auto parts stores, dealerships, department stores, independent tire dealers, and the Internet. When you do get price quotes, make sure you determine what's included, particularly the cost of installation and balancing (which, of course, you'll have to arrange yourself if you're buying tires on the Internet). Then follow these tips for getting the most out of your tires.

Read the Rubber

You'll see lots of sidewall gobbledygook on new tires, and it's hard to know what's important to you and what's a lot of hooey. Here are the codes you need to crack to get the most mileage for your money:

"DOT" identification number. This number is found around the inner circle of the tire's sidewall, and it tells you when the tire was manufactured. That's important to know before you plunk down your hard-earned cash because storage conditions and air quality can cause the material to deteriorate before the tires even hit the road. To determine the manufacturing date, look at the last four digits of the DOT ID. The first two digits indicate how many weeks into the year it was made, and the last two digits indicate the year it was manufactured. The number *2306*, for instance, means that the tire was manufactured in the 23rd week of 2006. A good rule of thumb is to not buy any tires that are more than three years old. Otherwise, you'll be paying your money and taking your chances.

Speed rating. Chances are that your car won't ever reach speeds of 186 miles per hour, so you probably don't pay much attention to the speed ratings of various tires, but you should! Tires that can endure extreme speeds are made of a softer rubber compound to grip the pavement, but unfortunately, that material deteriorates faster than tires made with a stiffer, less pliable material. Your best bet is to choose tires with a lower speed rating that'll really go the distance. Tires branded with the letters *Q, R, S,* or *T* can withstand speeds of 99, 106, 112, and 118 miles per hour, respectively. Any other letter indicates that the tire will survive at even higher speeds.

Tread-wear rating. This number tells you how long the tire treads should last when compared to other treads made by the same manufacturer. So a tire with a 300 tread-wear rating will last twice as long as a tire with a 150 tread-wear rating. The higher the tread-wear rating, the sturdier the tread material is.

When choosing the best tires for your car, consider what, where, and how you drive. Then check those factors against what your handy owner's manual says about your vehicle's tire requirements. If you want the lowdown on how the various brands of tires rate on traction, tread, safety, and overall performance, check out the National Highway Traffic Safety Administration Web site at **www.nhtsa.gov**.

A Working Re-Tirement

Not sure what to do with your old tires? I say, "Put them to work!" Use one or more to cushion your arrival home by attaching it to your garage wall; it'll soften the blow if and/or when you don't stop in time. You can turn the others into a tire swing, a raised bed for growing tomatoes, or even a sandbox that the under-seven set will just love!

DEALING WITH MECHANICS

Every day, we take a leap of faith by trusting folks who have more knowledge in a particular area than we do. But that doesn't mean we should surrender total control. Let's say that your doctor recommends surgery. You'd probably weigh the operation's risks and benefits, and the reliability of your doctor, before agreeing to it. You may even get a second opinion. Well, expensive car repairs deserve the same considerations. Even if you can't tell a lug nut from a walnut, don't sit on the sidelines and let your mechanic make all of the decisions. Here's what you need to know so you can take that leap of faith *and* stand your ground.

Learn the Language

Mechanics are only human. A misdiagnosis or a failed car repair happens to the best of them, but sometimes, the fault lies with you and/or a breakdown in communication. To bridge that gap:

1. Make it a point to actually *talk* to the mechanic. Most large auto dealerships and repair shops use a "whisper down the lane" approach to car repair—the customer explains the problem to the service adviser at the front desk, who then tells the mechanic. And things can easily get lost in translation. So save yourself some time and aggravation by having a one-on-one talk with the mechanic, if possible.

2. Don't diagnose the disease yourself and then request the treatment you think is best. Otherwise, you'll be on the hook for service that may not correct the problem. Remember: Too many cooks spoil the broth, and you want your broth to be in tip-top shape. So tell the mechanic what the symptoms are and how often they occur, and then leave the diagnosis (and the responsibility for fixing it) to him or her.

HOME REMEDY

Car parts have lousy timing; they always seem to work splendidly until their warranty expires. But listen up: If you're facing expensive repairs after the warranty has expired, you may still be eligible for some coverage. Some car manufacturers offer "After Warranty Assistance," or AWA, which pays for some or even, in rare cases, all of the repair costs. Not everyone qualifies (only loyal dealership service customers need apply), not every car is eligible (the vehicle must be properly maintained), and not every manufacturer offers an AWA program, but it's certainly worth looking into. So if you're facing costly car repairs, and the parts are just beyond the warranty period, ask your dealer if you're eligible for AWA.

3. Give the mechanic the specific whats, whens, and wheres of the problem. How? By writing things down as you notice them. Then, for instance, if your car stalls only on rainy days, or rattles only when you make a left turn, you'll know it. In this situation, any small detail could be a very important piece of the puzzle, so don't leave anything out.

4. Speak up. If you have any questions about the service you've received, use your copy of the written estimate (most states require that you receive one) and speak up, keeping the conversation focused. Mechanics, just like other businesspeople, want happy, satisfied customers, so it's in their best interest to work with you to keep you coming back. No matter how big the communication gap is between you and your mechanic, remember that *everyone* understands the language of money!

Don't Get Hooked on Dealers

Not every repair or maintenance check needs to be done by the dealership that you bought your vehicle from, or that sells your particular make and model. Now I'm not saying you should cut *all* the apron strings, but there are times when an independent auto repair shop is a much better way to go. Its mechanics can perform routine maintenance checks for as much as 30 percent less than the dealership, and most warranties won't be affected (but check your warranty, just in case). If your car needs a major repair job or there's a recall, then it should be serviced at a dealership. But once the warranty is up, all bets are off and you can take your business to the place that's going to give you the biggest bang for your buck!

Test-Drive New Mechanics

Every automobile owner should have a trustworthy mechanic, even if your car drives like a dream. Why? Because when your car suddenly starts having nightmares, you need to get it into reliable hands as soon as possible. The worst time to find a mechanic is when you need one NOW, because desperation almost always beats out logical thinking. So do a little investigating by asking friends and family about what kinds of experiences they've had with car mechanics, and who they would recommend. Then choose a winner based on the answers to these important questions:

1. Is the shop Automobile Service Excellence (ASE) certified and/or does it have any other certifications?

2. Does it offer warranties on its parts, and are those parts new, used, or salvaged?

3. Are the labor charges based on an hourly rate or flat fee? And what does the shop base those labor charges on?

4. Where is the shop located? For the sake of convenience, it should be close to home, work, or public transportation, or the shop should offer a free shuttle service to take you where you need to go.

5. Is the facility neat and orderly, and is the service staff friendly and courteous?

6. Is the waiting area clean and comfortable? This is no small matter if you have to wait while your car is serviced.

Once you've gathered this information, call your local Better Business Bureau to see if the shop has any complaints on record. If it does, then it's back to the drawing board. If it doesn't, then you've probably found yourself a winner.

SPEEDY CLEANUP

No matter how much you think you know, there are times when every vehicle needs the attention of a pro. Making major repairs to a complex piece of machinery takes time, knowledge, and the proper tools. And if you lack any of these, then drop those weapons, step away from the car, and take that seriously ill vehicle to the nearest trustworthy mechanic! But not every scratch, squeal, or scrape necessarily needs that level of attention. There are loads of simple, inexpensive remedies that you can use to treat all sorts of minor annoyances, including windshield dings, rust spots, and scratches. Here are a few of my favorite do-it-yourself fix-its—and don't worry, they're so easy, even a non–grease monkey can do 'em!

Be a Glass Act

Your windshield, car windows, and side-view mirrors all get plastered with plenty of traveling mementos—splattered bugs, small dents, mud, grease—the list goes on and on. Household glass cleaners aren't always up to the task of tackling tar, tree sap, and bug guts. Not only that, but many household glass cleaners contain ammonia, which will ruin tinted windows. So use my gentle homemade window wipers instead for these specific problems:

Bug splats. Pour some cola onto a sponge or an old pair of pantyhose, and wipe the glass clean.

Tree sap. Put a glob of mayonnaise over the sap, wait a few minutes, and then wipe it clean.

Small windshield dent. Drip a little clear nail polish into the hole, let it dry, and then add a few more drops. Repeat the procedure until the hole's completely filled.

Light window and mirror scratches. Squeeze a small dab of mildly abrasive toothpaste—not the gel kind—onto a soft, cotton flannel cloth. Carefully rub the scratches very lightly until they vanish.

Cigarette smoke–fogged glass. Wash the windows with a solution of 2 tablespoons of lime juice and 1 quart of water, using paper towels or newspaper to dry them.

Glue. Now's the time to use that household ammonia glass cleaner to remove any glue that's left from old tint film or inspection stickers. Spray it on and then wipe the glass with a paper towel immediately.

Window Wipe

When your car windows need a good general cleaning, mix 10 parts vinegar to 1 part water, and pour it into a spray bottle. Then spritz the glass and wipe it down with newspaper. You'll appreciate the crystal-clear results, even if you "don't do windows."

Wake Up Your Tires

When the rubber meets the road, it can be messy business indeed! Keeping tires clean is nearly impossible (unless you never plan to use them), but you can stop grime from marring your tires and scratching up the hubcaps. These timely tire treatments will keep them looking as good as new:

● Remove tar from whitewall tires by applying a paste-type car wax to the spots with a cloth or sponge, and then polishing it off with a soft cloth.

- Banish tree sap by rubbing on some mayonnaise, let it sit for a few minutes, and then wipe it off.

- Remove rust from chrome wheels by first washing the wheels with soap and water and drying them thoroughly. Then rub the rust with fine steel wool. Your wheels will soon be shining like the sun!

- Loosen up rusted-on lug nuts by soaking a cloth in cola, then holding it against the lug nut for a minute or two (or however long it takes).

Soapsuds for Cleaning

When your tires need a good all-over cleaning, don't use powerful detergents, which will only dry out the rubber. Use car-wash soap instead (you can find it at any auto supply store) because it gently cleans the tires without stripping out the moisture they need to keep on truckin'.

Add the Finishing Touch

As you might have guessed, car paint is one of the most resilient paints around. After all, it has to survive all of that horrible stuff people and Mother Nature throw its way. Unfortunately, finishes can't stand up to gravel, acid rain, tree sap, and fender benders without taking on a few battle scars, so treat the wounds left behind with these remarkable remedies:

Grease. Remove it with baby wipes. They'll clean up the mess in a flash, without harming the paint.

Acid rain. Minerals in acid rain can actually etch the finish if they sit on the paint too long. So when the car surface isn't hot, spray the areas with a solution made of equal parts distilled water and distilled vinegar. Wipe it off with a clean, dry soft cloth.

Scratches. Wipe down the area with soap and water, rinse and dry it well, and then apply a coat or two of clear nail polish to any scratches. The polish will keep the scratches clean and rust-free until you can get your car into a body shop.

Bumper stickers and glue. Saturate the sticker with nail polish remover. Then carefully scrape it, and the glue residue, away with a razor blade, sharp scraper, or old credit card.

Chrome rust and stains. Crumple up a piece of aluminum foil so the shiny side is facing out, dip it in cola, and gently scrub the rust and stains away.

FAST FORMULA

Road-Salt Remover

A wintry wonderland is lovely to look at, but ugly to drive in. If you live in snowy-winter territory, you know that a buildup of road salt on your vehicle will damage the finish over time. So keep this simple recipe handy, and use it every time you come home from a drive on sloppy, salt-treated roads.

1 cup of kerosene
1 cup of dishwashing liquid*
Water

Mix the kerosene and dishwashing liquid in a bucket of water, and use a sponge to rub away the salt deposits. (*Caution:* This stuff is flammable, so use it sparingly!)

* Do not use detergent or any product that contains antibacterial agents.

Keep the Interior Superior

Car passengers do more than just sit back and enjoy the view—they eat, drink, play, read, and even groom themselves. And nowadays, some vehicles come equipped with televisions and DVD players, so let's get this party started! If that's not an open invitation for stained and smelly car seats, then I don't know what is. Keeping your upholstery clean and protecting it from those messy moving violations is easy:

Coffee- and cola-stained upholstery. Rub the stains on vinyl and cloth coverings with baby wipes. (Seat belts require special care, so turn to page 94 for safe cleaning instructions.) *Note:* Don't use baby wipes on leather upholstery; many wipes contain alcohol, which dries out and may discolor leather.

Ink-stained fabric. Blot the splotches immediately and spray them with hair spray. Then blot them again. Repeat this process until the stains are gone.

Gummed-up fabric. Toss a few ice cubes into a plastic bag, and rub the bag over the gum until it hardens. Then scrape off the stiff gum using a credit card or plastic scraper.

HOME REMEDY

Try these inexpensive alternatives to pricey auto-store products to keep your car's leather upholstery nice, soft and supple:

- **Apply hair conditioner to a clean soft cloth, and rub down the leather. Then buff the area with another clean soft cloth.**

- **Wipe down the seats with a little milk, then polish them with a clean soft cloth.**

Water-spotted vinyl or leather. Cover the spots with a thick coat of petroleum jelly. Leave it on for a day or so, and then wipe it off with a clean soft cloth.

Stay in the Shade

No matter what kind of upholstery you have, it'll retain its color, shape, and good looks if you usually park your car in a shaded area. Over time, sunlight will dry out and fade any material, so keep the car's interior in the dark as much as you possibly can.

Clear the Air

Don't you wish that the new-car smell could hang around forever? Unfortunately, it doesn't and, over time, it's replaced by that old-car smell from food, cigarettes, pets, mildew, and God knows what else. Clear the air with these potent odor eaters:

- Pour a little bit of vinegar into a shallow bowl, and leave it in the car overnight. Just remember to take the dish out before you go for a spin, or you'll wind up with a car that smells like salad dressing!

- Cut off the foot of a pantyhose leg to make a pouch, and put a few chalk sticks inside of it. Cinch off the top of the pouch with a ribbon, rubber band, or what have you, and hide it under a seat. The chalk will absorb mildew-causing moisture.

Once the odors are gone, you can make your own air freshener with an empty lozenge tin and your favorite fragrant potpourri or strong-scented soap. Just poke holes in the lozenge lid, and then fill the bottom part of the tin with the potpourri or soap. Snap the lid closed, and shove the container under a car seat. That way, everything will be coming up roses, lavender, chamomile, or whatever!

DEALS ON WHEELS

The road to a great deal on a new or pre-owned car is full of hairpin turns. Financing, auto insurance rates, warranties, and, most importantly, price negotiations all make for some pretty tangled territory. And that's not to mention the mighty friendly salespeople who'll point you in the most expensive direction possible! But never fear—the safest route to buying a quality new or used vehicle is the one you map out yourself. Steering around dealership potholes is tricky, but it can be done with a little bit of preparation and haggling know-how. So buckle up and let's go for a spin!

Shop Smart

Remember that vehicles are meant to *serve* you—not inconvenience you with high insurance rates, uncomfortable seats, gas-guzzling accessories, and the like. Yes, the perfect auto should catch your eye, but it also needs to fit your budget and your lifestyle. You already know what pleases your fancy and your wallet; now answer these questions to find the vehicle that'll complement your lifestyle:

1. How much do you drive? If it's more than 30 minutes every day, then good gas mileage, safety features, and comfort should be your top priorities.

2. How much do you haul around? If you're a taxi service for lots of people, such as kids or clients, or you frequently fill your vehicle with sports gear, landscaping equipment, and other necessities, then you'll need all the cargo space you can get. So consider a good-sized minivan, SUV, utility truck, or four-door sedan.

3. What's your usual driving terrain? If your area gets blasted with snow, or if you live in mountainous or rocky territory, then you need a sturdy four-wheel-drive vehicle that'll withstand the elements. But if you live in sunny California, a nice little convertible may be just the ticket for you!

Stay Within Your Budget

For many folks, the make and model of the car they choose boils down to the sticker price. But there's more here than meets the eye—auto insurance, loans, and lease payments figure into the mix, too. A good rule of thumb is to keep your total monthly car costs at or below 15 percent of your monthly budget. Once you've tallied up all of the facts and figures, stick to this amount like white on rice! You'll meet lots of folks who'll want you to stretch that number until it snaps, but where will they be when those monthly bills come rolling in?

To find out if a particular make and model are in your price range, check out the latest *Kelley Blue Book* from your local library, or visit the Web site at **www.kbb.com**. You'll discover what the dealer's invoice cost is (the amount the dealership is charged for the vehicle, including shipping), which will give you a figure to work with when it comes time to negotiate. And, don't forget to figure in the high cost of insuring your new car, which can be anywhere from 8 to 12 percent of the purchase price! To put a lid on your coverage costs, drive straight ahead to the next tip.

Insurance Accidents Waiting to Happen

That small, plain car with the matching small, plain sticker price may look like the deal of the century, but it could cost you more to insure than a large, fully equipped vehicle. Why? Well, a heavier, sturdier car usually needs less repair work after a collision than a car that crumples like a tin can. Buying a new car will always jack up your insurance premiums, but these models and features will drive up those costs the least:

Family vehicles. It's a fact—minivans, station wagons, and large sedans are all involved in fewer crashes than smaller, sportier cars. And they also tend to cause less damage to other vehicles when involved in a collision.

Safety belts. Some cars are equipped with belt-crash tensioners, which reel in any seat belt slack right before the point of impact to lessen your body's forward motion. Less slack means more protection and less chance of injury.

Head restraints. All passenger cars are now built with front seat head restraints, but not all restraints are created equal. The most effective restraints are adjustable, so you can position them right where they need to be—close behind the back of your head. Just make sure that the head restraint can be locked in; some adjustable restraints aren't, so they can slip during a crash, which is precisely the time you need them to stay put!

Air bags. Front air bags are standard equipment in all new vehicles, but not every one has an advanced frontal air bag system, which detects how much protection is needed depending on the size of the passenger and the severity of the crash. And if you have a choice, side impact and rollover air bags will keep you and your passengers even safer.

Safety Pays

Most insurance companies offer discounts for safety features as well as antitheft devices, such

HOME REMEDY

Seat belts are by far and away the single most effective means of preventing injury and death in an automobile accident, so you want to keep them strong and properly maintained. That's why you should use only a simple mixture of soap and warm water to clean them. A more powerful cleanser could weaken the fabric of the belt. But if the buckle is sticky, you can use a more potent cleanser to clean it thoroughly, so it can lock in place securely. And if one or more belts are becoming frayed, don't even think about trying to reinforce them or replace them yourself. Take your car to a certified repair shop and have new belts installed, so you can feel confident that your loved ones are safely strapped in.

as an alarm system and window etching. But savings on these features and devices vary from state to state, so contact your insurance agent for further details. To find out if the car of your dreams is, in reality, an insurance nightmare, check out its crash-test rating on the National Highway Traffic Safety Administration Web site at **www.nhtsa.gov** and the Insurance Institute for Highway Safety Web site at **www.hldi.org**.

Keep Leases on a Tight Leash

Leasing a car isn't for everyone. Leases are best for folks who don't have much cash for a down payment, don't drive more than 15,000 miles per year, or who trade in their cars every few years. But those aren't the only considerations. You also need to be aware of what your options are when the lease ends—either buy the vehicle at the contracted price, or turn it in and pay some pretty hefty penalties based on its condition. If you travel a lot, aren't diligent about car care, and can afford a decent down payment, then buying a car is definitely the wiser way to go.

The good news is that you do have some wiggle room when it comes to negotiating the length of the lease and the down payment amount. But your best cost-saving strategy should be to bargain down the price of the vehicle, since this is what the payment amounts are based on. So the bottom line should be to never enter into a lease agreement until you've first negotiated the purchase price of the car.

Steer Clear of Financing Pitfalls

Dealerships are more than happy to design a car loan just for you, but don't let them do it! I know that those "low-interest" and "no money down" offers sound mighty tempting, but just remember one thing: The dealership will recoup its money somehow through the price of the car. No matter how you slice it, a dealership never loses out on those "great" offers. If you want to keep as much of your hard-earned dough as possible, then have your financing in place before you shop for a car. Follow these steps to hunt down the best loan for your new automobile:

1. Start your search with your local credit unions—they usually have the lowest rates in town. If you aren't a member of a credit union, find out if your job, church, school, community, or a professional organization is affiliated with one, and if so, join it now!

2. If you can't secure financing through a credit union, then your next best bet is to check out the interest rates local banks are offering. Start with your own bank: Since you're already a customer, you may qualify for a loan with a lower interest rate than those loans offered by other banks.

3. Once you've found the loan with the most attractive rate, ask to be pre-approved for automobile financing and get a document that spells out in writing the rate and loan amount you qualify for. Then when you're ready to negotiate the price of a car, show the salesperson this piece of paper and see if he or she can get you a better deal—but don't count on it!

Having said all this, there *is* one situation when financing through the car dealership could be to your benefit, and that's when the car manufacturer (*not* the dealership) offers special low-rate financing or cash rebates. You can truly save a bundle of money this way. But in most cases, you'll be ahead of the game if you negotiate the best purchase price possible with the dealership and leave the financing to outside financial institutions, where it belongs.

Make a Trade

Trading in your current car can take a chunk off the purchase price of a new car (assuming that your old one is fully paid for), but there are some disadvantages to going this route. On the other hand, selling your car privately isn't all wine and roses, either. So what's a car owner to do? Making the best choice starts with finding out just how much trade-in and private sale value your current car has. Check out the going rates in an up-to-date *Kelley Blue Book* at your local library, or go on their Web site at **www.kbb.com**. Community Web sites, such as **www.craigslist.org**, are also worth investigating. Then take a look at the classified ads in your local newspapers to see what prices car owners are asking. Now you've got some inkling of how much you stand to lose or gain, depending on how you get rid of your old car.

The bottom line is that a dealership will never give you top dollar for your trade-in. But in some circumstances, there are factors that may be more important to you than just getting the best price. Trading in your car makes sense when:

- Your vehicle needs a lot of work, and you don't have the time, money, or inclination to make it sale-worthy. A trade-in will at least save you the pre-sale repair expenses as well as the hassles that accompany them.

- Your vehicle needs some work that you could do yourself, but you have neither the time nor the desire to sell it privately.

- Time is of the essence and you need to sell your car now! (Private sales can take months.)

Sprucing Up

If you decide to use your car as a trade-in, you should invest a little time and elbow grease into making it look as cared for as possible; otherwise, you probably won't get a fair trade-in offer. So change the oil (if it hasn't been done in a while), give it a good once-over both inside and out, and repair any obvious, but minor, imperfections. Don't put too much money into a makeover, though, because you may not get that money back out of it. (You'll find plenty of cheap fix-it ideas on page 90.)

Make Me an Offer

Rest assured, you can make a tidy profit by selling your vehicle yourself, which you can then apply toward the price of another car. Just keep in mind that selling a car takes time, patience, and a certain amount of intestinal fortitude.

If you're up for it and fit into one of these situations, then let the bidding begin!

- Your vehicle is in excellent condition and you have the service records to prove it.

- Your vehicle isn't perfect, but you have the money to get it back into tip-top shape.

- You're not in any hurry and/or have no other auto-related commitments.

Use Your Senses

Sure, that shiny new automobile sitting in the dealership showroom looks beautiful, but how does it drive, feel, and sound? The point is that you've got to make sure the vehicle agrees with *all* of your senses before you take the plunge and make the purchase. Here are three ways your body can help you make up your mind:

See. Do the lines of the car please you? Does the color of the upholstery look good against

---

Quick Fix

Do you have a real clunker that won't fetch much money as a trade-in and certainly isn't worth the time or effort to patch up and sell privately? If so, then consider donating it and using the fair market value as a tax deduction. The tax break or refund you receive could be equal to the money you would have gotten for it if you sold it outright, but without all of the hassle. Check out Publications 4302 and 4303 on the Internal Revenue Service Web site at www.irs.gov to find out how to make a car donation work for you.

the exterior color? Is the cargo area spacious enough for passengers, groceries, sports gear, or anything else you'll need to transport? Are the front, back, and side views unobstructed?

Touch. Are all the seats comfortable? Do you like the feel of the upholstery? Are the instruments within easy reach of the driver's seat? Do the brake and gas pedals respond smoothly? Does the car seem to glide over the road, or do you feel every pothole? And does the car handle well in traffic and/or on the expressway?

Hear. Does the engine roar, or is it barely a whisper? Can you carry on a conversation, or is it drowned out by the din of the road noise? Is the stereo system nice and soothing, or loud and tinny? Crank it up and find out!

Take the Test

Believe it or not, I know some folks who test-drive a car by taking it around the block and then back to the dealer. Don't you be one of them! To make the most of your test-drive, plan on spending more than a few minutes in the car. Make U-turns, back up, drive over both paved and unpaved roads, open it up on a highway, and cruise quiet streets of nearby neighborhoods. Don't make your decision in one visit. Go back again and take it for two or three more spins to see how it handles at night and in adverse weather. All of this effort will pay off handsomely when you find just the right car at just the right price.

Choose a Used Beauty

Thanks to recent advances in the auto industry, cars are now built to last longer and perform better than ever before. So what does all that high-tech reliability mean for you? Simply this:

You now have a huge variety of top-quality pre-owned vehicles to choose from. The selection can be overwhelming, so keep these tips in mind when you're searching for that diamond in the rough:

- If you're buying from a dealer, seek out certification. Most dealerships offer warranties on certified pre-owned vehicles that have passed various inspections on all parts and systems on the car. If the dealership doesn't offer this type of warranty protection, find another one that does.

- Whether you're buying from a dealer or a private seller (see "Classified Information" on page 99 for more tips on buying privately), bring along your mechanic to give the vehicle the once-over. Most dealerships won't let vehicles leave their property without a chaperone, so bring a mechanic with you who'll inspect the automobile right there on the lot. It'll cost you some money, but an objective, professional point of view could stop you from falling for an overpriced clunker. And if the dealership won't allow a mechanic on its turf, then make tracks to the nearest exit.

- Before sealing the deal, study the vehicle's title. In most states, titles are required to list previous owners. Check out the number of previous owners. If the car has had, on average, more than one owner for every two years it's been on the road, then think twice about taking that baby home. So take a pass on, say, an eight-year-old car with more than four owners. Where there's smoke, there's fire, and lots of previous owners sure smell like lots of smoke to me.

- Check the VIN. The vehicle identification number (VIN) could hold the key to the car's skeleton closet. With it, you can review the vehicle's history of reported cases of damage, theft, or fraud. Just enter the vehicle's VIN on the CARFAX Web site at **www.carfax.com**. Keep in mind that this data includes *reported* cases only. Not every jurisdiction provides information to CARFAX, and not every owner reports an incident, so you still need to have the vehicle thoroughly checked out for any prior damage.

Let the Bargaining Chips Fly!

Over the years, car dealers have become more sensitive to customer satisfaction and less obsessed with moving a car off the lot. Why? Because the industry has found that car buyers who are stalked by pushy salespeople tend not to return. So we're now starting to see reputable dealerships that'll give you some space, and they're more likely to work *with* you, not *at* you. Today, buying a car isn't as unpleasant as it used to be, but when it comes to haggling on price, the rules themselves are as old as time.

HOME REMEDY

Here's a hot tip for you: Check out the local rental car agencies—not to rent a car, but to buy one! Rental cars are given top-notch care (for liability reasons), wear and tear is usually minimal, and many agencies will pass along the manufacturer's warranties to the buyer. And since rentals are considered past their prime after two years of use, you can get a fairly new car at a fairly reasonable price. So call the agencies in your area to find out where they put their "old mares" out to pasture.

Here's how to play and win the "survival of the fittest" game at the negotiating table:

Step 1. Let the dealer's invoice price (check it out at **www.kbb.com**), or the going price on pre-owned cars (also on the *Kelley Blue Book* Web site, as well as **www.craigslist.org** and the classified ads in your local newspaper) be the launchpad for your opening bid.

Step 2. If the car is used, play up any mileage issues, wear problems, dents, scratches, or other imperfections to lower the price.

Step 3. Don't negotiate a price for your trade-in until the price of your new car is set in stone. And let your used-car research from the *Kelley Blue Book*, craigslist, and/or newspaper guide you in your bidding.

Step 4. If and when you make a counteroffer, increase the amount by a small increment, such as $100. Anything else, and you're only bidding against yourself.

Step 5. If the best the salesperson can do is still well above the dealer's invoice price, ask him or her to write the price on the back of a business card, offer thanks for the time spent with you, and tell the person you need time to think about it. Then use that card as a bargaining chip at another dealership to determine if the folks there can cut you a better deal.

One point to remember: Negotiating should always be done in the most professional manner possible. That goes for you and for the salesperson, too. If the salesperson loses his or her temper during negotiations, then don't waste any more of your time. Cut your losses and find another dealership to work with. Trust me, there are plenty of them out there!

CLASSIFIED INFORMATION

Gone are the days when buying a used car from its owner meant settling for any old jalopy with an AM radio. Oh, you'll still find them around (and actually, those old cars can fetch top dollars), but today, newspapers and Web sites are bursting with "For Sale by Owner" ads touting quality used cars. Here's more good news—there's no middleman. Dealing directly with the owner eliminates all those outrageous manufacturing, dealership, and sales costs. Now here's the bad news—there's no middleman. So what do you do if you have a problem with the vehicle after you've bought it? Private cars are usually sold "as is" without the safety net of any warranties. If you end up with a clunker, your cost to buy and repair it can be equal to or greater than the price of a fully certified, pre-owned vehicle. Yes, buying a vehicle through a private sale has both its pluses and minuses. Follow these tips to end up on the winning side of the equation.

Put the Seller to the Test

One of the beauties of buying a car directly from the owner is that you can size up the situation from the comfort of your own home. All it takes is one phone call or e-mail, and you can get the answers to these revealing questions:

Why is the car for sale? This question gives you key information about both the car and the seller. Does the reason sound logical? Does it make sense? Does the seller sound like someone you could trust and do business with? Go with your gut instincts on this one.

How many owners has the car had? If there's been more than one, ask the seller for detailed information on the car's history. If he or she has none, then proceed at your own risk because buying this vehicle is a crapshoot.

Has the vehicle been in any accidents? Again, details are important. If it has, how extensive was the damage, and how much did it cost to repair it? Minor fender benders don't usually affect the performance of a vehicle, but a serious accident can have lingering effects, even if the repair was perfect, which it seldom is. Find out who did the repair and how recently it was completed. Pros will back up their work, but if the repair was the do-it-yourself kind, you should be wary.

How many miles does it have? If it's more than 20,000 miles per year, ask why it's so high. And ask whether it was primarily city or highway driving. Keep in mind that long commutes are generally much easier on a car than 20,000 miles' worth of short stop-and-go trips.

Write down all of the information the seller gives you, so if you decide to take a closer look and/or a test-drive, you can compare your notes to the actual condition of the car. And if the seller has been less than truthful with you over the phone or via e-mail, then you should bid him or her "good riddance."

Use Checks and Balances

Buying any type of major item is a gamble, but buying one without a warranty is a little like flying blind. Sometimes a private seller can transfer an extended warranty to the new owner *if* it's transferable (many of them aren't), but the seller isn't under any legal obligation to do so on privately sold cars. If, by a stroke of luck and good will, the owner does offer some sort of guarantee, make sure to get it in writing. In most cases, though, your garden-variety private car sales are on an "as is" basis. So give your potential vehicle a very thorough once-(or twice- or thrice-)over before striking a deal. It's easy to check all the obvious parts, but uncovering hidden problems can be a bit tricky. These simple tests will let the cat out of the bag, if there is one:

- Bounce each corner of the car. If it bounces more than two times, or if each corner bounces differently, then the suspension or shock absorbers may need work.

- Look at the car mats and the floor underneath them. Discolored and/or moldy spots could indicate a moisture problem. Stains on top of the mats or floor carpet may mean that the air conditioner or heater is leaking, so ask the seller for an explanation.

- Look at the exhaust smoke when the car has been idling for a while at normal temperature. If the exhaust is white or blue smoke, there could be an engine problem.

- Compare the tire treads on all five tires (don't forget that spare!). If the four tires on the car aren't equally worn from sidewall to sidewall, then that could mean the car was in an accident, or is misaligned. And if the spare tire shows signs of substantial usage, ask for the when and why details.

- Check the oil level *and* the color of the oil. Rub the dipstick on a rag to see if the oil is gummy, black, or gritty, any of which is a warning sign that the car hasn't been properly maintained. Beads of water in the oil could mean the head gasket needs replacing.

Quick Fix

Rust and accident damage to body panels are fairly easy to hide with auto-body filler. So take along a magnet when you inspect the car to test the bumper, panels, doors, and any other steel surfaces on the car. If the magnet doesn't stick in certain areas, then either the panel is made of fiberglass or some other nonmagnetic surface (such as aluminum), or someone could have used filler to repair rust or dents. Either way, it's a red flag that needs to be addressed. Note: Bring a small, thin piece of fabric to put between the magnet and the body panel so you don't scratch the paint.

- Ask to see all repair and maintenance receipts. These will not only tell you why and how often the car was serviced, but will also show how conscientious the owner was. If the owner whips out years' worth of receipts, then he's pretty responsible and trustworthy. If he can't verify the maintenance, walk away.

Take It to the Mechanic

Even if the used car looks immaculate, take it to your mechanic before you commit to any deal. Believe me, it's money well spent no matter how you look at it. If the car turns out to be a lemon, that small inspection fee saves you from spending thousands more to repair the vehicle. And if the car needs work, but it is still worth your while, show the seller the repair estimate and bargain for a lower purchase price. Finally, if the car is in great condition, the money you spent to verify it buys you peace of mind, which in my book, is priceless.

CHAPTER 6

World-Wise Traveling

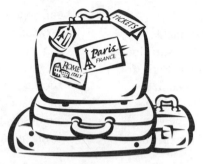

Soaring gas prices, inflated airfares, overpriced hotel rates—kinda takes all of the relaxation out of a vacation, doesn't it? Leaving your worries behind certainly is, well, worrisome. But don't throw in the beach towel just yet. You *can* trot the globe without losing your mind, or your retirement fund. Here's how to venture forth and get the biggest bang for your traveling buck!

FLYING LESSONS

It costs a pretty penny to fly the friendly skies, and many times, there is simply no other viable option. So you have to bite the bullet and pony up the cash. And the cost of airfare isn't the only price you pay—the time and aggravation factors of delayed flights, security checkpoints, waylaid luggage, and long lines have to be figured in as well. You have no other choice, right? *Wrong!* The terrific tips that follow will allow you to drop as few dollars as possible and enjoy the entire travel experience.

Travel the Web

These days, surfing the Internet is usually the surest road to lower airfares. It's not a quick fix, though, so be prepared to spend some time cruising around for the best deals on airline tickets. Start at the one-stop-shopping sites like **www.expedia.com** and **www.travelocity.com**. (You can find plenty of other online travel ticket companies via your favorite search engine. Just type in "airline tickets," and you'll have loads of sites to choose from.) But don't overlook individual airline Web sites, such as **www.united.com** or **www.delta.com**, especially if you're searching for last-minute deals. You're more likely to find low prices on flights taking off within the week on official airline Web sites than you would on travel ticket Web sites. When you're reviewing those sites, don't just peruse the standard fare listings—let the old creative juices flow. Here's what you should do:

Broaden your territory. Investigate flights to all major cities that are near your destination. For instance, if you're heading off to Cape Cod on vacation, don't just limit your search to Boston. Check out Providence, Manchester, and Hartford, too. You might find a lower fare flying into Providence, and the driving distance is about the same.

Pack it up. Oftentimes you can save big bucks by booking your plane tickets, hotel room, and rental car as a package deal. Nearly all airlines have partnership agreements with particular hotel chains, rental car agencies, cruise lines, and resorts, so take advantage of the deals when you can. Even if the Web site doesn't offer you a package deal, the partner companies will often reward you with frequent-flier miles, discounts, or other special offers when you use their services during your trip. You'll usually find these businesses listed in a special travel partners section of the Web site.

Reserve Wiggle Room

Flexibility will take you far—literally! No matter where you shop for your airline tickets, you'll almost always save more money if you can adjust your schedule a little bit. In fact, the more flexible your plans are, the less it'll cost you to ride the friendly skies. Check out these surefire ways to save money on your airfare:

1. Travel on the slowest, least-popular days and times. Tuesdays, Wednesdays, and Saturdays are usually the cheapest days of the week to fly, and early-morning and late-evening flights often cost less than those at more, um, civilized hours.

2. Travel off-season. Like every other business, airlines charge as much as the market will bear. So it only stands to reason that when everybody and his uncle are hankerin' to be in a particular place at the same general time (such as Easter vacation), then it's going to cost a pretty penny to get there. But you can get some big bargains if you head to your destination when most folks are either staying home, or going someplace else.

3. Sign up for free weekly e-mail announcements through individual airlines. In the middle of the week, you'll be notified of all last-minute price deals on tickets for the upcoming weekend. So if you have the luxury of traveling at the drop of a hat, then by all means, sign up!

There are plenty of deals to be found, but most low-priced airline tickets are non-refundable. So before you commit yourself to a flight, you should be reasonably sure that you'll be able to make it to takeoff.

Flying with Fido and Fluffy

Thousands of hotels, motels, resorts, and campgrounds (in all price ranges) welcome four-footed lodgers, but getting them from here to there can be a harrowing experience for both of you if you don't do your homework. Most airlines have a live-animal limit, so your first step to a hassle-free trip with your pet(s) is to make your reservations as early as possible. When you book your flight, be sure to ask these questions:

- What are the crate requirements? If your pet crate is too big, ask whether it can be upgraded to the passenger cabin if there's room. If you can upgrade your pet to the cabin, do you have to pay extra?

- What are the takeoff and landing temperatures? Make sure the temperature range is safe and comfortable for your pet, and that your pet is healthy enough to withstand that range. Federal regulations demand that animals not be exposed to temperatures below 45°F and above 85°F for more than four hours.

- What documents does the airline need to ensure that your pet is fit for flight, and when do they need them? Most airlines require rabies and vaccination certificates a week

---

HOME REMEDY

Even the roomiest, most cushiony airplane seat can seem like an instrument of torture after an hour or two of sitting in it. When your muscles start to ache, cramp, or stiffen up from lack of movement, a few simple stretches will loosen them up and get your blood flowing again. To give your neck a nice stretch, bring your chin down toward your chest and then slowly tilt your head toward your right shoulder, and then your left shoulder. To loosen up your shoulders, give them a few shrugs up, down, forward, and backward, holding each position for five seconds or so. To unclench calf and foot cramps, put the heels of your feet on the ground and then point your toes up. Use these stretches whenever you're short on space and long on time, and you'll feel a whole lot better!

---

to 10 days before takeoff, so contact your vet ahead of time to get all the necessary papers or vaccinations in order. Keep copies of the documents you send to the airline and bring them with you—you'll need them for your trip. Also, when you're talking to the vet, ask about tranquilizing your pet before the flight.

- If you and your pet are headed for foreign shores, contact the consulate or the embassy in that country as soon as possible to find out what the quarantine and vaccination regulations are. You'll find consular contact information on the Bureau of Consular Affairs Web site at **www.travel.gov**.

The American Kennel Club has a free booklet that's filled with tips on traveling with your canine cohort. To get a copy, log on to **www.akc.org**. Also, your local bookstore and the Internet have dozens of titles on traveling with your pet, so be sure to check them out. (To find out what to pack for your furry friend, see page 108.)

Charge!

Well, maybe. Those credit cards that offer frequent-flier miles for every dollar you charge can be mighty tempting. So can the ones that give you big discounts when you charge your airfare to the card. But think twice before you sign up for those cards because they'll land you some genuine bargains only if you pay your bill in full every month. If you routinely carry even a small balance, you'll probably wind up paying more in interest charges than you'll ever save on airfare.

Join the Club

Even if you don't fly very often, it generally pays to join a few frequent-flier clubs. It'll cost you nothing, yet you'll get regular mailings advertising special sales and programs, including money-saving deals on cruises, hotels, and rental cars. Plus, if you ever have a problem with an airline's customer service department, your frequent-flier membership will give you a little more leverage than you'd otherwise have.

Take It from Uncle Sam

No matter how little you pay for a plane ticket, it's not a bargain if your flight arrives several hours late, you're treated rudely, your luggage never shows up, or when it does, it looks like an 800-pound gorilla played with it. To set your mind at ease, before you book your next flight, log on to the Federal Aviation Administration (FAA) Web page at **www.faa.gov/index.cfm** to check out how each airline measures up

in performance. You'll get the lowdown on flight delays, overbooking of flights, damaged or lost baggage, treatment of passengers with disabilities, and all manner of consumer complaints about the major U.S. airlines. If the performance statistics of the airline you're considering look dismal, then walk away.

Pack Smart

You can't take it with you—or can you? Packing your carry-on luggage shouldn't involve guesswork. Since the list of restricted items is constantly changing, log on to the Transportation Security Administration Web site at **www.tsa.gov**, or call the airline ahead of time to find out what items are prohibited. And while you have someone on the line, find out what the baggage size and weight restrictions are (which can vary from one airline to the next) and if there are any charges associated with oversize carry-on bags. The list of banned items seems to change with the wind, but by using a little common sense, you can avoid security checkpoint snags by:

1. Choosing your traveling outfit carefully, so you'll sail right through the metal detectors. Even the tiniest bit of metal in such items as buttons, underwire bras, earrings, and barrettes will set the detectors off, and that means more delays.

2. Organizing your carry-on bag so the security X-rays can provide a clear picture of what's packed inside. Use clear zip-top plastic bags to hold your toiletries, medications, and other small containers together for ready inspection, if need be.

3. Keeping all of your medications in their original containers, so security officers can verify the prescription information on the

---

Quick Fix

If you have motion sickness or low blood sugar, or know that you'll need to catch some shut-eye on the plane, your seat assignment can mean the difference between a walk in the clouds or a nightmare at 10,000 feet! If motion sends your stomach spiraling, then reserve a seat close to the wings—this is the most stable area on the plane. If you suffer from low blood sugar and will need food pronto, sit near the galleys, where food is usually served first. And if you know you'll need to snooze during your flight, choose a seat in the front of the plane because it tends to be quieter, or the back of the plane, which is usually the least populated spot. With a little luck, you may even be able to sprawl out!

labels. Any suspicious items will cause you unnecessary delays.

4. Making sure all tickets, boarding passes, passports, IDs, and all of your other travel documents are handy and in order before you reach the security checkpoint. That way, when you are asked to show them, you won't lose precious time fumbling through your pockets or purse.

And my last bit of advice is to pack up some patience. It doesn't take up any space and it travels well no matter where you go. (For more packing tips, see page 107.)

CRUISE CONTROL

To some folks, the journey *is* the vacation, and nothing is more relaxing and adventurous than sailing the ocean blue. Everything is at your beck and call with transportation, lodging, meals, and entertainment all wrapped up into one big beautiful cruise ship. But high prices, crowded decks, sea sickness, and nasty weather conditions can capsize your expectations. So before you book your next cruise, heed these words and your trip will be smooth sailing all the way!

Cut the Deck Costs

You might think that cruises are too rich for your blood (and some of them may be), but when you actually break down the costs and compare them to all of the separate expenses of a vacation on solid ground, you may find that cruises are actually quite affordable. The price

per person for a typical cruise is about $100 a day, which covers food, lodging, transportation, and entertainment. Now compare that amount to what you would normally spend per day for the same accommodations and entertainment on land. Does $100 a day sound reasonable to you? If so, then perhaps an ocean adventure is in order.

The Early Birds Get the Boat

The cruise ship industry has grown by leaps and bounds over the past 20 years, and today you'll find a dizzying array of packages to meet every interest. But to find a cruise that fits your budget, you have to book early because the ships fill up quickly. Start your bargain hunting at least six months before you plan to ship off. You'll really save some dough if you book a cruise for the spring or fall, both of which are typically the slowest cruising seasons (except if you're headed to the Caribbean). The rates start to skyrocket during the summer, when kids have no school, and winter, when folks want to head for warmer shores.

If this is your first cruise, it's best to book your trip through a travel agent who specializes in cruises. A reputable agent will find a cruise that fits you to a "T" based on your budget, time constraints, and travel interests. Doing it yourself can be a challenge, but if you're up to it, then search the Internet for rock-bottom prices. There are boatloads of bargains on general travel Web sites such as **www.expedia.com** or **www.travelocity.com**. Also, include the cruise line Web sites (such as Carnival Cruise Lines or Royal Caribbean) in your search, so you can view the staterooms and entertainment and dining facilities. You'll also be able to check out the onboard activities, the variety of shore and land excursions for each destination, and even the menu selections. Almost all major cruise ship Web sites have last-minute package deals that you can reserve online—you may even find a better price here than on the travel Web sites.

Avoiding Weather Woes

Finding a fantastic bargain on a cruise during less popular off-seasons is fairly easy to do. But there are usually good reasons why those cruises aren't in demand, and a main one is the weather. Many folks would rather not head to the Caribbean during hurricane season, or to Alaska in December when the cold winds blow. So make sure you carefully consider climate conditions when you're choosing a *bon voyage* date, keeping these forecasts in mind:

The Tropics. Hurricane season runs from June to September in the Caribbean, with hurricanes being most active in August and September. Some islands in the south, such as Aruba and Barbados, are less likely to be blasted by hurricanes, but you never can tell. The summer months also signal the rainy season in the Caribbean and Hawaii, so pack some light rain gear if you're headed there during that time.

The Mediterranean. Summer is prime cruising time to the Mediterranean, so prices are bound to be high. You may find some good package deals for the fall and spring, which are actually more pleasant times to travel anyway (the onshore summer temperatures can be sweltering!). But no matter how high the mercury is expected to climb, don't make the mistake of packing just summer outfits. Bring heavier clothing, too—the evening temperatures at sea are always a bit nippy.

Alaska. Most Alaskan cruises run from May to September, when the amazing glaciers can be seen (they aren't accessible during the fall and winter seasons). If you plan to visit in May or June, don't forget your sunglasses! Alaska receives up to 17 hours' worth of sunlight every day during these two months, which makes it mighty tough on the eyes.

Just one final note: The larger cruise lines have the latest weather technology on board, so

---

FAST FORMULA

Chocolate Lip Balm

All of that sun, sand, and salty air can be devastating to your luscious lips. There are loads of lip balms on the market that you can spend your hard-earned money on, but why bother when making your own is so simple? And while you're at it, make a few extras for the chocoholics in your life.

2 tbsp. of petroleum jelly
1 vitamin E capsule
1 tbsp. of powdered chocolate milk mix (or to taste)*

Put the petroleum jelly into a microwave-safe container, and nuke it at 30-second intervals until it is melted. (Be patient—it might take several minutes.) Snip open the vitamin E capsule, pour the oil into the melted petroleum jelly, and then stir. Mix in the chocolate milk powder, return it to the microwave for another 30 seconds, and mix again until smooth. Let the mixture cool, and transfer it into small, clean, airtight containers. That's all there is to it!

* Or use vanilla or strawberry milk mix.

even if there's a nasty storm brewin', the crew will have plenty of advance warning to reroute the ship to calmer waters. The itinerary will naturally change, but I doubt if you'll hear too many folks complaining!

Treat Cabin Fever

You can really cut your cruising costs by sharing a cabin with one of your traveling companions instead of reserving your own individual cabin. Unfortunately, many cruise ship cabins aren't much bigger than a telephone booth, and there's barely room for one person as it is. Still, if your schedule is filled with lots of activities, you probably won't be spending much time in your cabin anyway—and if you do, what's the point of going on a cruise in the first place?

Location, Location

If you don't like the idea of sharing a cabin to save costs (see "Treat Cabin Fever" above), your next best strategy is to choose one in the "low-rent" district. That's because cabin fees are determined by location. Cabins on the inside deck are windowless, so they're cheaper than cabins with a view of the ocean. And depending on how the boat is outfitted, you may find a good deal on outside cabins with a lovely view of the...lifeboats. You'll still be able to see the ocean from your cabin, but for far less money than you would pay for a cabin with an unobstructed view.

Although price is an important consideration when choosing a cabin, don't let it be the *only* consideration, or you could be sacrificing comfort. Some cabins are close to the disco, the children's play area, or the elevator shafts, so if you like to sleep late (or sleep at all!), make sure your cabin is an inaudible distance from all the raucousness. Before you reserve a cabin, review the deck plan on the cruise line Web site so you'll know the lay of the land (so to speak) and where you'll be laying on that land.

Pack the Ginger

If the ocean blue makes you green in the gills with seasickness, there are two things you can do to quell the queasies. The first is to book a cabin at midship or on the lower deck because those quarters won't feel as rocky as the ones near the bow or on a higher deck. The other is to leave room in your luggage for some ginger. Studies have shown that $1/2$ teaspoon of this peppery spice works just as well as Dramamine® (an over-the-counter drug) to relieve motion sickness—and there are no known side effects. The powdered form of ginger will soothe your tummy the best, but if you forget to pack a stash of it, some ginger ale or ginger tea will calm your stomach, too.

LUGGAGE KNOW-HOW

Just about anyone who's taken more than a couple of trips—whether by plane, train, car, or boat—has at least one horror story to tell about luggage that's gone astray. At best, parting company (even for a short while) with your bags will put a damper on your trip. At worst, it'll put a big hole in your travel budget. And that's not to mention all of the aggravation you'll endure while you're supposed to be relaxing. That's why I've come up with some strategies for safeguarding my travelin' bags—and the house I've left behind.

Leave Home Without It

Even way back in Grandma Putt's day, things got lost on the road. So whenever she packed up her suitcase, she followed her rule for fret-free traveling: If losing a particular item would break your heart or your budget, leave it home. It's different for everybody, so you need to decide for yourself what those items are. In my case, it's the cuff links my grandchildren saved up to buy me last Christmas, which stay in my dresser drawer whenever I'm traveling (I take along a set that I won't miss if my bag takes off for never-never land). For you, it might mean leaving your favorite designer dress behind and taking a less treasured, less expensive stand-in.

Carry It On

All rules need to bend a bit, even Grandma Putt's. Sometimes it's just not possible to travel without a few things that would be hard, expensive, or impossible to replace. So if you're traveling by air or train or bus, for your peace of mind and your budget's sake, never check things like prescription medicines, eyeglasses, your address book, or any country's cash. Pack them

HOME REMEDY

Before you leave home on any trip, take a picture of the bags that are traveling with you. That way, if you and they somehow part company along the way and you need to fill out a missing-luggage report, you won't have to wrack your brain to remember exactly what they looked like. What's more, when your bags finally do show up, you'll be able to give the baggage-claim folks a positive ID in a hurry.

in your carry-on bag or your pocketbook, and keep them with you at all times.

Pocket It

It's not just checked baggage that can go astray. Although the chances are slim (as long as you're careful), your carry-on bag could be accidentally taken or even stolen—and if you have to evacuate the plane, train, or bus for any reason, you'll have to leave behind the bag and (yes, ladies) probably your pocketbook. So don't take chances. Always carry the following papers in your pocket, and leave a duplicate set at home with a trustworthy friend:

- A list of the contents and approximate value of your carry-on and checked bags.

- The numbers and denominations of your traveler's checks.

- Photocopies of your tickets, passport, visas, driver's license, and any essential prescriptions.

- Membership and credit card numbers or, if you've registered them, the phone number of the registration service.

- Any phone numbers and e-mail addresses that you may need on the road and may not be able to track down very easily.

Take a "Paws"

Packing for your four-legged friends that are traveling with you is all about comfort and safety. First, the comfort: Bring along their usual food bowls and one or two of their favorite toys. If they feel anxious in the new surroundings when traveling, those familiar items will put them at ease. Now, the safety: Take all the information, documents, and tools that are necessary to keep them healthy and restrained.

Make room in your carry-on bag for these safety essentials:

Leash and collar. Make sure they're good and sturdy, and the collar has current ID and vaccination tags on it.

Recent photos. In case the unthinkable happens, the authorities will be able to locate your pet a whole lot quicker if they have photos to work with.

Veterinarian's phone number. Take it along in case you need any pet-care assistance.

Vaccination records. Bring along copies just in case the hotel or boarding facilities need to see them.

Color It Safe

I have an old friend who spent years traveling the world for a big corporation. And you know what? Her luggage only got lost a couple of times, and she never once had a bag stolen or accidentally carried off by another traveler. Her secret, she says, was this: She always carried moderately priced and very brightly colored luggage for two reasons:

1. Because her bags were so eye-catching, no one could grab them by accident, no thief in his right mind would want to risk taking off with them, and if they do go astray, the baggage handlers would have no problem spotting and identifying such distinctive traveling gear.

2. Bright color aside, serious snatchers didn't bother with her bags for another reason: Though they were sturdy and good-looking, they were obviously not top-of-the-line models. To a thief's way of thinking, a fancy case with a big-name designer's initials all over it is bound to be full of expensive

goodies. Even if you picked up the designer luggage for five bucks at a tag sale, it all but jumps up and shouts "Take me!"

Double Your Chances

If your luggage gets lost or delayed in transit, then you'll have two wardrobe choices: Either live in your traveling clothes for God knows how long, or fork out your hard-earned cash for new ones. But it's easy to avoid the hassle if you're on the road with your spouse or a travelin' pal. Before you leave, each one of you should put one complete outfit in the other's suitcase. That way, even if one of your bags does go astray, it's not likely that both will, so you'll at least have a day's worth of garments to get you by.

Lock It Up

Here's a little traveling secret that could save you a lot of aggravation: Whenever you buy a new suitcase, the first thing you should do is throw away the lock that came with it. (Those things are about as secure as the front door on a dollhouse.) Then go to your local hardware store and buy a tiny—but serious-strength—padlock. It'll cost a couple of dollars, but it could save you hundreds of dollars and lots of time and worry if someone breaks into your hotel room, starts poking around, and decides to make off with some of your valuables. Of course, it goes without saying that you'll have to remember to lock your case when you leave the room! *Note:* If you're flying, your luggage locks should be TSA-approved so they can be opened by airport personnel. Pack away your padlock for use later at your destination.

Don't Put Out the Welcome Mat

Even if you've left your house in the hands of a trusted sitter, don't advertise your home address when you're on the road—it's like putting a "burglar-wanted" ad in the local newspaper. Professional crooks pick up leads anywhere they can find them—including luggage tags that they or their roving accomplices "just happen" to see in airports, hotel lobbies, train stations, or anywhere else that travelers gather. So use your head and outwit the sleazeballs: Instead of putting your home address on your luggage tags, use your business or destination address.

The same holds true for any reading materials you bring along. How many of us throw a handful of newspapers, magazines, or other reading material into our luggage to "catch up on" while on vacation? Well, that's fine and dandy, but before you start your trip, rip off the mailing label or anything else that contains your mailing address. That way, you can safely leave the magazine in your hotel room or out at the pool without a telltale address on it. It's just one more way to keep your home safe and secure while you're on the road.

WELL-GROUNDED ADVICE

So, your plane lands and you've finally arrived! Now you need to cover some ground *on* the ground—and if you're not careful, you can drop a whole lot of dough when you don't really need to. In this section, I'll show you how to rent a car without breaking the bank, so you'll have more greenbacks to spend on your holiday.

Think Small, Save Big

When you're price shopping for car rentals, don't overlook the small independent agencies. Their daily rates can be considerably cheaper than those of the larger rental agencies with

household names—sometimes up to 60 percent cheaper! And just because they sound generic doesn't mean their selection of cars is uninteresting. So how can they afford to offer such fantastic bargains? Well, they aren't located at an airport, so they aren't subject to the high taxes and fees paid by their well-known competitors, and they maintain a smaller fleet of cars. Of course, good deals usually come with certain restrictions, and the most common one here is mileage limitations. If you expect to be racking up some miles, you probably won't make out in the long run—the agency will charge you dearly for every mile over the limit.

Fortunately, independently run rental agencies must adhere to strict government regulations, so your chances of being scammed are small. But rip-offs do occur, so read your contract carefully and inspect the car thoroughly before you drive it off the lot. To find an independent car rental agency, check the Yellow Pages of the area you are traveling to by going online at **www.yellowpages.com**.

Oh, Taxi!

When you rent a car at most major airports, you're shelling out an extra 10 to 20 percent of your total bill just for the convenience of picking up a car at the airport. Even for a short weekend jaunt, that translates into a pretty penny. And for a one- or two-week vacation, that's a first-class budget breaker! So how do you avoid that surcharge? It's really quite simple: When you reserve your vehicle, ask where the closest off-premises office is, and arrange to pick up the car there. Then when your plane lands, hop a taxi or—cheaper yet—a shuttle or city bus, and go pick up your wheels off-site. (The only caveat is that the office must be close enough to the airport so that getting there won't cost more than the airport pickup fee, or be more hassle than it's worth.)

Check, Please!

Rental cars are an agency's bread and butter, so they're usually serviced frequently and kept in tip-top shape. Once a rented vehicle is returned, a reputable rental car agency will inspect it from top to bottom to make sure it hasn't been damaged before sending it off with another customer. But sometimes, blemishes caused by the previous driver are overlooked and that's precisely why you should give the car a thorough once-over before you drive it off the lot. Point out any dents, cracks, burnt-out lightbulbs, and other imperfections to the service agent and make sure that they're noted on your contract. Otherwise, you could be unfairly charged to repair the damage that was caused by the last customer.

While you're inspecting the vehicle, give these areas a good look-see:

Tires. Make sure they're sufficiently inflated (take a tire gauge with you, or ask to borrow one) and free of cracks, cuts, or bulges. If you have any doubts about the reliability of the tires, ask for another car.

⌛ *Quick Fix*

If you're planning on sharing the wheel of your rented automobile with your traveling companion, the agency will charge you extra for that second driver. But if your traveling companion happens to be your spouse or domestic partner, you're in luck! Many agencies will drop the fee if the second driver is your significant other. They don't usually volunteer this information, so you have to ask about it. And don't be shy—those second-driver fees can run up to $20 a day!

Lights. Switch on the headlights, turn signals, dome lights, and dashboard lights to see if they're burning brightly and working properly.

Windshield. Check for small cracks and nicks. Also, test the windshield wipers and washer fluid level.

Interior. Make sure any rips or stains on the seats, on the floor, or in the trunk are noted on your contract.

Trunk. Is there a spare tire, a jack, and a lug wrench in the trunk? If not, tell the agency that these tools are missing in action and request immediate replacements.

Unfortunately, even the best-looking cars break down. If this happens to you while you're on the road, immediately call the rental agency before doing anything else. If it wants to keep your business, the rental agency will arrange to have the car towed to its own repair shop and supply you with a replacement car ASAP.

Just Say "No"

Just like the rest of us, rental car companies are in business to make money—and believe you me, they make a bundle on the insurance they sell to folks who want to make sure they're covered "just in case" anything happens. Well, the fact is, you probably already have all the insurance you need, courtesy of your own auto insurance policy or credit card. Check on this before you leave home, and then politely decline the extra insurance coverage at the rental desk.

Gas Up and Go

Your contract will have a refuel option, which tells you how much per gallon you'll be charged to fill up your tank when you drop it off. This is almost always a bad deal, even if the price per gallon is cheaper than what you'll find at local gas stations. The rental company may charge you for an entire tank's worth of gas, even if the tank is half full. So avoid those obscene fuel prices, and fill up the tank with the lowest priced gasoline you can find right before you return the car.

LODGING FOR LESS

Although you could say that once you've seen one airplane seat, you've pretty much seen 'em all, that's certainly not the case when it comes to sleeping accommodations! There's a world of difference between bunking at a hotel, a bed-and-breakfast, a hostel, or a campground. But whether you prefer room service or sleeping under the stars, all lodgings have one thing in common: Their rates seem to bounce up and down like a beach ball. Here's how to catch those prices on the downward bounce, no matter where you choose to lay your weary head.

Be a Weekend Warrior

In most major cities, hotels make their money from business travelers who arrive on Monday morning and leave by Friday morning. So do big—and often fancy—motels that are near suburban campuses of major corporations. Rooms at these establishments usually carry hefty price tags from Monday through Thursday, but come Friday, it's a whole new ballgame. For a weekend stay, you can expect rates to drop by 35 percent or more for the same first-class accommodations. And quite often, these hotels will even throw in a whole slew of enticing

Quick Fix

A cabin in the woods can be a great summer getaway—and a terrific bargain, to boot—but sometimes, that rustic retreat lacks indoor facilities and is only equipped with a good old-fashioned "two-holer" out back. Well, here's a simple fix for reducing the, um, atmospheric aroma: Gather up some wood ashes from a campfire, and keep them in a bucket by the door, along with an old cup. Then, after each visit to the facility, make sure the visitor sprinkles a cupful of ashes in the hole. It won't exactly have things smelling like a rose, but it will certainly improve the air quality!

extras, such as free breakfast, free cocktails, free admission to the health club, or discounts at its dining room, nearby restaurants, or even theaters and nightclubs. So don't pass up this great opportunity—live it up!

Watch Out for Country Rates

While city hotels offer some mighty fine weekend deals (see "Be a Weekend Warrior" at left), once you get into the country, along any coast, and in any place that caters mainly to tourists, all bets are off. Outside of the city limits—in every accommodation price range—you'll generally get better rates during the week, when the hotels have plenty of rooms to spare, and not on the weekends, when vacationers are visiting. When you're bedding down midweek in the off-season, you can expect some real deals. So it pays to shop around!

Let's Swap

Here's one of the best ways to find comfortable

lodging free of charge: house swapping. It's not really a new concept—for years, savvy penny-pinchers have been trading digs with each other. Usually, though, they had to make the arrangements themselves, which involved word-of-mouth searches for willing swappers in the right locale with the same vacation schedules. Well, nowadays, there are plenty of registries that connect you with potential house swappers from all over the world. To explore the possibilities, crank up your favorite search engine and type in "house swapping" or "house exchanges." The basic details couldn't be simpler: You pay a sign-up fee (usually minimal), then fill out an online form describing your home and your local stomping grounds, and list the dates that it'll be available. Then you peruse the listings to find a domicile that strikes your fancy. You can settle into a beach house in Malibu, a condo in Manhattan, or a thatched cottage in the Irish countryside—the world's your oyster!

SIGHTSEEING INSIGHTS

If you ask half a dozen people what makes a great vacation, chances are that you'll get half a dozen different answers. That's why I'm not going to tell you where to go and what to do. I'll leave that up to the travel guides, and you'll have plenty to choose from at Internet travel sites and your local bookstores and library (just make sure the guides are current). What I *will* do is pass on some tricks for avoiding hassles and saving money on package tours, time-shares, and road trips, so you and your family can make the most of every moment—and every dime. Happy trails to you!

Peek Inside the Packages

To my way of thinking, there are certain times when a package deal makes great sense, even if you think you could shave a few bucks off the cost by going solo. Sign up for the tour if your travel plans match any of these three situations:

1. You want to explore a part of the world that's a lot different from ours, and you don't know the lay of the land. For instance, if you've never been to Russia, you don't know a soul there, and you don't speak a word of the language, go with a group. You're likely to see and learn a lot more than you would if you were stumbling around on your own. And you'll probably save some big bucks, besides! When you're there and the place catches your fancy, study up, make a few contacts, and then return on your own at a later time.

2. You find a tour that zeroes right in on a hobby or special interest of yours—or one that might launch you on a new one. Say you're a bird-watcher (or think you might like to be), and you come across a tour that's guided by an expert from the Audubon Society. Sure, you could probably explore the same places on your own for a lot less cash, but you'd lose the experience that amounts to an education-on-the-wing. (Sorry, I couldn't resist that cue!)

3. The tour takes you to places that you couldn't visit on your own at any price. For instance, outfits such as the National Trust for Historic Preservation run expert-guided tours that take you behind the scenes at museums, theaters, and historical sites, and include private homes and gardens where you'd never even get in the door unescorted. That type of exclusive access is definitely worth the price of admission.

Respect Your Elderhostel

If you're 55 or older and you don't know about Elderhostel, then you're missing out on one of the greatest travel bargains of the century! This not-for-profit group offers what it calls "learning adventures" all over the world, for groups of anywhere from 10 to 50 folks at a time. A free catalog lists 10,000 (count 'em!) treks, including everything from pottery classes in Santa Fe to museum binges in Paris and sightseeing tours of every place under the sun. Best of all, unlike most package tours, Elderhostel trips have no hidden charges—the amazingly low numbers you see in the catalog cover all costs. To find out more, call 800-454-5768, or log on to their Web site at **www.elderhostel.org**.

Find a Road Trip Buddy

For my money, there's no finer vacation than getting behind the wheel of a car and taking off on the highways and byways across the good old U.S.A. But with gas prices climbing ever higher, I'm always looking for ways to keep my costs under control. (That way, I can hit the road more often—for less dough!) One of the greatest ways to save money is to take a companion with you. If you're not blessed (as I am) with a spouse who loves the open road, then ask a friend to go along. Besides having someone to talk to, share the driving, and split the car expenses, you'll save big bucks on lodging. That's because in most places, a single room costs almost as much as a double one does. So get the double and share the room, which will translate into almost 50 percent savings for each of you!

Be Picky

Even if your potential travelin' buddy is your best friend, it pays to take a short trial jaunt before you head out cross-country. The last thing you want (or need) is to get a thousand miles from

Quick Fix

If you're heading to a popular national park during the summer, then be prepared to stand in long lines with about a hundred other park goers at the entrance...unless you take the "road less traveled." Most folks naturally flock to the main entrance, but some of the larger parks have secondary entrances that are rarely used. Before you leave for your trip, log on to the National Park Service Web site at www.nps.gov, and click on "Directions" to see if the park has a lesser-known entrance. That way, you can skip the throngs and enjoy the scenery.

home and find out, for instance, that your pal wants to go out drinking every night, when you'd rather eat sandwiches and play board games in the room. You could end up ruining a good friendship as well as a dream vacation—and maybe even having to shell out for a plane ticket home, to boot!

BEYOND OUR BORDERS

Pesos, pounds, or euros—no matter the name, it all means the almighty dollar to you and me. If you're bound for foreign shores, you'll find that many of the tips in this chapter will save you money regardless of where you're headed. Overseas travel, however, can present a whole new set of challenges that come in the form of driving laws, passports and customs, safe eating, and leisure practices. Throw in a few language barriers and before you know it, you've turned into the Ugly American. But you can travel the four corners of the globe without cutting corners on quality or fun. It just takes a little worldly wisdom. Here are some overseas pointers that'll save you time, miscommunication, red-tape messes, and money.

Don't Believe Everything You Read

Keep in mind that even the most up-to-date guidebook contains information that is at least a year old. That's how long it takes for all that material to get collected, written up, verified, printed, and delivered to the bookstores. Of course, you can still count on a good travel guide for a lot of the basics, like the address of Buckingham Palace or the height of the Eiffel Tower, which won't change from one year to the next. But other things can and do change; in 12 months, hotel and restaurant ratings can plummet, their prices can soar, or they can even go out of business. So if you want to get the lowdown on what's happening now, get your hands on some local newspapers and magazines, or check out relevant sites on the Internet. If you can't find what you want at your local library, try a large newsstand or a bookstore that caters to an international or expatriate crowd. Or go to the official travel Web site of your country of choice and you'll find up-to-date lodging, dining, and entertainment information.

Pinch Pennies with Plastic

There's no way around carrying some cash with you while you're sightseeing abroad. (Ever try using a credit card to buy a bottle of water from a street vendor?) But you should use your credit card or ATM card every chance you get in establishments that will accept them. Why? Because carrying plastic is not only safer than toting large sums of cash around with you, but you'll also automatically get the official exchange rate of the day. When you pay by cash, you get whatever rate the establishment happens to be using—and it's often less favorable than the official exchange rate. Just be sure to call your bank and credit card company before you leave to find out if your cards will be accepted overseas and your PIN will work over there.

Make It Official

You can gain entrance to just about any foreign land you desire with just one magic ticket: a passport. This little blue book opens doors worldwide, but getting one can seem like an overwhelming, time-consuming process. Actually, it doesn't have to be as complicated as most folks make it out to be. Here are three easy steps to getting your passport on time and hassle-free:

1. Get an official passport photograph. Many Federal Express facilities, office supply stores, and pharmacies provide passport photo services.

2. Bring two passport photos, your birth certificate, and a valid photo ID (such as a driver's license) to a designated passport acceptance facility and fill out a passport application. To find the nearest location, go to the Bureau of Consular Affairs Web page at **www.iafdb.travel.state.gov**.

3. Hand in your form and pay the fee (usually about $100). That's all there is to it!

You should start the process at least three months before your trip because it can take up to 10 weeks for a passport to arrive in the mail. (If you need a passport right away, you can speed things up by paying an extra fee of about $60.) Once you receive your passport, it's a good idea to make two copies of it. Keep one copy in your luggage or wallet, so if the original is misplaced or stolen, you can use it to prove your identity. Leave the other copy with a trusted (and reliable) loved one or friend as a backup, just in case the original and the copy can't be found. That way, your passport information is just a phone call away. Now you can globe trot to your heart's content!

Immunize Yourself

Among all the mementos you're planning to bring back from your trip, you're probably not counting on any parasites or viruses, but many travelers do end up with these "souvenirs." In fact, according to the International Society of Travel Medicine, half of all overseas travelers get sick during a two-week jaunt. So before you zip across the globe, make sure you're properly immunized against diseases and outbreaks that are rampant on foreign soil. You can find out which country requires what immunizations by logging on to the Centers for Disease Control Web site at **www.cdc.gov/travel**. If you need to be vaccinated, schedule your doctor's appointment at least four weeks prior to heading out, because some shots need that much time to take effect, and others are given over a period of days or weeks. And while you're there, make sure you're up to date on your routine vaccinations as well. Your doctor's office will give you documents to prove that you've had all the necessary shots. And just as you do with all of your other important travel papers, make copies of the documents and leave them with a trusted loved one for safekeeping while you're away.

Quick Fix

Beware of pickpockets—not just overseas, but over here, too! Visitors to foreign countries are especially vulnerable because they tend to be more easily distracted (after all, your mind is on your vacation!). So here's a neat idea that's downright ingenious: Bring along an inexpensive wallet when you travel, fill it with lots of those fake credit cards you receive in the mail, and tuck it into your back pocket or purse. Then if you're accosted, hand the "fake" one over to the perp. Keep your "real" money and credit cards safe and sound, tucked away in a money clip, pouch, or hidden pocket.

Do a Health Check

Before you leave on vacation, review your health insurance policy to see if you'll be covered overseas in case of a medical emergency. Some insurance policies will provide overseas protection for emergency care only, as long as the costs are considered reasonable and customary. But most policies won't cover health expenses caused by preexisting conditions. And even fewer will cover the exorbitant cost of an evacuation in case you need to be transported back to the States, which can run up to $100,000! So if you have a pre-existing condition, are planning to stay overseas for an extended period of time, or will be doing high-risk activities (such as skydiving or rock climbing), ask your insurance agent about supplemental travel health insurance. You can also find a list of insurance companies offering traveler's insurance on the Bureau of Consular Affairs travel Web site at **www.travel.state.gov/travel**.

116

Go Far with Car Deals

As with most things, timing is everything! And that's especially true if you want to get a bargain on a rental car overseas. The fees are usually less expensive when you book your wheels early, so do your price shopping and make rental arrangements at least two months prior to your trip, instead of waiting until you get there. You can start by contacting the major U.S. car rental companies, such as Avis and Hertz, since many of them also operate agencies overseas. When you're calling around, be sure to find out what the gas charges and late penalties are—some agencies won't volunteer this information until you show up. And reserve a fuel-efficient conservative compact car (or a car with a stick shift), instead of a luxury ride to save money on gas. Even though Americans grumble about the price of gas, our prices are far more friendly than fuel prices overseas. Besides, the gas-guzzling models are usually more expensive to rent anyway.

Be Part of the Crowd

Unfortunately, tourists are more vulnerable to crime than savvy natives are, and rental cars are just the type of tip-off that thugs are looking for. So take these precautions when choosing and driving your car and hopefully, you'll be able to blend right in with the locals:

- Choose a make, model, and color that's driven locally.

- Ask the rental agency to remove anything that identifies the car as a rental, such as a window decal or bumper sticker, if possible.

- Keep all car rental documents safely tucked away in the glove compartment or the trunk.

- If you're traveling when the temperatures are steamy, rent a car with air-conditioning so you can keep the car windows rolled up. Thieves have been known to snatch valuables through open windows, even when the car is moving!

When you're making your car rental arrangements, get specific information about the seating capacity and trunk size of the car. Overseas vehicles tend to be built smaller than vehicles sold in the United States, so you'll probably have to downsize your luggage—and maybe even drop a few pounds!

Get Some Driver's Education

Tooling around in a foreign country involves more than just driving on the right (or the left) side of the road. Each country has its own set of rules and regulations when it comes to driver's licenses, road permits, and car insurance. Knowing the rules of the road before you start your vacation will save you time, money, and possibly your life! So take these important detours before you leave home:

Driver's permit. Most English-speaking countries don't require an international driver's permit, but check with the American Automobile Association (AAA) or American Automobile Touring Alliance (AATA) ahead of time to find out. (These are the only two agencies authorized by the government to issue them, so beware of marketing scams!) If a permit is required, don't fret—obtaining one isn't hard or expensive to do. The cost is about $20. For more information, turn right onto the Internet and go straight to **www.aaa.com** or **www.travel.state.gov**.

Car insurance. Contact your insurance agent or auto insurance company to see if you're covered for an overseas car rental. Some insurance companies will extend coverage to neighboring countries, such as Canada and

Mexico, but others won't. Each country has a minimum amount of car insurance that must be carried. If you're not covered by your own car insurance and want to purchase some through the car rental agency, make sure it provides comparable coverage.

Driving laws. Brush up on local driving, parking, and seat belt laws, and obey them at all times. Some countries, for example, require drivers to flash their lights before passing another vehicle. Other countries won't allow drivers to travel on highways without a road permit.

You don't want to run afoul of the local constabulary because an expensive driving ticket will slow down the best-laid travel plans in a hurry! So learn all you can about driving abroad by checking out the U.S. Foreign Embassy Web site at **www.embassy.org** or the Overseas Security Advisory Council at **www.osac.gov**.

Turn a Phrase

It's two days before takeoff to a faraway land and you don't speak the language. At this late date, it's impossible to become fluent, but don't panic— you still have time to learn a few key words that'll make communication easier, and maybe even save a life! Here are a few important words you should concentrate on:

Greetings. "Hello," "Good-bye," and "Thank you."

Fast aids. "Help," "Hospital," and "Police."

Numbers. Learn the numbers 1 through 10, and more if you have time.

Restroom. "Bathroom," "Towel," and "Soap."

If you memorize these words and pronounce them with some fluency, the language barrier should be a few bricks lighter.

Be Wary of the Water

…unless it's chlorinated, that is. Montezuma's revenge is anything but sweet! If you aren't certain that the drinking water is safe, opt for tea or coffee made from boiled water, or beer, wine, or beverages (including water) that are bottled and capped. And always use soap and hot water to wash the outside of any containers that have been sitting in ice to kill waterborne bacteria. As for swimming, a chlorinated pool is your best bet. I know a dive into the pool isn't as romantic as wading in the clear blue sea, but neither is a wicked case of diarrhea. So unless you're absolutely certain that the waves haven't been contaminated with any kind of human, dog, or industrial waste, resist the temptation. If the lure of the ocean is simply too great, at least take some precautions— don a pair of nose plugs and avoid submerging your head underwater.

FAST FORMULA

Jet Lag Dip

Douse your jet lag blues with this pick-me-up bathtub formula. It'll give you the boost you need to get through those bleary-eyed days until your internal clock is reset.

1/2 cup of lime juice
1/2 cup of lemon juice
5–6 drops of lemon extract
1/2 cup of baking soda*

Mix all of the ingredients in a bowl, pour the solution into tepid bathwater, and ease into the tub. When you get out, you'll be ready for action!

Add baking soda only if you have hard water.

CHAPTER 7

Time to Get Fit!

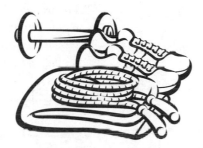

My prescription for good health is pretty simple—treat your body right and it will treat you right. In other words, the best cure-all is prevention. Now, I'm no doctor, but I'm a pretty healthy old bird (as was my Grandma Putt), so we both knew a thing or two about healthy living. Here are some how-tos I've learned that will help you get fit and stay that way, too.

SAY *SAYONARA* TO SMOKING

If you don't know by now that smoking is a major health risk, well, shame on you. And if you think that only applies to those pack-a-day puffers, think again. Research has found that smoking even as few as one to four cigarettes a day can have serious health consequences. Here's how to kick that nasty habit.

The Ugly Truth

There's a laundry list of reasons to quit smoking. Besides increasing the chances of getting lung cancer, emphysema, and other lung diseases, smoking raises your risk of heart attack and

stroke. And if you already have high blood pressure, you're in even more danger. Puffing on those sticks does an awful lot more though—and I mean "awful"! It increases the levels of LDL cholesterol (the bad kind) and reduces HDL levels (the good kind), which makes clotting in narrowed arteries more likely. Consider this for motivation: When you quit, your risk of heart disease drops rapidly, as does your cholesterol.
  Need to hear more?

Digestive demon. People who smoke are also more likely to get ulcers than those who don't indulge. If you've already got ulcers, tobacco tends to make the pain worse, and inhibits your body's ability to heal the damage. Got heartburn? It might be the smokes. The National Institutes of Health says that smoking is known to weaken the lower esophageal sphincter (LES), which lets stomach acid back up more easily.

Smoke gets in your eyes. Cigarette smoking increases the risk of developing age-related cataracts, and an article in the *Journal of the American Medical Association* says that quitting could reduce that risk. Smoking also increases your risk of developing macular degeneration by two to six times. Can you "see" why you should quit yet?

Diabetes danger. There's nothing sweet about it. Nicotine raises blood sugar levels all on its own, adding diabetes to its danger list. And here are just *some* of the other conditions diabetes can lead to:

- Heart attack
- Stroke
- Poor circulation
- Kidney disease
- Eye complications

Nothing to crow about. In addition to bringing on death, disease, and other forms of disaster, cigarette smoke is a major culprit in prematurely wrinkled skin! Not only does it damage skin cells, but smoking also causes you to spend hours every day squinting. That's why smokers usually have much more pronounced crow's-feet than other folks do. (Not to mention more wrinkles of all sorts.)

Ask for Help

It's definitely time to quit if you're still sucking down smoke. If quitting has been a losing battle for you so far, ask your doctor for advice. There are many new and effective ways to help you quit, and the sooner you do it, the better off you'll be. Look into all the aids to help you quit—from prescription medications and nicotine gum to group therapy. Your doctor can help you find the right method for you.

HOME REMEDY

Are you trying to quit smoking? This trick will help: Whenever you get the urge to indulge, suck on a lime. Besides curbing your desire for tobacco, it will replace some of the vitamins, phosphates, and calcium that smoking may have drained from your system. So pucker up!

Chew on This

When you feel like smoking, start chewing. I don't mean chewing tobacco (which is no better for you than cigarettes), but gum, licorice, or clover. It's basically trading a bad habit for a not-so-bad one. Chew gum only when you crave a cigarette. Any brand will do, but for an added benefit, choose one that is flavored with real peppermint because peppermint has been known to lessen the desire for nicotine.

If you're worried about putting on some pounds while trying to go smoke-free, chewing on a licorice stick is a healthy substitute. It's a natural, sugar-free sweetener that seems to satisfy the oral cravings smokers get when going "cold turkey." Or chew on fresh clover flowers, which satisfies the oral needs of smokers and is nicotine-free! Because red clover is a blood thinner, you should not use it if you are going to have surgery. Avoid red clover if you are pregnant.

Sip, Don't Smoke

While you're kicking the smoking habit, start drinking—herbal tea, that is. Choose one containing catnip, chamomile, hops, lobelia, or valerian. Each of these herbs is known to lessen the urge for nicotine and help you relax. Find yourself a comfy, quiet spot and enjoy the tea, especially when your stomach is doing flip-flops, or you feel a little anxious. One word of caution: Chamomile is a distant cousin of ragweed and chrysanthemums. So if you start to tear up and sniffle at the mention of these plants, you may want to avoid using chamomile just to be on the safe side.

Hop Off the Tobacco Train

Drinking beer will just make you feel like having a cigarette, so instead of downing a cold brew, have your hops hot. To make hops tea, put 2 teaspoons of dried hops fruits (or hops flowers) in a cup and pour boiling water over them. Let it steep for a good 15 minutes before drinking.

"B" Good to Yourself

If you've been smoking, you've probably run your stores of B vitamins into the ground. Make sure a good multivitamin containing B complex is on your grocery list if not already on your shelf. B vitamins are essential for cell formation and heart health, and can offer protection against the DNA damage that can lead to cancers. They work together to deliver a barrel of benefits to the body, such as bolstering your metabolism, enhancing your immune system, maintaining healthy skin and muscle tone, and helping to combat stress and depression.

Smoking dries out your lips and makes them more prone to chapping. Since it also robs you of your B vitamins, skin tissues in the corner of your mouth get weak, causing cracks or splits to appear. A daily dose of B vitamins should put your lips back in smacking order.

WEIGHTY MATTERS

With nearly two-thirds of all Americans currently overweight, it seems as though we are losing the battle of the bulge. And as you probably know by now, there are no quick fixes. The key is to get motivated and keep moving. If you're having trouble getting started, I've found that the best incentive is to remind yourself of all the unhealthy pitfalls of packing on extra pounds.

Less Is More

There's plenty of wisdom in this saying, especially when it comes to your weight. Just like smoking, weighing too much may increase your risk for developing a boatload of health problems. Here are a few conditions you'll avoid by shedding those extra pounds:

Heart disease and stroke. If you're overweight, you're more likely to suffer from high blood pressure, high levels of triglycerides (blood fats), and high LDL cholesterol (that's the bad kind). Losing 5 to 15 percent of your weight can lower your chances of developing heart disease or having a stroke. If you weigh 200 pounds, this means losing as little as 10 pounds. Weight loss may lower your blood pressure, triglycerides, and cholesterol level; improve how your heart works and your blood flows; and decrease inflammation throughout your body.

Cancer. It's not known exactly why being overweight may increase cancer risk, but that seems to be the case, according to the experts. Cancers of the colon, esophagus, and kidney, and uterine and breast cancers for women, are the ones showing up the most.

Diabetes. More than half of all Americans are overweight—and every extra pound raises the risk of diabetes by 4 percent! Fight back by deciding once and for all to lose those pounds, and make exercise an everyday event. A healthy weight and two 15-minute walks a day can make the difference between being able to do what you want in old age and living as an invalid.

Osteoarthritis. It's the "wear and tear" arthritis that occurs when the cartilage that protects your joints becomes thinner due to age and daily friction. It usually announces itself with pain and stiffness in the hips and knees. These happen to be weight-bearing joints, which is why experts warn that extra weight on the cartilage brings extra risk of arthritis—especially to people between the ages of 40 and 60. You're simply putting more biomechanical stress on the joints. So lighten up!

Asthma. Increasing numbers of adults—more women than men—are developing asthma, and researchers aren't sure of the exact reason. They suspect that along with the usual triggers (such as pollen, dust, and frigid air) that can inflame airways and cause them to fill with mucus, increased body weight—which can literally weigh on the chest wall, making it more difficult to breathe—could be the culprit.

Sleep apnea. With this condition, a person stops breathing for short periods during the night. Your risk for it goes up if you are overweight because you may have more fat stored around your neck, constricting the airway. A smaller airway can make breathing difficult or loud (from snoring), or cause it to stop altogether.

Erectile dysfunction. Sorry, guys, but this increases in direct proportion to your waistline. According to researchers, men with larger waistlines are more likely to experience problems than slimmer guys. In fact, men with waists of 42 inches are twice as likely to have erection difficulties as men with 32-inch waists.

Beware the Spare

Being apple-shaped can be rotten for your health. Even though your overall weight might be within the normal range, that extra fat

---

Quick Fix

Having denture pain? If you've gained weight recently, you may have found the reason. Gums can swell if you gain weight, and even small changes in the size and shape of your gums can throw your denture fit out of whack. Get in touch with your dentist, who will adjust your dentures to compensate for weight changes.

around the middle puts you at greater risk for serious conditions such as heart disease, stroke, diabetes, and breast and colon cancer. In fact, studies indicate that women who have spare-tire fat (whether they're overweight or not) have higher blood sugar levels, higher total cholesterol counts, and lower levels of the good HDL cholesterol than women who don't. This makes them worse off than overweight women without excess tummy fat. There's also evidence that carrying fat around your middle may increase estrogen activity in the body, which may explain why the incidence of breast cancer—considered an estrogen-fueled disease—is higher among women with belly fat than among those with overall fat, according to findings from the long-term Framingham Heart Study.

Try this trick: Take 1,000 milligrams of the supplement CLA (conjugated linoleic acid) with your meals. Although we're not sure how it works, CLA seems to trick the body into not storing fat! Some studies have shown that supplementing your diet with CLA is especially good at banishing belly fat. CLA is also found in dairy products; just be sure to stick to the nonfat or low-fat versions.

What Really Works

Experts agree—the bottom line to losing weight is calories. You either have to take less in or burn more. And the best way to manage your calorie count is to do both: eat less and exercise more. Here's how to do it:

Avoid fad diets. Sure, initially you may lose a lot of weight on those diets that are so popular, but the result is too often temporary. That can leave you feeling defeated or angry, and often you'll end up with a few extra pounds just for good measure.

Practice portion control. Studies show that larger portions do indeed mean larger bodies. But you can use these tricks to rein in both your portions and your pants size. When you go out, order an appetizer for the main meal or split an entrée with a friend, and get used to asking for doggie bags. At home, dole out pretzels or other snacks on a plate or in a bowl. Never put out the whole package because it's simply too easy to mindlessly dip your hand into a bag, and before you know it, the bag is empty. Serve meals on individual plates instead of putting out bowls family-style. And avoid giant platters—the temptation to fill them is too great. Read the serving sizes on packages. If the cereal box says a cup, get out a measuring cup, pour some cereal in, and learn just what a cupful really looks like.

Curb cravings scents-ably. Food cravings are often a reaction to stress. So when you're feeling tense, temper your taste buds and relax your mind with aromatherapy. Rub a drop or two of essential oil of peppermint (*Mentha x piperita*), chamomile (*Matricaria recutita*), or lavender (*Lavandula officinalis*) into your temples. Because essential oils can irritate sensitive skin, however, you may want to apply a thin layer of vegetable oil or lotion before putting on the essential oil.

Subdue your sweet tooth. When the leaf of an Indian herb called gymnema (which means "sugar destroyer" in Sanskrit) is chewed, it decreases the ability of the taste buds to detect sweetness. Gymnema capsules, which you can find at health-food stores, also make sugar distasteful. Take 200 milligrams twice a day, about half an hour before breakfast and then again before supper. Just one caveat: Gymnema can lower blood sugar too much, so consult your doctor before you take it.

Fill Up on Fiber

High-fiber foods not only slow down your food intake, but also enter your bloodstream in turtlelike fashion. This prevents your blood sugar from spiking and then dropping—along with your energy and your resistance to candy bars. For good sources of fiber, choose hearty, whole-grain bread instead of soft white bread; a mound of crisp greens sprinkled with crunchy carrots, broccoli florets, and sesame seeds instead of a greasy burger; or a bowl of steel-cut oat bran instead of sugary, melt-in-your-mouth cereal. You get the picture. Just make sure you include some fiber at every meal. The following foods top the list for fiber power, from most to least fiber-filled:

- Split peas
- Red kidney beans
- Raspberries
- Whole-wheat spaghetti
- Oat bran muffin
- Broccoli
- Oatmeal
- Green beans
- Brown rice
- Apple
- Popcorn, air-popped

Supplement with Psyllium

Taking a fiber supplement such as psyllium before meals could help reduce the number of calories absorbed by your body. Plus, psyllium helps you feel full and stabilizes blood sugar levels, which may help control food cravings. Check your supermarket, drugstore, or health-food store for psyllium powder, and take 1 to 3 tablespoons dissolved in water or juice three times a day before eating. Just be sure you swallow a full glass of water with your psyllium and drink 8 to 10 glasses of water throughout the day, since the extra bulk will pull water from your body.

Cook with Heat

Certain common kitchen spices may help raise both your body temperature and your metabolism, so you burn calories for fuel, rather than store them as fat. Plus, they may speed your digestion. These are my picks for adding good taste as well as fire:

- Cinnamon
- Ginger
- Mustard
- Red pepper

Red pepper, for instance, contains the compound capsaicin, which stimulates saliva, and that in turn can help the digestive process. People with sluggish digestion tend to gain weight, experts say. In fact, in one small study, dieters who added 1 teaspoon of red-pepper sauce and 1 teaspoon of mustard to every meal raised their metabolic rates by 25 percent. Perhaps what these tasty spices do best, though, is make food savory, so you need less fat (such as oil) to make it palatable, and you can feel satisfied with smaller portions. To start, sprinkle some red pepper on your baked potato or some grated ginger on your veggies instead of butter.

Go Bananas

Besides being a good source of fiber, a banana that's a bit underripe—that is, still a

FAST FORMULA

Get Your Red Hots Here!

This savory sauce makes an excellent fat-burning meal topper. Grow your own tabascos, or substitute dried ones that have been rehydrated. Other small, hot, fresh red chilies can be substituted for the tabascos.

1 lb. of fresh red tabasco chilies, chopped
2 cups of distilled white vinegar
2 tsp. of salt

Combine the chilies and the vinegar in a saucepan and heat. Stir in the salt, and simmer for 5 minutes. Remove from the heat, cool, and place in a blender. Puree until smooth, transfer to a glass jar, and let steep for two weeks in the refrigerator. Remove, strain the sauce, and adjust the consistency by adding more vinegar, if necessary. Then try it on meat, fish, poultry, and vegetables.

Yield: 2 cups

little green at the tip—produces half the glycemic response of a ripe banana and is less likely to spike your blood sugar, which will keep you feeling full longer.

Feel Full with Fennel

You may be familiar with fennel seeds being a top digestive aid, but did you know the ancient Greeks fawned over fennel as a weight-loss aid? Its Greek name, *marathron*, comes from a verb meaning "to grow thin." In Europe during medieval times, hungry churchgoers would chew on fennel seeds during sermons to keep their stomachs from rumbling!

Perk Up with Primrose

Evening primrose oil is in the spotlight lately for its possible role in dieting. Its stimulating effect on the body may actually help convert fat into energy. Now, wouldn't that be a welcome treatment for losing those unwanted pounds! But extracting oil from evening primrose is too difficult a job to try at home; I know—I've tried. This is one herb I recommend you buy at a health-food store or drugstore. The best way to take evening primrose oil is in capsule form. The recommended daily dose is 1,000 to 2,000 milligrams, or three to six capsules. Count your lucky stars because this is one of the safest herbs found in Mother Nature's medicine cabinet.

Go Green

There's been exciting news lately about green tea having fat-burning properties. A study conducted by American and Swiss scientists at the University of Geneva showed that people who were on a green tea diet were more likely to use up more fat than those not on a green tea diet. Two 375-milligram capsules of it a day were used in the test, but you could start by choosing a reputable brand of organic green tea at a health-food store or natural grocery, and drinking a cup every day.

Help for Mood Munching

Moods can cause a lot of overeating. Fortunately, Mother Nature provides us with herbal helpers for times like this. If you tend to reach for "comfort food" when you're feeling stressed, anxious, or down in the dumps, give these a try:

Kava calm. If, like so many of us, emotional upheaval has you reaching for sweets or other foods, a cup of warm kava tea is just the thing to calm your nerves. Grate 1 to 2 teaspoons of dried kava root into a cup of

FAST FORMULA

Eat Better with Bitters

Herbs that tone the digestive system can help normalize your eating patterns. If you overeat, try this bitters formula warm before meals.

$1/2$ tsp. of dandelion root (*Taraxacum officinale*)

$1/2$ tsp. of centaury (*Centaurium erythraea*)

$1/2$ tsp. of chamomile (*Matricaria recutita*)

$1/2$ tsp. of fennel (*Foeniculum vulgare*)

1 cup of hot water

Steep the dandelion, centaury, chamomile, and fennel in the water for 20 minutes; then strain. Drink $1/4$ to $1/3$ cup warm before meals. *Caution:* Dandelion is rich in potassium and should not be taken with potassium tablets. Also, people with ragweed allergies should steer clear of chamomile.

boiling water. Cover, then let steep for a good hour. Strain, and then sip up to 2 cups a day. But be forewarned: Kava is mighty bitter. If your tongue feels a bit numb, there's no cause for alarm. For most folks, it takes awhile to acquire a taste for kava, so you may want to add some honey, or try tinctures or capsules instead.

Nervous Nellie cure. Try drinking an herbal tea containing wood betony (*Betonica officinalis*) to quell nervous energy. It is both a nerve soother and a digestive tonic that can be used long term, with no adverse effects. Make a tea using 1 teaspoon per 1 cup of hot water. Strain. Drink 1 cup twice daily.

Lemony lift. If a gloomy mood has you headed for the junk food aisle, lemon balm and its mood-lifting properties could get you back on the right diet track. Mix 2 cups of fresh chopped lemon balm leaves with $1/2$ cup of olive oil and three garlic cloves (peeled and crushed) and presto—pesto! Keep it handy to dribble over broiled or grilled seafood or poultry.

GET MOVING

Now I know you're going to say you're too busy, but I bet if you look…let's say…under the couch you sit on to watch TV, you can find enough time to get the exercise you need to lose weight! In fact, studies show that adding just 30 minutes of walking per day is enough to prevent weight gain and encourage moderate weight loss. (If you're reluctant to take the first steps because a chronic condition such as arthritis or back pain is causing you to wince, see page 129 for helpful ways to sidestep the pain.)

Quick Workouts Count, Too

The great news about daily exercise is that you don't have to get it all in one shot. Research says that three brisk 10-minute walks per day are just as effective as a daily 30-minute walk. Just five times a week will do the trick, and it won't cost you a thing. Other great low- or no-cost workouts include:

- Bike riding
- Jogging
- Jumping rope
- Swimming

Do Those Chores!

Make a workout of household chores. Mow the lawn, weed the garden, rake the leaves, or shovel the snow. Even indoor activities such as vacuuming and scrubbing count as a workout if they increase your heart rate. Just put on some peppy music to help you move along.

Tricks of the Trade

Sometimes you need an extra push to get moving. I know. I've been there, done that. Here are two ways to keep your exercise plan on the right track:

1. Try the buddy system. Studies show that teaming up with a loved one—human or canine—when exercising will increase the amount of weight you lose. So enlist family, friend, or Fido and get going!

2. Reward yourself. We all need an incentive to keep up our motivation—just make sure it's not an edible one. Think along the lines of a movie, a new book, a new tool set, or a pair of shoes. And there's always a pat on the back from me!

Work Up to Working Out

Unfortunately, so many of us are injuring ourselves while trying to get in shape that emergency rooms are filled with wounded exercisers. Trouble is, most of us don't bother to warm up and work our way into an athletic activity gradually. Experts advise we heed these six rules when jumping into a fitness routine:

Rule 1: Warm up. Muscle tissue becomes less flexible as we age. Warm up by walking for a few minutes, then slowly begin stretching your back and legs. These few minutes of mild exercise will give your muscles a chance to get ready for more intense movement.

Rule 2: Work up to it gradually. Try not to cram all your action into one or two days. Increase your activity in increments of no more than 10 percent a week.

Rule 3: Perfect your technique. Some sports injuries happen because you're not making the right moves. Tennis elbow, for example, can develop when you're not using the racket properly. If you're intent on playing a game you don't know, get some coaching—even if it's only from a video or a book.

Rule 4: Treat your feet to the right stuff. Do you need basketball shoes, running shoes, walking shoes, or cross-trainers? They all look pretty much the same, yet each meets a different need. So when you plan to devote time to a sport, find out what shoes are best. Ask other players, the coaches, and the folks at your local sporting goods stores. The proper footwear will protect you from trips, falls, and injuries to your Achilles tendon, legs, and feet in general.

Rule 5: Wear a helmet. Here's a scary fact: Did you know that adults are twice as likely as kids to die from a head injury? If you ride a bike, swing a bat, or in-line skate through town, always wear the headgear.

Rule 6: Hydrate. When you exercise, drink lots of water to prevent dehydration and replenish the fluids and nutrients you lose during workouts. Have a glass of water before you begin, and take a break every 20 to 30 minutes for more. This is especially important for people with diabetes.

"E" for Exercise

Want to stop muscle pain before it starts? Take vitamin E before you exercise. This powerful antioxidant can offset muscle damage caused by exertion. Ask your doctor how much is right for you.

Listen to Your Body

If you've already made the move to an exercise regimen and are suffering more than your fair share of muscle aches, spasms, or cramps, listen up. Lucky for us, most muscle aches get better by themselves in 48 hours with rest. But some aches and pains persist. And because they do, they may be symptoms of a systemic illness, such as the flu or Rocky Mountain spotted fever. For that reason, if the aches don't ease up after 48 hours, or if you also have symptoms such as a fever or headache, you should call your doctor. And never brush off unexplained arm or chest pain as a muscle cramp. It could be signs of a heart attack, so

---

HOME REMEDY

Watermelon is like a natural sports drink. It boosts your energy and keeps your blood sugar (your brain's only food) at normal levels, so you'll be physically coordinated and able to think straight. But you don't want to cart around sloppy watermelon slices to your workouts! Instead, take advantage of its healthful properties by making your own very portable watermelon refresher. Simply scoop a cup of cut-up seeded watermelon into a sports water bottle and freeze it overnight. Then take it to the gym the next day, or bring it along on your daily walk. By the time you work up a sweat, the frozen melon will have defrosted enough to be a nice, cool slush that you can sip and savor.

---

get medical attention immediately to be on the safe side.

Relief for Muscle Misery

If you're suffering from the usual muscle aches and pains caused by overuse, here's some help:

Give it a rest. If your muscles ache because you spent the day in the gym after a winter on the couch, head back to its soft embrace for a day or two. Bed rest, followed by gradual exercise, will improve most muscle aches.

Hit all the hot spots—with cold. A cold pack can ease the pain of muscle aches, but use it for just 15 to 20 minutes at a time. The effects of cold last longer than heat because your body takes longer to warm up than it does to cool off.

Soak that ache. Applying heat can also soothe sore muscles. While relief from heat won't last as long as cold, it does help for one hour or more. Moist heat penetrates more deeply than dry heat, so stand in a hot shower or soak in a tub. Epsom salts baths relieve the pain of almost any sports injury. Add 1 to 2 pounds to a tub of warm water, and soak those aches and pains away. If you opt for an alternative heat source, such as a heating pad, microwave heat pack, or a hot compress, leave it on the sore muscle for no more than 20 to 30 minutes at a time. And let your muscles cool down for one to two hours before you reapply heat.

Wrap it up. Try a hot vinegar wrap to soothe sore muscles. Heat equal parts of water and vinegar, soak a towel in the mix, and wring it out. Apply the towel as a hot compress to the sore area, leaving it in place for five minutes. Then follow with a cold compress (a wrung-out towel that's been soaked in cold or ice water until it's well chilled). Repeat the cycle three times, ending with the cold compress. Then cover the area warmly, and rest.

Mind your minerals. Your muscles need minerals to function properly. If you have cramps, they may be due to a lack of nutrients, so taking a swig of a sports drink before and during exercise could prevent them from occurring (or recurring).

DON'T BE SIDELINED!

Arthritis, back pain, intermittent claudication, and varicose veins—if you suffer from one of these chronic conditions and think exercise will just make it worse…think again! Not only will moving your body ease the pain, but it could also rid you of the problem altogether. To keep yourself in the game, consider the suggestions here for ending your discomfort.

When Your Joints Are Out of Joint

Are your hinges so creaky in the morning that you feel like the Tin Man without his trusty oilcan? Do your fingers, knees, and hips get so stiff that even simple activities, such as working in the garden, make you feel as if you're doing hard time in the mines?

Mother Nature doesn't mess up very often, but she sure could have done a better job of joint design. By age 40 or 50, many of us begin to notice some joint tightness. It's usually caused by osteoarthritis, the "wear and tear" arthritis that occurs when the spongy cartilage that covers and protects the bones of our joints becomes thinner as a result of age and daily friction. Osteoarthritis usually announces itself with pain and stiffness, especially in weight-bearing joints such as your hips and knees. Read on to learn how to safely exercise and ease arthritis pain.

Move and Lose

Of course, you should call your doctor at the first sign of joint pain. It's always possible that you have rheumatoid arthritis or another kind of joint disease. In most cases, though, your joints are simply wearing out a bit. But don't get panicky and throw a lot of money at the problem right away. In many cases, you can use simple, inexpensive remedies to eliminate most—if not all—of your pain. Start with these two:

1. Exercise as much as you can. When you sit still, the synovial fluid between your joints can become as stiff as molasses in a Maine winter. Although you may not feel like walking when your joints are stiff, it's actually the ideal way to keep the synovial fluid warm and flowing—and your weight in check so you don't overload your joints. If you have too much knee or ankle pain to walk, ride a stationary bike. Set the seat high, so you don't have to bend your knees as much.

2. Cut those calories. The next time your bathroom scale sneaks up a hair, don't fret about your fanny—it's your knees that deserve your pity! Each time you gain a single pound of body fat, experts say, it feels like four times that much on your knees. The strain is especially hard on your muscles and tendons—your built-in shock absorbers. The good news is, studies show that if you lose as few as 11 pounds, you can reduce stiffness and pain in your knees by half. Now that's what I call relief!

129

Rx to the Rescue

What's the best pill to reach for when you need arthritis relief—ibuprofen, acetaminophen, or naproxen? There's no clear answer. You'll just have to try different painkillers until you find the one that works best for you. If you're going beyond the guidelines on the label, or you have any chronic health problems besides arthritis, consult your doctor first.

When you do take medications, it's best to take any arthritis drug before noon. Since the pain and inflammation tend to be worst in the late afternoon and evening, you can get a jump on them by starting your treatment in the morning or at midday.

Hide the High Heels

Any woman who regularly wears heels higher than 2 inches—whether they're stilettos or wide-heeled pumps—is twice as likely to develop arthritis than a woman who doesn't. Heels shift your body weight away from your ankles and onto your hips and the inner part of your knee joints, and arthritis is often the result.

Arthritis Antidotes

Grandma Putt knew a thing or two about stiff, achy joints. And now science has proven many of her home remedies to be right on target. Here are a few that work as well now as they did back in Grandma's day:

Get action with attraction. Although scientists aren't sure why, studies show that wearing knee wraps embedded with magnets may help you get out of a chair more easily, walk faster and less stiffly, and even sleep better. Attracted to the possibilities? Look for wraps with "unipolar" magnets, then place the positive end of the magnet directly over your sore knee. You should feel relief within 30 minutes.

Oil your joints. Trout, salmon, and other cold-water fish contain an abundance of omega-3 essential fatty acids, which ease swollen, stiff joints by reducing both inflammation and cartilage destruction. So serve these fantastic fishes often.

Pepper the pain. A quick way to ease arthritis pain is to apply a topical cream that contains capsaicin, the hot chemical compound that's found in red pepper. You get local numbing of nerve endings along with a warming effect. Most drugstores carry the cream, which comes in concentrations from 0.025 to 0.075; if you have sensitive skin, try a lower strength first. Follow the label directions, and be careful not to get it near your eyes or on any areas of broken skin. And make sure to wash your hands after using it.

Add some arnica. To soothe aching joints, add a few drops of arnica oil to your favorite healing salve. Try using a warming wintergreen, lavender, or rosemary salve as a base, since all three can help increase circulation to the painful area. For every 2 teaspoons of salve, add 3 or 4 drops of arnica oil. Apply to sore joints three or four times per day. Arnica is for external use only, and don't use it on broken skin.

HOME REMEDY

Cabbage leaves have been used for centuries to soothe inflammation. A sturdy, outer leaf is just the right shape to place over a bent knee or an elbow. Blanch a leaf or two, then apply it, warm or cool, to inflamed joints. Wrap it with gauze or an elastic bandage to hold it in place.

Fortify with D

New evidence links low levels of vitamin D to the progression of osteoarthritis. One study showed that people with too little vitamin D in their diets were more likely to develop osteoarthritis and three times more likely to have any existing arthritis get worse. Although your body produces vitamin D when you're exposed to sunlight, it's also a good idea to drink milk that's fortified with this important vitamin.

Needle Your Knees

Does the thought of having slender needles eased under your skin make you queasy? Truth is, there is no pain involved in acupuncture, and it just might soothe the pain of arthritis. Research directed by the National Institutes of Health indicates that people with osteoarthritis of the knee who receive acupuncture have less pain and better function than people who receive standard care—even weeks after the treatment. Ask your doctor to recommend a reputable acupuncturist near you.

Running Hot and Cold

When an arthritic joint is inflamed, it may be painful, swollen, or even hot. Put some ice on that fire. Ice is very good for inflammation and swelling, so put an ice pack on the sore joint for about 20 minutes at a time. Repeat the treatment once an hour, continuing for as long as it seems to help.

When your joints are achy, but there's no swelling, heat works better than cold. It feels good, for one thing, and it promotes the flow of healing nutrients into the joint. Moist heat seems to work best, so use a warm compress instead of a heating pad. Soak a small towel in hot water, wring it out, and drape it over your painful joint. When the towel cools, soak it again and reapply it.

Try an Herb from the East

The herbs guggul, boswellia, gokshura, and madder are commonly used in India to relieve joint pain, and there's good evidence that they work. They all have anti-inflammatory properties. These and other anti-inflammatory herbs are available in supplement form in health-food stores. Follow the directions on the label, and be sure to let your doctor know you're taking them.

Licorice, Anyone?

Licorice root is a friend indeed when your arthritis flares up, because it can counteract the inflammation. Licorice root is available in capsules and tablets at health- food stores (don't bother with licorice candy, which contains little or no real licorice). Since a substance in licorice called glycyrrhizic acid can cause high blood pressure in some people, look for deglycyrrhizinated licorice (DGL) products, then follow the label directions.

Lay Off the Lattes

If you drink more than four cups of coffee a day, you're doubling your risk of developing arthritis. Caffeine not only alters the mineral balance that's needed to make cartilage, but it can also dry up the fluid required to keep cartilage and joints lubricated. So instead of reaching for that third cup of joe, fill up on good ol' H_2O. Like most people, you probably don't drink enough water, and that could be making your arthritis symptoms worse. Drink at least eight full glasses every day—and don't wait until you're thirsty. By the time you feel thirsty, your body's water levels have already dropped too low.

Boron Beats Pain

What do raisins, pears, apples, and other fruits, as well as nuts and beans, all have in common?

Well, besides being healthy snacks, they all contain the trace mineral boron. That's good news for those of us with arthritis, because experts say that boron can relieve joint pain and stiffness and actually appears to protect against arthritis.

Rebuild with Glucosamine

One of the most effective treatments for osteo-arthritis is glucosamine sulfate, a supplement produced from shellfish. It combats cartilage-destroying enzymes and halts cartilage loss in the knees and hips. Start with 500 to 1,000 milligrams three times a day (you'll find the supplements at your local drugstore or health-food store). It takes two to four weeks to get relief from pain—and twice that long to ease functioning in your joint. *Caution:* Avoid glucosamine sulfate if you have a seafood allergy.

Oh, My Aching Back

Sooner or later, just about everyone gets it. And it isn't just the freight lifters among us who are getting nailed. Sure, you can injure your back on the job or in a car crash, but by far the most frequent cause isn't anything catastrophic—it's everyday weakness and inflexibility in the muscles that support the back. And the weaker your muscles (especially those in your upper back, hips, and hamstrings—the muscles at the backs of your thighs), the more apt you are to hurt your back. A sudden, uncharacteristic movement—such as swinging a golf club—strains the stiff muscles, tendons, and ligaments, damaging tissue and causing swelling and intense aching. And living under the burden of chronic emotional stress can create muscle tension, which, in turn, can block blood flow to the muscles and create more spasms and pain. The more pain, the more stress. It becomes a vicious cycle.

Daily exercise can reduce stress as well as keep your muscles strong and limber—and that's exactly what you need to keep the pain at bay. Back pain that's severe or doesn't start getting better within a week or two should always be checked by a doctor. For garden-variety backaches, though, here's what you need to do.

Keep Moving

The worst thing anyone with an achy back can do is to sit still. In fact, resting for more than a day or two reduces muscle flexibility and strength and can lead to further disability. On the other hand, movement keeps blood flowing into the site, waste products flowing out of it, and muscle spasms to a minimum. Let your pain be your guide. You may not want to move your piano, but it's okay to lift a bag of groceries. The best advice? Do everyday activities as you can tolerate them.

Stretch and Flex

Even if your back pain has you lying on the floor, you can still stretch your arms and legs, which elongates the tissues in your back and draws healing blood and oxygen to the area. Just remember to stay relaxed, cushion your back with a pad, and use slow, gentle movements as you extend your arms over your head and stretch your legs along the floor. Hold each stretch for about a minute, then relax.

As your back pain eases, you need to continue to work those muscles so you can return to normal activities. Try this exercise, which requires the use of a large exercise ball (available at sporting goods and department stores):

Step 1. Lie face down across the ball with your hands and feet on the floor.

Step 2. Lift one arm and then the other as high as you can, raising your torso from the

FAST FORMULA | Drink Ginger-ly

Ginger is a mighty powerful anti-inflammatory—just what you need to take the edge off of arthritis pain. Here's how to make a healing ginger tea.

1 tsp. of grated ginger
1 cup of water
Honey, to taste

Boil the water, pour it into a mug, and stir in the ginger. Steep for 10 to 15 minutes, then strain. Sweeten with honey. Drink 2 cups a day, and your knees may soon begin to feel as nimble as that other famous Ginger's.

ball. Pause for a count of 10, then return both hands to the floor.

Step 3. Place both hands behind your head and lift your torso as high as you can. Hold for five counts, then release.

Step 4. Repeat the sequence as many times as is comfortable.

Put Cold to Work

Ice is a great analgesic and is preferable to aspirin or other nonsteroidal anti-inflammatory drugs such as ibuprofen, which, in large doses, can upset your stomach. Simply fill a paper or foam cup with water and freeze it, then peel away the rim to expose the ice surface. Grasping the cup, lie on your side, then apply the ice directly to the painful area in a circular motion. Limit the massage to about five minutes, and don't place the ice directly on the bony portion of your spine.

Lie Down and Say "Ahh"

According to studies from the Group Health Cooperative in Seattle, the need for pain medication for back spasms and tight muscles can be cut in half by weekly massages. As a general rule, a muscle spasm should relax when the therapist massages it. If it persists, you probably have some inflammation, too, and in that case, massage may not be the best therapy for you.

Salute Your Inner Soldier

Stand at attention to keep back pain at bay. Shoulders back, chest out, stomach in, chin up! That's good posture as well as a good drill for a new army recruit. Correct posture means that your body is aligned, so it puts less strain on your lower back.

Take Thyme to Relax

Remember, stress can be what's causing your back pain, so it's important to unwind. Here's one way to get the job done: Toss a handful of dried thyme into the tub as you run hot water for a bath. Soak for 10 to 15 minutes, letting the aromatic oils in this herb wash your stress—and any aches and pains—down the drain.

Sit Smart

One way to relieve back stress is to keep your feet flat on the floor if you sit at a desk all day. Your arms should be positioned so your elbows form right angles. Set your computer monitor at eye level. Your chair seat should be deep enough to support your hips, but the front edge should not touch the backs of your knees. The chair back should have an angle of about 10 degrees and cradle the small of your back comfortably. If it doesn't, add a wedge-shaped cushion or lumbar pad there.

133

Take a Load Off Your Shoulders

Ladies, listen up. When you carry a shoulder bag, you tend to tense your shoulder to keep the bag from slipping off. This scrunched-up posture causes all kinds of muscle strain and related pain. Check out purses by designers such as Liz Claiborne® and Calvin Klein®, who are heeding the message with new lines of short-handled carryalls. When you can't sling a bag over your shoulder, you'll be more inclined to switch the weight from hand to hand.

Five Ways to Ease the Ache

Stretches, cold packs, improving your posture—all will go a long way toward relieving an aching back. Here are a few more suggestions you might want to try:

Bathe with Epsom. A traditional Epsom salts bath can help ease back spasms and relieve pain. Add 2 cups of the salts to a hot bath, sink down, and feel the relief. Afterward, place an ice pack on your back for no more than 20 minutes.

Knock down swelling. Studies have shown that aspirin, ibuprofen, and similar drugs often work as well for back pain as more powerful prescription drugs. They help in two ways: They're analgesics, which means they work directly on pain, and they have anti-inflammatory effects, which reduce swelling. Acetaminophen is fine for pain, but it has little or no effect on inflammation.

Get in the swim. Swimming is one of the fastest ways to take the kinks out of aching back muscles. For one thing, merely submerging yourself in warm water will help reduce muscle tension. More importantly, the water supports your weight, which allows you to exercise without putting additional strain on your back.

Baby it with bromelain. This anti-inflammatory enzyme, derived from the pineapple plant, may be especially helpful for relieving pain related to inflammation. Try formulas that include bromelain, papain, and trypsin—all enzymes that help calm down the chemical pathways that cause pain. As long as you're not taking blood thinners, check at a health-food store for supplements, then follow the label directions.

Sleep sideways. The best sleeping position for people with back pain is to lie on their sides with a pillow between their knees. If you're comfortable only when you sleep on your back, at least put a pillow under your knees to reduce the arch in your back and relieve some of the strain.

Walk Away from Leg Pain

We all know about heart attacks, but have you ever heard of a leg attack? Well, the same thing that causes ticker shock can also jam up the

Quick Fix

Have you ever wondered why traditional pubs have foot railings that run the length of the bar? It's because bar owners want you to stand there—and buy drinks—as long as you can. Standing with one foot raised greatly reduces pressure on back muscles, so it's a good position when your back is hurting. When you're standing for more than a few minutes, look for any raised surface—a curb, a chair rung, or anything else that's at least a few inches above the ground—that you can use to keep one foot higher than the other.

legs—specifically, buildups of cholesterol and other fatty substances that restrict blood flow. If a blood vessel in your leg is narrowed by fatty sludge, the muscle that depends on that vessel won't get enough blood or oxygen. This may not be a problem when you're just sitting around, because the muscle isn't demanding very much blood. When you're active, though, it calls for more fuel than it's able to get. The result: a painful cramp that forces you to stop moving and rest the muscle. The condition is called intermittent claudication because it comes and goes. It also usually follows a distinct pattern. The pain comes on when you walk or are otherwise active, and it goes away when you relax. Another telltale sign is the regularity of the attacks. You may feel pain whenever you're 100 feet into your daily walk, for example, or 20 minutes into your weekly bike ride.

Keep in mind that anything that affects the circulation in your legs could also be causing problems in your heart or other parts of your body. But that doesn't mean you have to risk bankruptcy to find relief. Along with a doctor's care, the following tips can make a real difference.

Get Pumping

Exercise is good for your heart, and it's just as good for improving circulation in beleaguered leg muscles. Get 20 minutes of exercise every day. Experts say it's the most important thing you can do. The type of exercise is up to you; swimming, cycling, and walking are all great choices. The goal is to get your heart rate up and to break a sweat. If you haven't been exercising regularly, talk to your doctor before starting a new regimen. Then do it!

Stop and Go

Attacks of intermittent claudication can be intensely painful because your leg muscles are literally starved for blood and oxygen. For almost instant relief, stop whatever it is you're doing. The pain will probably go away in a minute or two, but don't use it as an excuse to call it quits altogether. Once the pain is gone, start exercising again. There's no harm in continuing once the pain goes away.

Eat Heart Smart

The same type of diet that's recommended for preventing heart disease will also go a long way toward protecting your legs. Quit eating fatty foods, eat five servings of fruit and vegetables a day, use olive oil in place of butter, and load up on legumes and whole grains. Eating a healthier diet will keep all of your blood vessels, including those in your legs, a whole lot healthier. While you're focusing on a healthier diet, try some of these:

- Chomp a clove. Garlic is both a clot buster and a cholesterol reducer. Its heating properties also make it a great circulatory tonic because it gets the blood moving to where it needs to be. Eat one raw clove per day to help alleviate claudication.

- Get help from hawthorn. Hawthorn, lime blossoms, and ginger are recognized for their ability to reduce the stickiness of blood platelets and enhance circulation. As long as you're not taking any other medications, use them together, or choose just one. To use together, mix equal parts of dried hawthorn, lime blossoms, and ginger, add 1 heaping teaspoon of the mix to 1 cup of hot water, steep for 15 to 20 minutes, and strain. You can drink 2 or 3 cups of this tea per day.

- Dine on fin cuisine. Salmon, tuna, and other cold-water fish are loaded with omega-3 fatty acids. These healthful fats help prevent blood clots and may lower cholesterol. Try to eat at least two or three servings of fish a week.

- Drink green. If you have intermittent claudication, make your tea the green kind. It's a great source of bioflavonoids, which are natural chemical compounds that make blood vessels stronger and less vulnerable to blockages and pain. You can buy green tea bags in most stores where tea is sold; just steep a tea bag in a cup of hot water for 10 minutes, then enjoy. Aim for a cup or two every day.

Add Some E

Vitamin E is a vasodilator, meaning that it opens narrowed blood vessels and allows more blood to flow through. It can allow people to walk farther without pain. The recommended dose is 400 to 800 IUs daily, but check with your doctor before taking vitamin E.

FAST FORMULA

Leg Wrap

Herbalists use yarrow and peppermint to improve circulation. Visit your local health-food store to pick up the ingredients so you can improve yours, too.

2 tbsp. of dried yarrow
2 tbsp. of dried peppermint
2 cups of hot water
Gauze, cheesecloth, or muslin

In a teapot, steep the herbs in the hot water for about 15 minutes. Strain out the herbs, and put the teapot in the refrigerator to chill. Meanwhile, gather enough gauze, cheesecloth, or muslin to wrap your lower legs. Soak the cloth in the chilled liquid, wrap it around your legs, and rest with your legs elevated for about 20 minutes. Do this once a day for several weeks, and the discomfort should dissolve.

In addition to E, keep magnesium on hand. It relaxes smooth muscles in artery walls, and it's helpful in lowering blood pressure. Check with your doctor first, then take 300 to 600 milligrams daily.

Varicose Veins: An Uphill Climb

Do your legs start hurting as the day goes by? Do you find yourself wearing long pants even on 95°F days? Maybe you're one of the millions of Americans with varicose veins—and no matter what you hear, they're not just a cosmetic problem.

Even though nearly everyone has some varicose veins, there's a lot of confusion about what they really are. A varicose vein is simply a blood vessel that doesn't have quite enough strength to push its cargo of blood uphill and back into circulation. After a while, the accumulated blood causes the vein to swell, resulting in a varicose vein.

Varicose veins can make your legs feel tired and achy. That's the most common problem, but there's also a risk that the poor circulation that accompanies varicose veins can cause ulcers on your lower legs. Less often, the swollen veins can promote the formation of blood clots that are potentially serious. Surgery and other techniques can remove them. In most cases, however, you can bolster your veins with some simple home strategies that cost little or nothing to use. Here are a few things to try:

Exercise often. Having varicose veins isn't an excuse for not exercising. In fact, it's all the more reason to be active. The more fit you are, the better your circulatory system will be able to cope with the diminished capacity of your leg veins. It's best to do an exercise like yoga, swimming, or walking, which doesn't put excessive pressure on the lower extremities.

Firm up with stockings. Snug-fitting hose, called compression stockings, are available from drugstores and medical-supply stores. They provide extra support to the walls of blood vessels in the legs, which helps keep blood moving upward. Your doctor should write a prescription for the right kind of hose for you. Over-the-counter compression stockings work well, but they may not provide the exact amount of pressure that you need. And while compression stockings are designed to put your veins under pressure, other garments that put pressure on your legs can interfere with circulation. So avoid tight pantyhose, girdles, and other kinds of restrictive clothing.

Raise your legs. The blood in your legs has to fight gravity to climb all the way back to your heart. Why not reverse the situation and let gravity work for you? To do it, raise your feet above the level of your heart for a couple of hours each day, or sit with your legs propped up on pillows. About 10 minutes after you elevate your legs, the ache will go away.

Point your feet. Sleeping with your feet raised a few inches will give your veins a boost all night long. You can prop your feet on a flat pillow, or put some boards under the foot of your bed. Check with your doctor first, though, since this sleeping position may aggravate some health problems.

Beat the Heat

You don't want your legs to get too hot when you have varicose veins, because it could result in tissue-damaging inflammation. So be sure to avoid long, hot baths and other activities that make your legs hotter than usual.

Get Soaked

You can improve the pumping action of leg veins with a technique called contrast hydrotherapy, in which you alternate between hot and cold treatments. First, soak a cloth in hot water, wring it out, and place it over the area where you have varicose veins. Leave it in place for three minutes, then replace it with a cold cloth for 30 seconds. Repeat the cycle two or three times, always ending with the cold cloth.

Cool It

Cold witch hazel is a cool solution to aching veins. Chill a cup of witch hazel in the refrigerator for about an hour, then soak a washcloth in the liquid, and apply it to the parts of your legs that hurt. Keep the compress in place for about 15 minutes while also elevating your legs. Witch hazel has astringent properties, which means that it improves blood flow and eases pain. Believe me, you'll soon be saying "aaahhhh."

Rub 'Em Right

There's nothing like a massage for soothing tired legs (or tired anything, for that matter). Besides making you feel good, massage can improve your circulation, which is a big plus if you have varicose veins. To help ease the ache even more, add a few drops of comfrey oil to a few tablespoons of olive oil, then give yourself a soothing oil massage. The comfrey will boost circulation and help the discomfort fade a lot faster.

Take Extra C

Your body uses vitamin C to strengthen blood vessels. Unless you have stomach or kidney problems, take 500 to 1,000 milligrams of vitamin C two or three times daily. Since taking this much vitamin C may cause diarrhea, it's a good idea to start with the lower dose and gradually work up from there.

Fight Back with Flavonoids

Strong, healthy veins are less likely to become varicose. One way to strengthen yours is to get more bioflavonoids in your diet. These natural plant chemicals, found in most fruits and vegetables, make the vein walls stronger and better able to push blood uphill. Most researchers recommend at least five servings of fresh fruit and vegetables a day.

SPRAINS AND STRAINS

Okay, here's a test: What's the difference between a sprain and a strain? Answer: A sprain is an injury to the ligaments that support your joints, and a strain is a pulled or overexerted muscle. A sprain usually occurs from overextending or twisting your arm or leg beyond its normal range of movement and tearing or seriously stretching a ligament. You end up with pain when you move the limb, as well as swelling and pain in the involved joint. It feels tender to the touch, and you'll probably get black and blue. And exactly like a strain, it hurts like the dickens.

If you are uncertain if an injury is a sprain or a break, the American Medical Association advises always treating it like a break until you get medical help. Then, when you know it's a sprain or a strain, follow this advice.

RICE Is Nice!

The first thing you should do is remember RICE, which stands for Rest it, Ice it, Compress it, and Elevate it. In other words, stop the activity, and rest the injured body part. Apply ice wrapped in a towel or a cold compress to decrease swelling. Wrap the injured limb in an elastic bandage or a splint or sling. And then keep the injured part

elevated above the level of your heart. Don't use heat until at least 24 hours after the injury, when the swelling is gone. And by all means, seek medical attention if the pain or swelling is severe.

Pack It Up

For a cooling, heating, and healing experience all wrapped into one, add essential oils to your cold pack. First, fill a bowl with ice-cold water. Sprinkle several drops of essential oil into the water—try camphor, eucalyptus, chamomile, or rosemary. Next, soak a clean washcloth in the bowl, and wring it out well. Lay the washcloth over the sprained area, and cover with an ice pack. Limit the ice phase to 10 to 20 minutes to avoid frostbite!

Banish Pain

Bromelain and turmeric are powerful partners when it comes to reducing inflammation and pain. Take 250 to 500 milligrams of each between meals, three times daily. *Caution:* People with sensitivities to pineapple should avoid bromelain.

Get Close to Comfrey

Comfrey (*Symphytum officinale*) wraps work wonders for speeding recovery of a sprain. Blanch two to four leaves, and place over the sprain. These can be worn all day underneath an elastic bandage. Ointments containing comfrey root are great blister beaters, promoting speedy healing of the little devils. And for a great muscle mender, fill a 12-ounce glass jar with freshly chopped comfrey leaves, then cover completely with a mixture of olive oil and the oil from a vitamin E capsule. Put the jar in a sunny indoor spot for a week, shaking it a couple of times a day. Strain the oil and put it into a clean glass bottle, then add 15 drops of juniper and wintergreen oils. You can rub the liniment into sore muscles whenever you feel the need. Store in a cool place or in the fridge.

CHAPTER 8

Eating Right

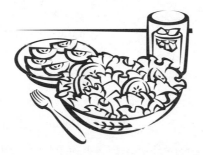

Don't worry. I'm not going to lecture you about your diet. Well, maybe just a little. Here goes: YOU ARE WHAT YOU EAT! It's true; science says so. And I know that changing old habits is not an easy thing to do. Sure, it was hard to give up all my old favorites, but once I learned how eating right "does a body good," it was easier to make the switch. Here's how to make sure you get all the food your body needs each and every day.

CLIMB THE PYRAMID

The U.S. government's got a new food pyramid. Experts say it better reflects everything we know up to this point about how food affects our bodies and minds. Here's how much we need and why.

Gobble Up Whole Grains

With the recommendation for 6 to 11 servings a day, you may wonder why pasta, rice, whole wheat, and other grains are so important. For one thing, they're absolutely jammed with fiber. They're nutritional powerhouses that provide key vitamins, minerals, and other chemical compounds you need for good health. Best of all,

grains do all this without overloading your body with excess calories by helping to:

Lower cholesterol. Generous amounts of whole grains in your low-fat diet lower both your total and LDL (or "bad") cholesterol levels. Just 1 cup of oatmeal a day can reduce your cholesterol levels pretty quickly, according to the American Heart Association.

Prevent stroke. Homocysteine, an amino acid your body makes as it digests protein, has been linked to stroke and heart attacks. One way to lower homocysteine levels is to increase your intake of foods that are high in B vitamins, specifically folate, B_6, and B_{12}, which you can get from whole grains.

Reduce blood sugar. Studies have shown that a natural, whole-foods diet that is heavy on grains is far more likely to help stabilize blood sugar than one that includes fast food and refined sugar.

Prevent constipation and diverticulosis. The insoluble fiber in whole gains and vegetables adds bulk to stools, which helps prevent constipation. At the same time, a diet rich in grains decreases pressure on the colon and reduces the risk of diverticulosis—high-pressure "blowouts" in the colon wall.

Manage stress. Grains can help you deal with the stresses of a life in overdrive. They're packed with pantothenic acid, a B vitamin that's necessary to keep your adrenal glands working well when your body is stressed.

Prevent folate-deficiency anemia. Folate (folic acid) is a B vitamin that builds red blood cells and comes from not only whole grains, but also from dark, leafy greens, citrus fruits, and beans. Women who are pregnant or breast-feeding are most likely to come up short on folate, which isn't stored in the body and needs to be replenished daily. And studies show that vitamin B_6 and folate may help prevent heart attacks.

Quick Fix

Got asthma? Then eat your All-Bran®! It's loaded with magnesium, which doctors say can keep your asthma attacks in check. It turns out that magnesium in whole grains and other foods, such as spinach, peanuts, and lima beans, is like a sedative for your bronchial tubes. Sort of like slipping them a "magnesium Mickey"!

Stay Lean with Protein

Protein keeps our engines running. We need two to three servings a day of foods in this group—meat, poultry, fish, eggs, beans, nuts, and seeds. But choosing the wrong ones could put the brakes on good health. You'll want to limit the amount of foods you eat from this group that are high in saturated fat and cholesterol.

Say "no" to:

- Fatty cuts of beef, pork, and lamb

- Regular (75 to 85 percent lean) ground beef

- Regular sausages, hot dogs, and bacon

- Luncheon meats like regular bologna and salami

- Poultry like duck

Say "yes" to:

- Boneless, skinless chicken breasts and turkey cutlets

- Round steaks and roasts (round eye, top round, bottom round, round tip), top loin, and top sirloin

- Lean pork choices such as pork loin, tenderloin, center loin, and ham

Eat Your Veggies—and Fruits!

Are you eating three to five servings of vegetables and two to four servings of fruits *every day*? No? Then get going! Eat them any way you like—fresh, frozen, canned, or dried—they're all good for you. All fruits and vegetables contain antioxidants, which are chemicals that counteract the oxidative wear and tear that's always going on in our bodies. And we know that the more we get of these, the more likely we are to ward off diseases such as cancer, heart disease, stroke, diabetes, kidney stones, and macular degeneration. But variety is as important as quantity. No single fruit or vegetable provides all of the nutrients you need to be healthy. A simple way to make sure you get what you need is to "follow the rainbow." The compounds that will keep you the healthiest are also the compounds that are responsible for the color of fruits and vegetables. So fill your plate with greens, oranges, purples, reds, and yellows. And remember, even though 100 percent fruit and vegetable juices count toward your daily goal, juice won't give you the fiber that whole veggies and fruits will.

If you're trying to lose weight, feel free to up your intake of fruits and veggies in order to quell hunger pangs. All produce is low-calorie and brings no cholesterol to the plate!

Go Nutty

Many of us stick to meat and poultry for our protein portions every day, and that's a shame. Including fish, nuts, and seeds as protein sources in your diet can provide those "good" polyunsaturated and monounsaturated fats that we've heard so much about. Nuts, especially walnuts, contain omega 3-fatty acids, which have been linked to lowering levels of total and "bad" cholesterol (low-density lipoprotein, or LDL, cholesterol) while raising levels of "good" cholesterol (high-density lipoprotein, or HDL, cholesterol). Protein, B vitamins (niacin, thiamine, riboflavin, and B_6), vitamin E, iron, zinc, and magnesium are also valuable nutrients this group offers. Cooking with olive, canola, sunflower, peanut, and other vegetable oils is another great way to get the benefits of these nutrients. So use them instead of butter, lard, and margarine.

Discover Dairy

When I was a kid, every day after school I would sit down to a snack that always included a nice tall, cold glass of milk. And I still enjoy a glass every day. It's a good habit to have, because the average person needs 1,200 mg of calcium daily (1,500 mg for postmenopausal women) to maintain strong bones and prevent osteoporosis, a serious bone-thinning disease that affects millions of women and is a leading cause of hip and spinal fractures. Getting the calcium you need from the recommended two to three dairy servings per day isn't hard, if you include cheese and yogurt along with your milk. Just be sure to choose low- or nonfat versions. Whole-milk dairy products will only load you up with more fat than you need, while the sugars in the sweetened milks and yogurts will put empty calories where you don't want them. And don't think you're getting a calcium boost from cream cheese, cream, or butter, because you're not. Each has little or no calcium.

The benefits of dairy products go beyond bone health. Take a look at what they can do:

Lower high blood pressure. Potassium prevents thickening of the artery walls and works with sodium, an electrolyte, to regulate your body's fluid levels. That's important because too much fluid in your arteries can raise your blood pressure. Studies have shown that people who get enough potassium can sometimes get their blood pressure back to normal levels. The potassium in that glass of milk will help you do it.

Stop weight gain. Recent studies are suggesting that consuming three servings of dairy a day, in a healthy diet, can fight obesity by regulating our fat metabolism. A cup of low-fat yogurt, a glass of reduced-fat or skim milk, and 1 ounce of low-fat cheese are all it takes.

Prevent colon cancer. A review of 10 studies done in 2004 says that a higher consumption of milk and calcium is associated with a lower risk of colorectal cancer. So drink up!

Zinc About This...

For a healthy sex life, men, get plenty of zinc. The prostate needs this mineral to produce semen. And, true to its legend, the good old oyster really is just "shuck-full" of zinc. Try this quick recipe to restore the roar.

6 oysters, shucked, washed, and drained
1/2 cup of flour
2 eggs, beaten
1 cup of bread crumbs
2 cups of peanut oil

Heat the peanut oil in a heavy frying pan. One by one, dip the oysters in flour, then egg, then roll them in the bread crumbs. Fry until golden brown.

Even out mood swings. There's good news for women approaching menopause: About 2,000 milligrams of calcium a day may help even out mood swings.

Ease muscle cramps. Here's why they happen: Your muscles move in response to nerve signals they get from the minerals that surround your muscle cells. An imbalance in these minerals can interrupt the flow of signals and cause cramps, so give your body what it needs by including plenty of dairy in your diet. It'll provide you with those muscle-loving minerals calcium, chloride, sodium, potassium, and magnesium.

Conquer PMS. A calcium deficiency could be the key to why some women suffer from premenstrual syndrome. In one recent study, women who boosted their intake of this mineral had half the number of symptoms

they had before they increased their calcium consumption.

Stop migraines. When calcium is combined with riboflavin (and both of these are plentiful in dairy products), migraines take a vacation.

Dull sugar cravings. Calcium can help relax a stressed nervous system and nip sugar cravings in the bud.

Soothe sciatica. Calcium and magnesium are like a magic bullet for sciatica because they help relax tight muscles.

Vitamins Are Vital

A daily multivitamin and mineral supplement offers a kind of nutritional backup, like health insurance in a pill! It shouldn't replace healthy eating, or make up for poor eating, but it can fill in the gaps in your nutrient bank when you need it. There's no need for an expensive name-brand or designer vitamin; a standard, store-brand, RDA-level one is fine. Look for a vitamin that meets the requirements of the USP (U.S. Pharmacopeia), an organization that sets standards for drugs and supplements. You'll find the USP designation on the box or bottle.

Water, Water Everywhere

The earth's surface is mainly water. Most of your body weight is water. Your skin, heart, and other organs are awash in water. Get the picture? Without water, your body simply can't function—and even a short-term drought caused by not drinking enough water can have long-term consequences. Here's what doctors say chugging 8 to 10 glasses a day can remedy:

Constipation. All experts agree that the simplest way to wake up your colon when you're constipated is to drink water—lots and lots of it. When stools in the colon absorb water, they become larger, softer, and easier to pass. So try to down 10 glasses within 24 hours.

Cranky gut. You need to give up milk and other dairy products when your intestines are under the weather. Likewise, you'll want to avoid citrus and vegetable juices, alcohol, and caffeine, which also make things worse. Instead, drink plenty of water—as much as you can hold.

Dehydration. When you exercise, drink lots of water to prevent dehydration and replenish the fluids and nutrients you lose during workouts. Have a glass of water before you begin, and take a break every 20 to 30 minutes to drink some more. This workout wisdom is especially important for people with diabetes.

Diarrhea. According to the Centers for Disease Control and Prevention, if you have severe diarrhea, you should take in only fluids (such as water or sports drinks) and salty crackers until it's under control.

Headaches. Before you reach for an aspirin, ask yourself how much water you've had today. For many of us, a headache is the first symptom of dehydration (even before thirst!), so drink a glass or two of water before you pop that pill.

Dry skin. You need lots of water to keep all parts of your body working well, including your skin. It's really quite simple: The more water you drink, the more water is available to pump up and out to your epidermis. So don't be stingy; drink at least 8 to 10 glasses a day, and carry a water bottle with you when you're exercising or out in the heat.

Pneumonia. You should never be more than an arm's length away from a glass of water while you're recovering from pneumonia—and you need at least eight glasses a day. Drinking lots of water dilutes all the mucus your lungs produce when you have pneumonia. So if you stay hydrated, you'll breathe easier, and your lungs will recover more quickly.

UTIs. The more water you drink, the more bacteria will be flushed from your bladder, which can help prevent urinary tract infections (UTIs). Drinking plenty of water can also help you feel better if you already have an infection. In addition to flushing out bugs, water helps dilute pain-causing substances in the bladder. Doctors recommend drinking at least 2 quarts a day.

Water a Toothache

I know this sounds crazy, but a toothache can get a lot worse when your mouth is dry. So until you can get to your dentist, keep the H_2O handy at all times and drink up to keep things hydrated.

SOME HEALTHY SNACKING SOLUTIONS

You are what you eat—and that doesn't just apply to your three square meals a day. Snacks count, too! Snacking seems to be our national pastime, but it's a sport that is weighing heavily on its fans, literally! Experts agree that snacking and on-the-go eating are major causes of soaring obesity rates. Many snack foods are loaded with refined carbs and sugars, and most times, they seem to be the easiest things to grab. But if you stop and take a second to look around, you'll find much better alternatives.

My Favorite Munchies

It took a while for me to throw away those bags of chips and cookies and stock up on healthier fare. But once I started, I found I really didn't crave those greasy, salty, and sweet snacks anymore. Don't know where to begin? Try a few of my favorites:

- Air-popped popcorn
- Angel food cake with berries
- Apple wedges and peanut butter
- Baked chips—tortilla, soy, sweet potato, and rice
- Celery and low-fat cream cheese
- Cheese (Just make sure it's low-fat; if not, limit yourself to 1 ounce.)
- Cut-up veggies with low-fat ranch dressing
- Fruit—any kind
- Low-fat, unsalted whole-wheat pretzels
- Whole-wheat crackers

Yahoo for Yogurt

We're all screaming for ice cream, when we should be yelling for yogurt. Tangy tasting yogurt makes a perfect snack. Why? Because apart from its load of essential nutrients, yogurt contains beneficial bacteria that not only keep you healthy, but can also reverse conditions that have already taken hold. Here are a few remarkable reasons why you should include yogurt in your daily diet:

Protect your bones. When calcium is needed to accomplish certain bodily functions, such as cell regeneration, your body searches for it. If you haven't consumed enough, it's withdrawn from your bones, so you can see why it's important to take in ample amounts.

The daily calcium requirement is 1,200 milligrams for adults, or 1,500 milligrams for postmenopausal women. One cup of yogurt provides 275 to 325 milligrams of calcium.

Stop the gas. Live-culture yogurt can reduce gas because it breaks down milk sugars and keeps a balance of healthy bacteria in the digestive tract. So eat it often for better digestive health.

Avoid lactose intolerance. If you're lactose intolerant, you may be able to eat fermented dairy products, such as yogurt and kefir, without problems.

Fight anemia. Yogurt contains lactic acid, which promotes iron absorption from other foods. It's a good choice if you have iron-deficiency anemia.

Soothe vaginitis. The *Lactobacillus acidophilus* organisms in yogurt crowd out the bad bugs that cause vaginitis, and restore the acid-alkaline balance (pH) of the vagina. Eat more yogurt to help prevent future infections.

Thwart IBS. Yogurt helps balance bacteria in the digestive tract and reduce the cramps, diarrhea, and other symptoms of irritable bowel syndrome (IBS). Look for brands of yogurt that contain active cultures of beneficial *L. acidophilus*.

Ease surgical side effects. A common side effect of surgery is the loss of the "good" bacteria that live in your digestive system. Anesthesia destroys them, and the antibiotics that we often have to take after surgery can also kill them. Protect yourself by eating a serving or two of live-culture yogurt daily.

Strengthen immunity. Yogurt may rev up your entire immune system. A review of studies at

Tufts University suggested that people with compromised immune systems, especially older folks, may increase their resistance to certain diseases by eating yogurt. If you find that you get sick more often than you'd like, make yogurt your No. 1 daily snack.

Reduce cancer risk. Animal research suggests that the organisms in yogurt may decrease the risk of breast, colon, and liver tumors that are triggered by carcinogens—those nasty cancer-causing chemicals.

Nuts to You

A lot of people avoid nuts because these crunchy snacks are among the most concentrated sources of fat in the plant world, with up to 25 grams in $1/3$ cup. Don't let this hold you back, though, because the fats in nuts are better for you than those in meat, and there's good evidence that nuts are among the most powerful foods you can eat. Have a handful a day to reap the rewards without excess fat and calories! Here's what "shell power" can fight:

Asthma. Nuts can help you breathe easier if you have asthma because the magnesium they contain acts like a sedative for your bronchial tubes.

Dandruff. One of the B-complex vitamins, biotin, is essential for healthy hair and can help discourage dandruff. To get enough in your diet, eat a handful of nuts a day.

Depression. Nuts contain tryptophan, an amino acid that is converted into serotonin, which is an important mood regulator for your body. In one study, when women who were depressed feasted on tryptophan-rich foods like nuts, their depression eased without the help of medication!

FAST FORMULA

Quell Queasiness

Stomach going topsy-turvy on you? Mix up this creamy concoction to settle things down in a hurry.

$1/2$ cup of plain yogurt
2 pinches of cardamom
$1/2$ tsp. of honey

Mix all the ingredients in a cereal bowl, and eat slowly. Repeat a few hours later, if needed.

Ear noise. Low levels of magnesium may constrict inner-ear arteries and lead to tinnitus, which is that annoying ringing or other "ghost" noise in the ears. You may find that the sounds diminish when you start eating more nuts, which are rich in magnesium.

Gum disease. The vitamin E in nuts fights cell damage caused by free radicals. The more E you get, the less risk you have of getting serious gum disease.

Heart disease. Many of us don't get nearly enough selenium, a trace mineral that appears to play a role in keeping arteries clear. Nuts are loaded with it, and unlike selenium supplements (which can be dangerous), they're perfectly safe!

High cholesterol. Studies have shown that both walnuts and almonds can lower cholesterol, and a report in the Journal of the American Dietetic Association revealed that pecans can, too. The theory is that the monounsaturated fat in nuts can protect against heart disease.

Joint pain. Nuts—along with beans, raisins, pears, apples, and other fruits—all contain the

145

trace element boron, which can relieve pain and joint stiffness and actually appears to protect against arthritis.

Leg swelling. If your legs or feet swell, you may need to balance your electrolytes, such as potassium and magnesium, which counterbalance sodium and help reduce excess fluid in your body. For potassium, have grapes, orange juice, vegetable juices, and bananas. For magnesium, nuts will fill the bill.

Macular degeneration. Nuts are loaded with vitamin E, a nutrient that appears to reduce the risk of macular degeneration, which is the leading cause of blindness in older people. Eating nuts regularly will help keep your vision sharp year after year.

PMS. Many women crave sugar and chocolate when they're premenstrual. While a sweet treat may be a quick pick-me-up, the sudden rise in blood sugar is bound to be followed by a crash that will make you miserable. If you do indulge your sweet tooth, include some protein (chocolate with nuts, for example) to reduce the sugar's negative effects.

Weak bones. To keep your bones healthy and strong, you need magnesium. Nuts are one of the best food sources, along with potatoes, seeds, legumes, whole grains, and dark green vegetables.

Peanut Power

Grandma Putt loved to indulge us with her homemade peanut butter. Little did she know she was spreading good health! Peanuts are packed with a miracle elixir called coenzyme Q10 that brings oxygen to the heart and, if you have heart problems, may even help curb the damage caused by a lack of oxygen.

SUPERFOODS TO THE RESCUE

It's a bird…it's a plane…it's the "superfoods"! These are special members of the good nutrition club that go beyond the call of duty to deliver more than their fair share of protection against disease. By substituting superfoods for some of the mainstays in your diet, you're doing the most you can to ensure that you feel better and look great. Try to eat at least one serving of the following every day: berries, walnuts, avocados, olive oil, spinach, apples, beans, oats, tea (green or black), and dark chocolate. Read on to find out why.

Better Health Is in the Bag

Coffee is the favored pick-me-up in this country, but worldwide, green and black teas are by far the most popular beverages—and not only because they offer such a wide variety of tastes. Hundreds of scientific studies have shown that tea can play a key role in stopping heart disease and dozens of other common health threats. Why, it even helps prevent wrinkles! Check out the latest findings:

- Preliminary studies show that green tea gives the body a metabolic boost. In other words, it helps your "engine" run faster, so it burns more calories. If you're trying to lose weight, you may want to drink a few cups of tea daily.

- Green tea contains tannins, which are chemical compounds that kill decay-causing bacteria in your mouth and stop them from producing glucan, the sticky substance that helps acid-generating bacteria stick to your teeth. Drink a cup of green tea after every meal for best results.

- Drinking even a single cup of black or green tea a day may preserve bone density, especially if you sip it daily for 10 years, according to studies that looked at the tea-drinking habits of women ages 65 to 76. In contrast to coffee, which increases calcium loss in urine, the natural phytoestrogens in tea may help bones remain thicker.

- Here's good news for all you sneezers and wheezers: Green tea contains epigallocatechin gallate, a compound that studies show blocks the allergic response in human cells. While researchers don't know how much you need to drink to stop the allergic reaction, you might try drinking a cup of green tea before heading outside.

- In countries where people drink lots of green tea, folks rarely get certain kinds of cancers. Tea leaves are rich in polyphenols, special cancer-battling compounds that help cancer drugs attack bad cells and spare healthy ones. And a recent study found that giving green tea to mice protected them against cancers of the skin, lung, esophagus, stomach, small intestine, colon, bladder, liver, pancreas, prostate, and mammary glands.

- Green tea protects the liver, so that it's able to function optimally as your body's detoxification center. Try to drink three to five cups every day.

- If you have intermittent claudication (leg pain caused by poor circulation), make sure your tea is the green kind. Its bioflavonoids make blood vessels stronger and less vulnerable to blockages and pain. So try to drink at least a cup or two each day.

- Research suggests that drinking several cups of black tea a day can help you recover more quickly from the stresses of everyday life. How? By reducing levels of cortisol—the stress hormone.

- Green tea is among the best sore throat remedies around because it's loaded with bioflavonoids, which help quell irritation and inflammation. If green's not your cup of tea, try chamomile—it's a traditional herbal remedy for sore throat pain.

Blueberries—More Than Just Dessert

You may think that blueberries are nature's incentive to take long, rambling walks with a berry-picking basket under your arm, but they're actually among the most potent food remedies on the planet. With every bite, you get a burst of intensely flavored juice, along with some impressive health benefits. Work 1/2 cup into your diet each day, and they'll help hold the following ailments at bay:

Allergies. Why load your body with antihistamines, which frequently cause side effects, when you can naturally fight allergies with blueberries? They contain

Quick Fix

For a shorter hospital stay, tell your friends and family to hold off on those get-well cards and flowers—have them bring a box of blueberries instead! These tasty morsels can help you heal after surgery. They help reduce inflammation, mend damaged tissue, and strengthen tiny blood vessels traumatized by the operation. Here's to a "berry" speedy recovery!

chemical compounds that inhibit the release of histamine, which is the body chemical that causes congestion.

Bad memory. Eating $1/2$ cup of blueberries a day may clear the sludge from your memory banks and improve your balance and coordination, reports a Tufts University study. Blueberries are reported to have the highest antioxidant content of any fruit or vegetable.

Bruises. Blueberries are loaded with vitamin C and chemical compounds called bioflavonoids, which will help bruises heal faster and make your blood vessels stronger and better able to resist future damage.

Heart problems. The bioflavonoids in blueberries work to strengthen your cardiovascular system. They also help prevent the molecular damage that makes cholesterol more likely to form thick sludge on artery walls and prevent heart-nourishing blood from getting through.

High blood pressure. Studies show that the fiber in fruit apparently works even better than the fiber in vegetables and grains to lower systolic blood pressure. Blueberries are an especially good example, so use them to top your morning oatmeal or cold cereal.

UTIs. Blueberries provide the same anti-infection protection as their crimson cousins, cranberries, when it comes to keeping bacteria from binding to the bladder wall and causing urinary tract infections (UTIs).

O Is for Oatmeal

A few hundred years ago, most people had never tasted oatmeal because oats were given almost exclusively to horses. In some parts of the world, though, this nutritious grain made the journey from the stable to the kitchen table—and our health today is better for it. Oats are a great source of fiber and a good source of many other nutrients, including protein, vitamin E, zinc, selenium, copper, iron, manganese, and magnesium. Here are four reasons why doctors call this a superfood:

1. Oatmeal is a great source of soluble fiber, which is the kind you want more of when you're trying to lower your cholesterol. Soluble fiber reduces LDL cholesterol (the bad kind) without lowering HDL cholesterol (the good kind). Just 1 cup a day can reduce your cholesterol levels pretty quickly.

2. Oatmeal is just the ticket when you're dealing with constipation. It contains a gummy type of fiber called mucilage that soaks up water, which makes stools larger and softer. So be sure to start the day with a bowl of oatmeal—it'll make stools easier to pass, with a whole lot less straining.

3. Oatmeal is packed with insoluble fiber. The American Cancer Society says this fiber contains cancer-fighting properties because it attacks certain bile acids, thereby reducing their toxicity.

4. The soluble fiber in oats slows down the digestion of starch. This is a boon to diabetics because, when you slow down the digestion of starch, you avoid the sharp rises in your blood sugar level that usually occur following a meal.

One Fabulous Fat

About 50 years ago, scientists first noticed that people in Greece and other Mediterranean countries had heart disease rates that were a fraction of those for us here in the United States. Was it the wine they drank? The produce they ate? All that exercise going up and down hills? The answer to each of these questions was yes—but there was something else—olive oil. It turns out that this oil can almost literally turn back the clock on disability and disease. Here's how it helps:

Halts mental decline. A daily splash or two of olive oil will help keep your mind healthier. An Italian study found that cognitive impairment was less common among elderly people who ate a Mediterranean diet, which includes lots of olive oil, a monounsaturated fat. As their "healthy fat" intake increased, their risk of memory problems declined.

Prevents heart attack. The risk of heart attack among people who live in the Mediterranean region is half that of Americans, although they actually eat a bit more fat than we do. The reason is olive oil. People who eat a lot of olive oil tend to have lower levels of harmful LDL cholesterol, while maintaining higher levels of beneficial HDL.

Cures constipation. Taking 1 to 3 tablespoons of olive oil acts as a mild laxative and can help get you moving again—without resorting to more powerful drugs.

Strong to the Finish

Spinach is a veritable powerhouse of phytonutrients, which are plant chemicals that scour the arteries, protect the heart, and lower blood pressure—and that's just for starters. What else can spinach do for you? Just a whole lotta good. Take a look:

- Spinach is a great source of potassium. According to the FDA, diets rich in potassium and low in sodium may reduce the risk of stroke—so eat lots of spinach salads!

- A magnesium deficiency can cause constipation, so make like Popeye and eat your spinach because it's rich in this mineral. If you have chronic constipation, you may also want to check with your doctor about taking magnesium supplements.

- Spinach can protect your heart. It's packed with coenzyme Q10, a hardworking compound that appears to help bring oxygen to the heart. It may even prevent damage caused by a lack of oxygen.

- Green leafy vegetables, such as spinach, are like nature's sunglasses—just what you need if you spend a lot of time outdoors. They're rich in a chemical called lutein, which is also part of the pigment in the macula of the eye. This pigment helps filter out the light implicated in macular degeneration, and it also fights the destructive effects of oxidation.

- Low blood levels of vitamin E are associated with higher rates of angina, which is chest pain due to impaired circulation to the heart. You need the antioxidant power of vitamin E to prevent damage to your arteries. While it's tough to get enough vitamin E from foods, spinach is a good source. Eat some daily to keep your ticker humming right along.

HOME REMEDY

Women: Stock up on spinach and you just may get through your next period without the pain of cramps. Spinach is chock-full of cramp-busting electrolytes such as magnesium, potassium, and calcium. So down a daily spinach salad or stir-fry a bunch of baby spinach leaves for a nutritious meal—and smoother sailing around that time of the month.

- Spinach provides lots of magnesium, a mineral that relaxes smooth muscles, including those that encircle blood vessels. To keep your blood pressure in check, eat plenty of spinach and other produce every day.

- Research shows that spinach is loaded with plant chemicals that can help restore memory. To help keep your mind sharp, make sure spinach is on your menu several times a week.

- Nature has created a remarkable array of anticancer compounds in all fruits and vegetables. But who's the leader of the pack? I'll give you one guess—spinach!

Get Crackin' with Walnuts!

Unless you buy them shelled, walnuts aren't the easiest (or neatest) snack in the house, but they're definitely one of the healthiest. Studies have shown that people who eat a lot of walnuts feel better and may even live longer than those who don't. It's due to those valuable fatty acids that all nuts have, but walnuts are tops. Ailments they alleviate include:

Brain fog. Regularly eating walnuts is a great way to enrich your diet with omega-3 essential fatty acids. Those are the "good fats" that reduce the inflammation that can hijack your focus and memory.

High cholesterol. Scientists report that people who eat walnuts tend to have lower cholesterol and healthier hearts. The theory is that the monounsaturated fat in nuts can protect against heart disease, but their mineral content—magnesium and copper—may help guard the heart as well. About $1/4$ cup of nuts per day is the recommended serving.

Heart disease. Doctors have known for a long time that the Mediterranean diet, which is brimming with fat (along with boatloads of fish, fruit, and vegetables) is very good for the heart and arteries. Now there's evidence that you can make a good diet even better by substituting a handful of walnuts (8 to 11 a day) for some of the oil in that diet. According to a study reported in the Annals of Internal Medicine, walnuts can lower cholesterol even more than olive oil can, and they reduced the risk of coronary heart disease by 11 percent. In other research, walnuts incorporated into the Mediterranean diet reduced bad cholesterol by almost 6 percent more than the basic Mediterranean diet did. A handful of nuts a day is enough to provide that critical protection.

Itchy skin. If your skin gets itchy in winter, you probably need more fatty acids in your diet. So dig the nutcracker out of the junk drawer and enjoy a few walnuts. Your skin will probably feel better within a few weeks.

Health from the Garden of Eatin'

An apple a day really *could* keep the doctor away! Emerging research may breathe new life into the old cliché: Scientists have recently learned that apples contain a host of nutrients and phytochemicals that could very well leave doctors with a little more time on their hands. Here are a dozen things apples can do:

1. Lower cholesterol. They contain pectin, which is a type of fiber that binds to cholesterol and keeps it from getting into the blood. In one study, pectin lowered participants' cholesterol by as much as 16 percent!

2. Cool down hot flashes. Munch on apples, and you'll have fewer blasts from your internal furnace during menopause. Why? Because they contain naturally occurring

plant sterols called phytoestrogens, which aren't as powerful as human estrogens, but have a similar effect. So they may help cool down annoying hot flashes that are triggered by fluctuating hormones.

3. Beat queasiness. There's a good reason why doctors often recommend applesauce for people whose stomachs are flip-flopping. Along with other bland foods, such as plain rice or toast, apples are easy to digest and they give your body the nutrition it needs while your stomach is recovering.

4. Improve allergies. Eating an apple a day is an easy way to help you survive allergy season. Apples contain quercetin, a potent bioflavonoid-antihistamine combo that reduces allergy symptoms.

FAST FORMULA

A Moving Mix

This combo of apple-sauce, prunes, and bran is a favorite on hospital menus where "getting things moving" is often a problem. The soluble fiber in apples keeps stools soft so they pass more easily, the bran provides bulk from insoluble fiber and decreases pressure on the colon walls, and we're all familiar with the powers of prunes as a natural laxative!

4 to 6 prunes, chopped
1 tbsp. bran
$1/2$ cup applesauce

Mix up a batch and eat it before bedtime to get things going in the right direction the next day.

---

5. Ease arthritis. The next time your joints are aching—or better yet, before the pain starts—eat a few apples. They contain the trace element boron, which can relieve joint pain and stiffness and actually appears to protect against arthritis.

6. Fight fatigue. Don't let fatigue make your metabolism drag; just load up on apples. They provide malic acid, which helps your cells get energized.

7. Soothe irritable bowel syndrome, or IBS. They're among the best remedies for IBS because they're loaded with fiber, which helps tame intestinal spasms and encourages regular bowel movements. They're also easy to snack on as you go about your daily activities.

8. Lower stroke risk. A study showed that men and women who ate an apple every day had a lower risk of ischemic stroke (the kind caused by a blood clot blocking an artery in the brain) than those who didn't.

9. Deter cancer. If cancer runs in your family, you should definitely make an effort to eat more apples. The quercetin they contain appears to fight cancer, possibly by deactivating carcinogens.

10. Deal a blow to diabetes. You can't go wrong with apples if you have diabetes. They contain the soluble fiber pectin, which slows the absorption of nutrients into the bloodstream, helping to keep blood sugar under control.

11. Stave off gum disease. Apples contain compounds that inhibit the gum-destroying enzymes secreted by oral bacteria. So crunch an apple a day to help clean your mouth between brushings.

12. Blast high blood pressure. Move over, bananas; apples contain potassium, too! Potassium prevents thickening of the artery walls and works in conjunction with sodium, an electrolyte, to regulate your body's fluid levels. Those levels are important because excess fluid in your arteries can elevate your blood pressure.

Know How to Pick 'Em

When selecting an apple, make sure it passes the thumb test—if a gentle squeeze produces a dent, it's too soft. You don't want any bruises or cuts, either—just tight, pretty skins. And even though there are no "bad apples" nutritionally, did you know that the smaller they are, the better they taste? Two other apple-icious tips are:

Keep 'em chilled. Room temperature will make apples go mushy fast, so put them in the fridge as soon as you get home. They'll stay nice and crisp for up to six weeks.

Spice 'em up. For a little variety in your apple-a-day routine, try one cooked. Just take a large Rome Beauty, core it, and fill the center with a mixture of raisins, chopped pecans, ground cinnamon, and brown sugar. Microwave for about five minutes, until the apple is tender. It smells divine and tastes sublime.

Avocados Are A-OK!

It's easy to understand why avocados have gotten a bad reputation. For one thing, they contain more calories than just about any other fruit. They're also loaded with fat, with up to 30 grams each. But don't let any of this scare you off—eaten in moderation, avocados are among the best foods for preventing disease, and they have some extra benefits that put them in the superfoods category. When eaten in moderation, they can help prevent:

Cancer. Animal studies have shown that the plant compound beta-sitosterol, which is found in avocados, inhibits the growth of cancerous tumors. Not a bad reason to put these green wonders on your menu.

Fatigue. If you've been tired and achy lately, whip up a salad that includes plenty of avocado. It's a good source of magnesium, the mineral used by cells to stave off fatigue and ease muscle pain.

High blood pressure. It's hard to resist baked chips and guacamole—and why should you? The avocado in guacamole is packed with potassium, a mineral that helps keep all the other minerals in your body in balance. It is also vital for lowering blood pressure.

High cholesterol. Researchers at the University of California, Los Angeles, have found that avocados (at least those grown in California) boast 76 milligrams of beta-sitosterol in a 3 $^1/_2$-ounce portion. This plant compound can inhibit the absorption of cholesterol from your intestines, so you'll have less in your bloodstream, which will reduce your risk of heart disease.

Mental problems. Avocados are a good source of folate (folic acid), which is a B vitamin that's essential for mental health. In fact, according to one study, if you don't get enough folate, your brain could degenerate.

Obesity. An 18-month study at Brigham and Women's Hospital in Boston compared a diet rich in unsaturated fat with a low-fat diet. Those on the high-fat plan were allowed about 45 grams of fat a day, mostly from foods such as avocados, nuts, and olive oil. The group on the low-fat diet received only 25 grams a day. A year later, the low-fat group had a net loss of 6 pounds, while the high-fat folks had a net loss of 11 pounds!

Disease-Lickin' Legumes

Beans are the ultimate power food, low in fat and high in protein, vitamins, and minerals. That's reason enough right there to add more beans to your diet, but here's something else: Study after study has shown that beans are loaded with biologically active substances that can, quite literally, save your life. Here's how:

- A study of 12,000 Americans aged 25 to 75 showed that people who ate a variety of legumes several times a week had a 19 percent lower risk of heart disease than those who ate legumes less than once a week. Researchers believe that both the protein and fiber in legumes may help hearts stay healthy.

- Beans are a nearly perfect food when you have back disk pain. They're jam-packed with protein, the nutrient that your body needs to repair damaged disks and ligaments. Also, unlike meat, dairy products, and some other high-protein foods, beans don't stimulate the production of pain-causing inflammatory chemicals in your body.

- Quite simply, beans are Mother Nature's laxative. So eat 1/2 cup a day to keep constipation at bay.

- There is a movement among desert Native Americans to return to their original diets, which typically included a lot of beans. These low-fat, low-sugar, high–complex carbohydrate foods are more healthy than today's highly processed, packaged foods. Studies in Arizona and Australia have shown that people on such a diet have more stable blood sugar levels than most of us who eat a "normal" diet.

- You may need to eat more beans if you have the annoying ringing in your ears that's known as tinnitus. Beans are rich in magnesium, a

---

HOME REMEDY

Good news for men: If erections don't come as easily or as quickly as you'd like, beans are, indeed, "the magical fruit." They contain an amino acid—arginine—that helps blood flow freely to all the right places.

---

mineral that can promote better circulation in the inner ear.

- If you have herpes, eat more lentils, black beans, and other legumes. They're loaded with lysine, which is an amino acid that seems to help discourage herpes outbreaks.

- If your life is in overdrive, it's vital to include beans in your diet. They provide a bushel of pantothenic acid, which is critical for keeping your adrenal glands up to snuff when they're maxed out and depleting your energy.

- Just 1/2 cup of cooked beans kicks in 3 to 6 grams of fiber, both the insoluble type (a colon cancer fighter) and the soluble type (a cholesterol controller). A study at the University of Kentucky found that eating 1 cup of canned beans in tomato sauce daily for three weeks lowered cholesterol in middle-aged men by about 10 percent.

- Beans release carbohydrates into your bloodstream slowly and can keep your energy humming at peak capacity. If you want to fight fatigue, beans will sustain you longer than a food such as a potato, which quickly releases its carbohydrates into you bloodstream.

- If you find that you keep getting cold after cold after cold, add more beans to your diet. They're loaded with zinc, a mineral that appears to prevent colds, either by stopping the cold virus from reproducing, or by increasing the body's immune response.

- On the scale of gas-producing foods, beans are almost off the chart. What you may not know is that these foods cause trouble mainly for people who don't eat them very often. Adding beans to your menu more frequently will often cut down on excess emissions—and that's good news for everyone!

Get Your Just Desserts

When it comes to dessert, chocolate is probably the one sweet that most women (and men!) can't do without. You obviously don't want to eat too much—it's not exactly light on fat or calories—but a little taste now and then can do wonders for your health. Just be sure your choice is dark chocolate, and not milk or white chocolate. Only the dark version contains high enough levels of the plant phenols that have health benefits. So what can dark chocolate do for you? Check it out:

Clear brain fog. If you have trouble focusing—and have a hankering for chocolate—chances are that your brain really needs it. Chocolate contains phenylethylamine, methylxanthines, and caffeine, which together can improve concentration. A 1.75-ounce bar of dark chocolate will do the trick.

Keep cholesterol in check. Drinking a frothy cup of hot chocolate made with pure cocoa powder does more than stave off winter's chill: Cocoa is rich in flavonoids, which have been shown to prevent oxidation of LDL cholesterol. When LDL cholesterol is oxidized, it clings to arteries and increases the risk of heart disease and stroke. Studies also show that chocolate helps raise levels of HDL cholesterol, the beneficial type that helps remove the bad LDL

cholesterol from the body. And you don't need much—one 8-ounce serving of hot cocoa a day will do it.

Build magnesium levels. *The Journal of the American Dietetic Association* reports that some people may crave chocolate to compensate for a magnesium deficiency. When you're stressed, your body uses more magnesium than it would normally, which depletes your supply. So go ahead, have a little chocolate and replenish your magnesium. A 2-ounce serving of dark chocolate contains about 50 of the 200 to 400 milligrams your body needs every day in order for your muscles to function properly.

Lower stress. Research has shown that chocolate helps release endorphins, which are chemicals produced in the brain that play a key role in controlling mood. People with higher levels of endorphins feel less stressed and more relaxed and confident.

Ease PMS symptoms. When premenstrual syndrome gets you down, give in to your chocolate cravings. Create a cocktail to fight the symptoms by adding 1 tablespoon of fat-free chocolate syrup to a glass of calcium-rich, fat-free milk. You'll feel better in less time than it takes to wash the glass.

PRACTICE STEALTH HEALTH

By now, I hope you've read enough to convince you of the benefits of healthy eating. But don't be surprised if you come up against some resistance when you go about changing your family's diet. Finicky eaters (like kids) and those who are reluctant to give up their bad habits may put up a fight. Sometimes, we have to be a little bit sneaky when it comes to taking care of our loved ones. That's where "stealth health" comes in—my tips and tricks to sneak in the good stuff wherever you can. As I always say, "What they don't know will only help them!"

Secret Recipes

You can probably think of many others, but here are some of my favorite tricks for sneaking in some extra goodness to your old standby sauces, soups, and sandwiches:

- Add finely chopped spinach to a taco. It looks like green chilies, and no one will even taste it.

- Make guacamole with a smaller amount of avocados, substituting smashed cooked peas for some of the avocado. It'll make the dip low fat and pack it with protein and phyto-power. Eating the guacamole with baked tortilla chips instead of the fried ones will also keep the fat content under control.

- Shred carrots or zucchini into meat loaf, casseroles, quick breads, and muffins.

- Toss chopped vegetables in pasta sauce or lasagna.

- Order a veggie pizza with mushrooms, green peppers, and onions, and ask for extra veggies.

- Prepare ground beef for chili by draining off all the fat after browning the beef. Then rinse it under cool running water to remove even more fat. Add beans—such as dark or light red kidney beans or pinto beans—to boost the fiber without any additional fat. Chop up and throw in as many different types of veggies as you can. Or you can substitute ground turkey

Quick Fix

You can start eating healthier by changing your shopping list.

- *Buy whole-wheat bread and pastas instead of white (there are now brands that are truly whole wheat, but retain their white color!).*

- *Choose low-fat or nonfat milk, cheese, and ice cream in place of whole-fat varieties.*

- *Look for whole-fruit spreads instead of sugar-laden jelly.*

- *Use "good" cooking fats, such as canola oil, olive oil, and trans fat–free margarines, instead of regular margarines, butter, and lard.*

- *Replace ground beef with ground chicken or turkey.*

- *Choose eggs enriched with omega-3 fatty acids in place of regular eggs.*

for the beef, or go the soy route, using textured soy crumbles instead of ground beef. Another option is to use half soy crumbles and half ground beef.

- Make guilt-free nachos by cutting soft flour tortillas into wedges and crisping them in a 400°F oven for four minutes. Then top with lots of veggies: tomatoes, onions, shredded carrots, lettuce, and green and yellow pepper strips. Instead of hamburger, use fat-free refried beans and sprinkle with low-fat shredded cheddar cheese. You'll save more than half the calories without sacrificing the taste.

- Use pureed, cooked vegetables, such as potatoes, squash, or cauliflower, to thicken stews, soups, and gravies.

- Add crushed pineapple to coleslaw, or include mandarin oranges or grapes in a tossed salad.

- Try meat dishes that incorporate fruit, such as chicken with apricots, or pork tenderloin topped with peaches.

- Add 1 cup of pureed black beans to brownie batter. You'll add as much fiber as in a slice of whole-wheat bread.

It's in the Bag

Grandma Putt always knew a good idea when she heard one, and she would've put this tip at the top of her list. Always keep your freezer stocked to the hilt with bagged fruits and veggies; they are just as nutritious as fresh ones and will always be there when you need them.

Halt the Salt!

If you want to reduce the amount of salt in your diet, you can try salting herbs the way my Grandma Putt used to do. It's an old-fashioned way of culinary herb preservation that works delightfully well with chives. First, harvest your chives, then wash and let them dry completely. In a glass jar, pack alternate layers of chopped chives and salt. For best results, make sure that the first and final layers of salt are thicker than the middle layers. Put the lid on the jar and place it on a cool, dry shelf in your kitchen, within arm's reach of the stove. Then, instead of using the salt shaker when recipes call for salt, reach for the chive shaker. You'll cut your salt intake in half without sacrificing any flavor!

Icy Goodness

During the dog days of summer, nothing beats a cool, refreshing flavored ice to cool things off. But instead of offering up those empty-calorie ice pop treats, buy 100 percent fruit juice and make your own. You can use plastic ice pop holders or simply pour the juice into ice cube trays and freeze them.

Sneak It In

Here are two quick and easy ways to sneak in healthy alternatives to the usual family fare. You'll be serving up some good nutrition right under their noses!

- Replace your favorite buttery spread with one of the new brands, such as Smart Balance®, that contain no trans fats, but do have a healthy dose of omega-3 fats. If it's good enough for the country's top chefs, it's got to be a family palate pleaser!

- Switch to light or reduced-fat mayonnaise in place of regular mayo in salads and on sandwiches, then watch the calories disappear like magic!

Flax Your Flapjacks

Flaxseeds are a great source of fiber and omega-3s. Grind them finely and add to your favorite pancake or waffle recipe—or even into a pot of oatmeal. No one will be the wiser, just a whole lot healthier!

Shake Things Up

If your family members tend to skimp on their fruit intake, here's an easy way to make sure they're getting their share: Take nonfat yogurt and any kind of berry or fruit (the more, the merrier) and blend away. Serve it up in parfait glasses or dessert bowls, and they won't be able to resist!

Dip This Way

Kids love to plunk their carrot and celery sticks into a creamy dip. But instead of using sour cream as the base for a flavorful dip, substitute a mix of low-fat tofu and fat-free cream cheese.

SUPER RECIPES WITH SUPERFOODS

A number of foods offer extra health benefits (see "Superfoods to the Rescue" on page 146). It's not hard to add these superfoods to your daily diet with the delicious recipes here.

RISE AND SHINE

Vanilla-Almond Oatmeal

When I was a child, butter and brown sugar flavored my oatmeal. It sure did taste great, but there are healthier ways to eat oatmeal. You can, for example, trade the unhealthy fat in butter for the healthy fat in nuts. Then switch the refined sugar for some intriguing spice.

$^1/_2$ **cup of instant oats**
2 **tbsp. of golden seedless raisins**
1 **cup of fat-free milk**
1 **tsp. of honey**
$^1/_2$ **tsp. of vanilla extract**
1 **tbsp. of toasted slivered almonds**
$^1/_8$ **tsp. of ground nutmeg**

In a microwave-safe cereal bowl, combine the oats, raisins, and milk. Microwave on high for 3 to 4 minutes, or until the oats are cooked. Stir in the honey, vanilla, and almonds. (If the oatmeal is too thick, thin with warm water.) Dust with the nutmeg.

Yield: 1 serving

Nutritional data per serving: Calories, 375; protein, 17 g; carbohydrate, 60 g; dietary fiber, 5 g; total fat, 8 g; saturated fat, 1 g; cholesterol, 4 mg; sodium, 131 mg; vitamin A, 15% of Daily Value; vitamin C, 5%; calcium, 36%; iron, 13%; vitamin D, 25%; potassium, 22%.

Lemon-Blueberry Muffins

Blueberry muffins have been a favorite of mine since I was a little kid, and Grandma Putt made the best muffins in town. But now I like them to be really hearty and not quite so sweet. If that suits you, try these favorites.

2 **cups of Arrowhead Mills Multigrain Pancake & Waffle Mix®**
$^1/_2$ **cup of nonfat dry milk**
1 **tsp. of grated lemon peel**
1 **tsp. of baking powder**
$^1/_4$ **cup of honey**
1 **egg**
$^1/_2$ **cup of canola oil**
$^3/_4$ **cup of water**
2 **cups of fresh blueberries, washed and patted dry**

Preheat the oven to 400°F. Lightly coat a 12-cup muffin pan with nonstick spray. In a large bowl, combine the pancake and waffle mix, dry milk, lemon peel, and baking powder. Stir until well mixed. Add the honey, egg, oil, and water. Stir with a fork just until mixed. Fold in the blueberries. Spoon the batter into the pan and bake for 15 to 20 minutes, or until a toothpick inserted in the center of a muffin comes out clean. Loosen the muffins with a knife, remove from the pan, and cool on a rack. Serve with a kiss of butter and a drop of honey.

Yield: 12 servings

Nutritional data per serving: Calories, 211; protein, 4 g; carbohydrate, 28 g; dietary fiber, 3 g; total fat, 10 g; saturated fat, 1 g; cholesterol, 16 mg; sodium, 149 mg; vitamin A, 4% of Daily Value; vitamin C, 22%; calcium, 13%; iron, 4%; vitamin E, 11%; omega-3 fatty acids, 86%.

Peanut Butter Oatmeal

This may be the ultimate breakfast for lowering your cholesterol, keeping your blood sugar under control, and keeping hunger at bay until lunchtime. Think of it as a hot peanut butter and jelly sandwich!

- $^1/_2$ **cup of old-fashioned oats**
- 1   **cup of fat-free milk**
- 2   **dried apricots, cut into sixths**
- 1   **tsp. of honey**
- 1   **tbsp. of chunky peanut butter**
- $^1/_4$ **tsp. of ground cinnamon**

In a microwave-safe cereal bowl, combine the oats, milk, and apricots. Microwave on high for 3 minutes. Stir in the honey, peanut butter, and cinnamon.

Yield: 1 serving

Nutritional data per serving: Calories, 385; protein, 18 g; carbohydrate, 57 g; dietary fiber, 6 g; total fat, 12 g; saturated fat, 2 g; cholesterol, 4 mg; sodium, 207 mg; vitamin A, 25% of Daily Value; vitamin C, 5%; calcium, 34%; iron, 17%; vitamin D, 25%; potassium, 25%.

Honey-Banana Oatmeal

I like to fill up on a good hearty breakfast whenever I can. So when my innards are grouching and grumbling, I soothe them with this delicious, nutritious meal.

- 1   **packet of plain instant oatmeal**
- 1   **cup of fat-free milk**
- 1   **medium banana, diced**
- 1   **tbsp. of honey**
-      **Dash of ground cinnamon**

In a microwave-safe cereal bowl, combine the oatmeal and milk. Microwave on high for 2 to 3 minutes, or according to package directions. Stir in the banana and honey, and dust with the cinnamon.

Yield: 1 serving

Nutritional data per serving: Calories, 365; protein, 14 g; carbohydrate, 75 g; dietary fiber, 6 g; total fat, 3 g; saturated fat, <1 g; cholesterol, 4 mg; sodium, 413 mg; vitamin A, 61% of Daily Value; vitamin C, 22%; calcium, 48%; iron, 38%; folate, 33%; magnesium, 26%; potassium, 28%.

Walnut Corn Muffins

What could be better on a cold, rainy day than hot corn muffins fresh from the oven? They're warm, comforting, and good news for your body!

- 1   **package (7 oz.) of corn muffin mix**
- 1   **egg**
- $^1/_2$ **cup of water**
- 1   **tbsp. of walnut oil**
- $^1/_4$ **cup of chopped walnuts**

Preheat the oven to 400°F. Lightly coat a 6-cup muffin pan with nonstick spray. In a small bowl, combine the muffin mix, egg, water, oil, and walnuts. Stir with a fork just until blended, then spoon into the pan. Bake for 20 minutes, or until a toothpick inserted in the center of a muffin comes out clean. Remove from the pan and cool on a rack (if they last that long). Enjoy with a cup of tea.

Yield: 6 servings

Nutritional data per serving: Calories, 190; protein, 3 g; carbohydrate, 25 g; dietary fiber, 1 g; total fat, 9 g; saturated fat, 1.5 g; cholesterol, 31 mg; sodium, 230 mg; vitamin A, 1% of Daily Value; vitamin C, 1%; calcium, 7%; iron, 6%; omega-3 fatty acids, 70%.

Super Cereal Bowl

A hearty, carry-you-till-lunchtime breakfast is at your fingertips...and there's no cooking needed! It's as easy as 1-2-3-4.

1. Measure one serving of whole-grain cereal into your bowl. The fiber and phytochemicals in whole grains fend off diabetes. Look at the label. "Whole grain" (of some kind) should be the first ingredient.

2. Add some fresh, dried, or canned fruit. Its fiber and antioxidants protect your heart, memory, and eyesight. Begin with a banana, then get creative with blueberries, strawberries, mangoes, dried apricots, raisins, mandarin oranges, or tropical fruit.

3. Top with 1 to 2 tablespoons of nuts or seeds. Healthy fats in these foods keep you fortified until lunchtime and add major minerals that work minor miracles in your body. Consider adding walnuts, pecans, hazelnuts, almonds, peanuts, or even macadamias.

4. Pour on the milk. Along with bone-building, fat-fighting calcium, you'll get blood pressure protection, too. Fat-free or 1%, chocolate, evaporated, buttermilk, lactase-loaded Lactaid®, and calcium-fortified soy milk all do the milk magic trick.

Ready to try a super cereal bowl? Here are some combinations:

- Kick-start: Kix® cereal, blueberries, toasted pecans, and 1% milk.

- Total Control: Whole Grain Total®, sliced banana, chopped walnuts, and fat-free milk.

- Get Movin': Bran Chex®, chopped prunes, sliced almonds, and Lactaid.

It's gonna be a great day!

Waffles with Autumn Sauce

When you want to get more carbs, pile on the fruits, vegetables, and whole grains and ease up on the fat. This spicy breakfast really gets the job done. As a bonus, replacing typical pancake syrup with this fruit sauce more than doubles your breakfast fiber.

2	medium apples, cored and coarsely chopped
1/4	cup of dark seedless raisins
1/2	cup of ruby red grapefruit juice blend with calcium
1/2	tsp. of pumpkin pie spice
1	tsp. of molasses
4	frozen whole-grain waffles
2	tbsp. of sunflower seeds

In a medium saucepan, combine the apples, raisins, grapefruit juice, spice, and molasses. Bring to a boil. Reduce the heat and simmer, uncovered, for 10 minutes, or until the apples are tender and the sauce is thick. Toast the waffles and place two on each of two large plates. Ladle one-fourth of the sauce onto each waffle and garnish each with sunflower seeds. Serve with glasses of cold milk.

Yield: 2 servings

Nutritional data per serving: Calories, 381; protein, 9 g; carbohydrate, 77 g; dietary fiber, 9 g; total fat, 8 g; saturated fat, 1 g; cholesterol, 5 mg; sodium, 740 mg; vitamin A, 1% of Daily Value; vitamin C, 42%; calcium, 29%; iron, 43%; vitamin B_6, 44%; vitamin E, 18%; potassium, 19%.

LUNCH BREAK

Mighty Minestrone

This is not your grandmother's soup—it takes less than 30 minutes to make! Besides being warm and zesty, this bean-filled beauty is packed with all the "hearty" ingredients your body could ever hope for. Just add a green salad and a slice of 7-grain bread for healthy perfection.

1   tbsp. of dehydrated onions
4   oz. of gemelli pasta
6   cups of water
2   cups of frozen mixed vegetables
1   can (14 $^1/_2$ oz.) of diced
      tomatoes with basil,
      garlic, and oregano
1   can (15 $^1/_2$ oz.) of red kidney
      beans, rinsed and drained
1   can (15 $^1/_2$ oz.) of chickpeas,
      rinsed and drained
1   tbsp. of olive oil

In a large pot, combine the onions, pasta, and 4 cups of the water. Bring to a boil, reduce the heat, and simmer for 8 minutes. Add the mixed vegetables, return to a simmer, and cook for 5 minutes. Add the tomatoes (with juice), kidney beans, chickpeas, oil, and the remaining 2 cups of water. Simmer for 15 minutes.

Yield: 14 servings

Nutritional data per serving: Calories, 124; protein, 5 g; carbohydrate, 23 g; dietary fiber, 5 g; total fat, 2 g; saturated fat, 0 g; cholesterol, 0 mg; sodium, 365 mg; vitamin A, 9% of Daily Value; vitamin C, 10%; calcium, 4%; iron, 9%; folate, 14%.

Grilled Swiss with Spinach and Mushrooms

Grilled cheese goes gourmet—who says great cooking has to be hard? Not me!

2   slices of rye bread
1   tbsp. of creamy dill mustard
2   thin slices (1 oz.) of reduced-fat
      Swiss cheese
$^1/_2$ cup of sliced mushrooms
$^1/_2$ cup of baby spinach, washed and
      spun dry

Heat a nonstick skillet over medium-high heat. Lightly coat one side of each slice of bread with nonstick spray. Spread the opposite sides with the mustard. On one slice of bread, layer the mustard side with one slice of the cheese, $^1/_4$ cup of the mushrooms, the spinach, the remaining $^1/_4$ cup of mushrooms, and the remaining slice of cheese. Top with the second slice of bread. Place in the skillet, cover, and reduce the heat to medium. Cook for about 3 minutes, or until the bottom is brown. Turn the sandwich, cover, and cook for 2 to 3 minutes, or until brown. Place on a plate and let cool for 1 to 2 minutes. Cut in half diagonally.

Yield: 1 serving

Nutritional data per serving: Calories, 260; protein, 14 g; carbohydrate, 37 g; dietary fiber, 4 g; total fat, 6 g; saturated fat, 1.5 g; cholesterol, 10 mg; sodium, 498 mg; vitamin A, 12% of Daily Value; vitamin C, 9%; calcium, 33%; iron, 14%; vitamin B_1 (thiamine), 20%; vitamin B_2 (riboflavin), 28%; vitamin D, 10%; vitamin E, 6%; folate, 21%; potassium, 10%.

Double Duty

Not only does olive oil replace saturated fat in the minestrone soup recipe, but it also helps your body absorb cancer-fighting lycopene from the tomatoes. It's a delicious deal!

Tuna Pita with Avocado

Tired of tuna with mayo? Try mashed avocado instead. Its rich, creamy texture adds just the right touch to a sandwich that's packed with the vitamins and minerals your body craves. And stuffing it in a whole-grain pita pocket will help keep diabetes off your family tree.

1   **can (6 oz.) of water-packed white albacore tuna, drained**
1   **avocado**
1   **lime wedge**
2   **small whole-wheat pita pockets**
2   **leaves of red-leaf lettuce**

In a small bowl, mash the tuna and avocado. Squeeze the lime over the mixture and stir until blended. Toast the pitas until puffed. Split the pitas and spread half the tuna inside each pocket. Stuff with a lettuce leaf, and enjoy!

Yield: 2 servings

Nutritional data per serving: Calories, 271; protein, 24 g; carbohydrate, 21 g; dietary fiber, 5 g; total fat, 11 g; saturated fat, 1 g; cholesterol, 36 mg; sodium, 488 mg; vitamin A, 10% of Daily Value; vitamin C, 11%; calcium, 4%; iron, 12%; vitamin B_3 (niacin), 34%; vitamin B_6, 20%; vitamin D, 34%; vitamin E, 11%; folate, 11%; magnesium, 17%; potassium, 18%; omega-3 fatty acids, 87%.

Bean Burrito with Avocado

It used to be that vegetarian meals were bland, boring, and rather blah. But these days, eating veggies doesn't have to be ho-hum. In fact, this delicious dish is really yummy and bursting with heart-healthy stuff. So don't make just one—triple or quadruple the recipe, heat up a stack of tortillas, and let everyone dig in!

1   **large corn tortilla**
$1/_8$ **avocado**
$1/_3$ **cup of cooked black beans**
2   **tbsp. of Mexican-style corn**
1   **tbsp. of sliced black olives**
2   **tsp. of mild chipotle taco sauce**

On a paper plate, microwave the tortilla on high for 20 to 30 seconds, or until warm. Mash the avocado in the center of the top half of the tortilla. Top with the beans, corn, olives, and sauce. Fold the bottom half of the tortilla over the top half. Fold in the sides, then fold in half.

Yield: 1 serving

Nutritional data per serving: Calories, 305; protein, 11 g; carbohydrate, 48 g; dietary fiber, 7 g; total fat, 9 g; saturated fat, 1.5 g; cholesterol, 0 mg; sodium, 679 mg; vitamin A, 2% of Daily Value; vitamin C, 5%; calcium, 12%; iron, 16%; folate, 26%; omega-3 fatty acids, 12%.

Did You Know?

A whole-wheat pita delivers four times the fiber, three times the magnesium, twice the zinc, and more heart-smart vitamin E and potassium than a white pita. A real nutritional bargain!

SUPPER'S READY!

Beans 'n Greens 'n Pasta

Here's a simple supper using leftovers from a too-large restaurant meal. But you don't need restaurant leftovers to make this dish. Just use frozen mixed greens and canned beans instead.

1	**cup of cooked pasta**
¹/₂	**cup of cooked greens (such as collards, spinach, or kale)**
1	**cup of cooked dried or rinsed and drained canned cannellini beans**
2	**tbsp. of olive oil**
2	**tbsp. of freshly shredded Parmesan cheese**
	Salt and freshly ground black pepper to taste

Place the pasta in a medium bowl. In a nonstick skillet, sauté the greens and beans in the oil until heated through. Ladle over the pasta. Sprinkle with the cheese, salt, and pepper.

Yield: 1 serving

Nutritional data per serving: Calories, 496; protein, 15 g; carbohydrate, 40 g; dietary fiber, 5 g; total fat, 32 g; saturated fat, 6 g; cholesterol, 9 mg; sodium, 312 mg; vitamin A, 124% of Daily Value; vitamin C, 59%; calcium, 35%; iron, 31%; folate, 55%.

See What I Mean?

Certainly, spinach is the vanguard of vision protection. It also builds bone and helps blood clot properly, so serve this salad often.

Talkin' Turkey Tacos

I really love meat. But fatty meats can drive up cholesterol and clog my arteries. So in the interest of protecting my heart, my wife Shirley has started talking turkey to me. Why? Because ground turkey breast is heart-healthy and nearly fat-free.

1	**lb. of ground turkey breast**
1	**small onion, chopped**
1	**tsp. of olive oil**
³/₄	**cup of Taco Bell Pour 'n Simmer Taco Seasoning Sauce®**
4	**oz. of shredded reduced-fat four-cheese blend**
2	**medium tomatoes, chopped**
2 ¹/₂	**cups of shredded iceberg and romaine lettuce**
1	**avocado, chopped**
10	**soft taco shells (small tortillas)**

In a large nonstick skillet over medium-high heat, brown the turkey and onion in the oil. Stir in the sauce and simmer for about 3 minutes. Place in a serving bowl and keep warm. Meanwhile, place the cheese, tomatoes, lettuce, and avocado in individual serving bowls. Wrap the taco shells in plastic wrap and microwave on high for 1 minute, or until warm. Place on a serving platter, then step back and let everyone create their own special tacos.

Yield: 10 servings

Nutritional data per serving: Calories, 204; protein, 19 g; carbohydrate, 18 g; dietary fiber, 4 g; total fat, 6 g; saturated fat, 2 g; cholesterol, 42 mg; sodium, 351 mg; vitamin A, 4% of Daily Value; vitamin C, 15%; calcium, 14%; iron, 10%; vitamin B_3 (niacin), 20%; vitamin B_6, 17%; folate, 12%; potassium, 10%.

SUPER SIDES

Spinach Asiago

Quick as a wink, you can serve up this colorful side dish that's pretty to look at and offers powerful protection for your eyes—not to mention that spinach also serves up hefty doses of folate and vitamin E to safeguard your heart.

1   bag (10 oz.) of baby spinach, washed but not dried
1/8   tsp. of salt
      Freshly ground black pepper to taste
1/2   yellow bell pepper, thinly sliced into 1-in. strips
2   tbsp. of shredded Asiago cheese

In a large, deep skillet over high heat, sprinkle the wet spinach with the salt and black pepper. Top with the yellow pepper. Cover and bring to a boil. Reduce the heat to medium and steam for about 5 minutes, stirring occasionally, until the spinach is wilted and the peppers are crisp-tender. Spoon into a serving bowl and garnish with the cheese.

Yield: 4 servings

Nutritional data per serving: Calories, 40; protein, 4 g; carbohydrate, 5 g; dietary fiber, 3 g; total fat, 1 g; saturated fat, <1 g; cholesterol, 3 mg; sodium, 92 mg; vitamin A, 62% of Daily Value; vitamin C, 98%; calcium, 12%; iron, 14%; folate, 32%; vitamin E, 10%; magnesium, 20%; potassium, 16%; omega-3 fatty acids, 12%.

Berry Memorable Spinach

You can balance the often-bitter taste of spinach by simply stirring in a sweet, flavorful fruit. Just about anything goes. You can try blueberries, strawberries, oranges, cranberries, or mangoes when they're in season. Otherwise, out of season, you can substitute frozen spinach and frozen fruit for the fresh stuff.

1   bag (10 oz.) of fresh spinach, washed, with heavy stems removed
1/4   tsp. of salt
1   tsp. of butter
1/2   cup of fresh blueberries, washed and patted dry
1   tbsp. of toasted pine nuts

Place the spinach in a deep, heavy saucepan with just the water that clings to the leaves after washing. Sprinkle with the salt. Cover and bring to a boil. Reduce the heat and cook for 5 minutes, stirring occasionally, until wilted. Drain, place in a serving bowl, and toss with the butter. Stir in the blueberries and garnish with the pine nuts.

Yield: 4 servings

Nutritional data per serving: Calories, 43; protein, 2 g; carbohydrate, 5 g; dietary fiber, 2 g; total fat, 2 g; saturated fat, <1 g; cholesterol, 3 mg; sodium, 201 mg; vitamin A, 39% of Daily Value; vitamin C, 31%; calcium, 6%; iron, 10%; vitamin E, 7%; folate, 28%; vitamin K, 284%; potassium, 10%.

Autumn Harvest Applesauce

Try a heaping spoonful of this spicy fruit treat topping on pancakes or waffles.

- 4 **large Red Delicious apples, washed, cored, and cut into chunks**
- 4 **large Bosc pears, washed, cored, and thinly sliced**
- 1 **cup of fresh cranberries, washed and sorted**
- 1/2 **cup of coarsely chopped walnuts**
- 1 **tsp. of pumpkin pie spice**
- 1/2 **cup of water**

In a heavy saucepan, combine all the ingredients. Cover and bring to a boil. Reduce the heat to low and simmer, stirring occasionally, for about 15 minutes, or until the apples and pears are fork-tender.

Yield: 8 servings

Nutritional data per serving: Calories, 170; protein, 2 g; carbohydrate, 32 g; dietary fiber, 6 g; total fat, 6 g; saturated fat, <1 g; cholesterol, 0 mg; sodium, 0 mg; vitamin A, 1% of Daily Value; vitamin C, 19%; calcium, 3%; iron, 4%; potassium, 8%.

Sesame Spinach Salad

The eyes have it when it comes to this ultra-simple but simply delicious salad.

- 10 **oz. of spinach**
- 1 **can (8 oz.) of sliced water chestnuts, rinsed and drained**
- 1/2 **cup of Asian-style dressing with ginger and sesame**
- 1 **tbsp. of toasted sesame seeds**

Wash the spinach and spin dry. Remove the heavy stems and tear the leaves into bite-size

SALAD SMARTS

Apple and Orange Kohl Slaw

Turn almost any cabbagey vegetable into "cole" slaw.

- 2 **cups of shredded peeled kohlrabi**
- 2 **cups of shredded peeled Fuji apples**
- 1/4 **cup of orange juice**
- 1 **tbsp. of walnut oil**
- 1/4 **cup of orange-flavored dried cranberries**
- 2 **tbsp. of coarsely broken walnuts**
- 1/4 **tsp. of salt**
  Freshly ground black pepper to taste

In a medium bowl, combine the kohlrabi, apples, and orange juice. Stir well to blend. Add the oil, cranberries, walnuts, salt, and pepper. Refrigerate until ready to serve.

Yield: 6 servings

Nutritional data per serving: Calories, 95; protein, 1 g; carbohydrate, 15 g; dietary fiber, 4 g; total fat, 4 g; saturated fat, 0 g; cholesterol, 0 mg; sodium, 106 mg; vitamin A, 1% of Daily Value; vitamin C, 55%; calcium, 1%; iron, 2%; copper, 5%; potassium, 7%; omega-3 fatty acids, 48%.

pieces. In a large salad bowl, combine the spinach, water chestnuts, and dressing. Toss until well coated and sprinkle with the sesame seeds.

Yield: 12 servings

Nutritional data per serving: Calories, 15; protein, 1 g; carbohydrate, 4 g; dietary fiber, 1 g; total fat, 2 g; saturated fat, 0 g; cholesterol, 0 mg; sodium, 175 mg; vitamin A, 20% of Daily Value; vitamin C, 14%; calcium, 0%; iron, 17%; vitamin E, 3%; folate, 15%; potassium, 5%; omega-3 fatty acids, 4%.

Three-Bean Slaw

The sweet slaw dressing in this salad will help you entice reluctant vegetable eaters. Try it on your hang-back family and friends.

2   **cups of shredded red cabbage**
2   **cups of shredded green cabbage**
1   **cup of shredded carrots**
1   **cup of rinsed and drained canned black beans**
1   **cup of rinsed and drained canned pinto beans**
1   **cup of rinsed and drained canned chickpeas**
1   **cup of well-drained juice-packed crushed pineapple**
$^1/_3$ **cup of apple cider vinegar**
$^1/_3$ **cup of sugar**
$^2/_3$ **cup of low-fat mayonnaise**
    Salt and freshly ground black pepper to taste

In a large bowl, combine the red and green cabbage, carrots, black beans, pinto beans, chickpeas, and pineapple. Set aside. In a small bowl, combine the vinegar, sugar, mayonnaise, salt, and pepper. Use a wire whisk to blend into a smooth sauce. Pour the dressing over the vegetables. Refrigerate for 4 hours or overnight to let the flavors blend.

Yield: 16 servings

Nutritional data per serving: Calories, 91; protein, 3 g; carbohydrate, 18 g; dietary fiber, 3 g; total fat, 1 g; saturated fat, 0 g; cholesterol, 0 mg; sodium, 321 mg; vitamin A, 20% of Daily Value; vitamin C, 21%; calcium, 3%; iron, 5%; folate, 7%; potassium, 5%.

Pumpkin-Seed Salad

In any other book, you'd find a spinach salad packed with bacon and eggs. But not in this one! We're going for more veggies and fruits—and pumpkin seeds for a totally awesome taste.

4   **cups of baby spinach, washed and spun dry**
2   **cups of red bell pepper chunks**
2   **tsp. of olive oil**
2   **tsp. of red wine vinegar**
    Salt and freshly ground black pepper to taste
$^1/_2$ **cup of fresh pineapple chunks**
2   **tbsp. of hulled pumpkin seeds**

In a large salad bowl, combine the spinach and peppers. Add the oil, vinegar, salt, and pepper and toss until well blended. Garnish with the pineapple and sprinkle with the pumpkin seeds.

Yield: 4 servings

Nutritional data per serving: Calories, 99; protein, 3 g; carbohydrate, 13 g; dietary fiber, 3 g; total fat, 4 g; saturated fat, 1 g; cholesterol, 0 mg; sodium, 27 mg; vitamin A, 63% of Daily Value; vitamin C, 255%; calcium, 4%; iron, 9%; vitamin B$_6$, 13%; vitamin E, 7%; folate, 19%; magnesium, 15%; potassium, 12%.

Food for Thought

When you add crunch to your salad with pumpkin seeds instead of croutons, you boost the trace minerals magnesium, potassium, copper, and zinc. So seize the seeds!

Four-Bean Tossed Greens

In addition to just tasting so darn good, this salad sneaks in a boost of folate, which is crucial for the development of new body tissue and is a nutrient that is especially important for pregnant women. So go ahead and enjoy this tasty salad—whether you're pregnant or otherwise!

1	cup of rinsed and drained canned red kidney beans
1	cup of rinsed and drained canned chickpeas
1	cup of rinsed and drained canned soybeans
1	cup of rinsed and drained canned black beans
1	cup of canned or frozen yellow corn
2	tbsp. of light ranch dressing
$^1/_2$	cup of sliced celery
$^1/_2$	cup of diced red bell peppers
4	cups of mixed salad greens
2	tbsp. of light vinaigrette dressing

In a medium bowl, combine the kidney beans, chickpeas, soybeans, black beans, corn, and ranch dressing. Stir until well mixed. Set aside. In another medium bowl, combine the celery, peppers, greens, and vinaigrette dressing. Toss until well coated. Divide the salad mixture among four luncheon plates. Pile equal portions of the beans on top of the greens. Serve with hot rolls and cold white wine.

Yield: 4 servings

Nutritional data per serving: Calories, 356; protein, 20 g; carbohydrate, 50 g; dietary fiber, 14 g; total fat, 10 g; saturated fat, 1 g; cholesterol, 2 mg; sodium, 1,022 mg; vitamin A, 27% of Daily Value; vitamin C, 87%; calcium, 15%; iron, 33%; folate, 54%; potassium, 28%.

MUNCH ON THIS

California Guacamole

Those Californians—they always seem to get it right before the rest of us. And whether it's a Super Bowl party or a quiet dinner on the deck, their guacamole with chips really hits the spot. This healthier version, sans mayo, is compliments of the California Avocado Commission. It packs the kind of fat your heart adores. So love it, and don't leave it!

2	ripe California avocados
3	tbsp. of fresh lemon juice
$^1/_2$	cup of diced onions
3	tbsp. of chopped tomatoes
$^1/_2$	tsp. of salt
2	tbsp. of minced fresh cilantro

Cut the avocados in half, remove the pits, and scoop out the pulp. In a medium bowl, drizzle the avocados with the lemon juice, then mash. Add the onions, tomatoes, salt, and cilantro and stir until blended. Serve with baked tortilla chips.

Yield: 12 servings

Nutritional data per serving: Calories, 55; protein, <1 g; carbohydrate, 3 g; dietary fiber, 2 g; total fat, 5 g; saturated fat, <1 g; cholesterol, 0 mg; sodium, 101 mg; vitamin A, 2% of Daily Value; vitamin C, 8%; calcium, 1%; iron, 2%; vitamin B_6, 5%; vitamin E, 2%; folate, 5%; potassium, 6%.

Quick Trick

Need chips? Stack 10 corn tortillas and, using a sharp chef's knife, cut them into sixths. Spread in a single layer on cookie sheets, and mist lightly with olive oil spray. Bake at 450°F for 5 minutes, or until crisp and beginning to brown.

Cheese 'n Garlic Popcorn

Believe it or not, popcorn, because it uses the entire corn kernel, is a whole grain. Whoopee! But how do you get from a heart stopper loaded with salt and butter to a lip-smackin', finger-lickin', heart-lovin' treat? It's easy. Just do as I do and whip up a batch of this delicious snack whenever guests arrive, or just to serve to the family while you're enjoying that late-night movie. I guarantee that you'll end up eating the healthiest popcorn in town.

- $^1/_2$ **cup of popping corn**
- 1 **tbsp. of olive oil**
- 1 **tsp. of garlic powder**
- 2 **tbsp. of grated Parmesan cheese**

Preheat an air popper by plugging it in and letting it run for about 3 minutes. Add the popcorn and pop it into a large bowl. Place the oil in a mister and mist the popcorn, tossing constantly to coat. Sprinkle with the garlic powder and cheese and toss again. Then dig in!

Yield: 4 servings

Nutritional data per serving: Calories, 136; protein, 4 g; carbohydrate, 19 g; dietary fiber, 3 g; total fat, 6 g; saturated fat, 1 g; cholesterol, 2 mg; sodium, 58 mg; vitamin A, 1% of Daily Value; vitamin C, 0%; calcium, 4%; iron, 3%; vitamin B$_1$ (thiamine), 8%; vitamin E, 2%; potassium, 2%.

Fantastico Olive Oil Dip

Mangia…pane e olio d'oliva…'e fantastico!— "Eat bread with olive oil…it's fantastic!" Some folks like to dip their fresh bread in plain olive oil, but I prefer this extra-savory version. By the way, when you dip into olive oil instead of slathering your bread with butter, you get one-quarter of the saturated fat and eight times the vitamin E. Be still, my heart!

- 1 **cup of extra-virgin olive oil**
- 1 **tsp. of dried basil**
- $^1/_2$ **tsp. of crushed red pepper**
- $^1/_4$ **tsp. of dried oregano**
- $^1/_2$ **tsp. of salt**
- 1 **garlic clove, pressed**

In a cruet with a stopper or other container with a tight-fitting lid, combine the oil, basil, pepper, oregano, salt, and garlic. Refrigerate overnight or longer. At mealtime, pour a small amount of the flavored oil into a dipping dish. Return the cruet to the refrigerator. (Discard any leftover room-temperature oil.) Serve with crusty Italian bread.

Yield: 48 servings

Nutritional data per serving: Calories, 40; protein, 0 g; carbohydrate, 0 g; dietary fiber, 0 g; total fat, 4.5 g; saturated fat, <1 g; cholesterol, 0 mg; sodium, 24 mg; vitamin A, 0% of Daily Value; vitamin C, 0%; calcium, 0%; iron, 0%; vitamin E, 3%; omega-3 fatty acids, 3%.

The Inside Skinny

Misto® and other brands of oil sprayers are available at kitchenware stores. You fill them with the kind of oil you like, then get a little exercise pumping up the pressure to create a nonaerosol spray that's perfect for spritzing on salads, popcorn, you name it.

I'LL DRINK TO THAT!

Top-Shelf Smoothie

Just when I think there's nothing good left in the house to eat, I remember my top shelf, where I stash a few nutritional nuggets for safekeeping. Here's what I usually find.

1   box (8 oz.) of orange juice
1/3   cup of nonfat dry milk
1   tbsp. of chocolate-hazelnut spread
1   tbsp. of unsweetened cocoa
         powder

In a blender, combine the orange juice, dry milk, chocolate spread, and cocoa. Blend until smooth and creamy. Pour over ice for a tasty afternoon pick-me-up.

Yield: 2 servings

Nutritional data per serving: Calories, 287; protein, 13 g; carbohydrate, 46 g; dietary fiber, 3 g; total fat, 8 g; saturated fat, 2 g; cholesterol, 5 mg; sodium, 136 mg; vitamin A, 14% of Daily Value; vitamin C, 270%; calcium, 37%; iron, 8%; folate, 12%; potassium, 22%.

Apple Pie Sipper

Mmm...smell the cinnamon. Yum. It's enough to tempt even the crankiest tummy into enjoying a little liquid refreshment. And in addition to taming your tummy, the insoluble fiber in applesauce helps lower your cholesterol.

1   cup of Stonyfield® fat-free plain
         yogurt
1   cup of natural berry-flavored
         applesauce
2   tbsp. of apple jelly
1/2   tsp. of ground cinnamon

In a blender, combine the yogurt, applesauce, jelly, and cinnamon. Blend on high for about 1 minute, or until well blended. Pour into a 16-ounce glass and sip through a straw.

Yield: 1 serving

Nutritional data per serving: Calories, 328; protein, 8 g; carbohydrate, 56 g; dietary fiber, 3 g; total fat, 0 g; saturated fat, 0 g; cholesterol, 0 mg; sodium, 150 mg; vitamin A, 1% of Daily Value; vitamin C, 92%; calcium, 47%; iron, 4%; potassium, 6%.

Blueberry-Basil Smoothie

In the heat of July, try to remember to whirl up this cold and creamy treat. The basil gives it just a hint of something different. See if your friends can identify your secret ingredient.

1   cup of Stonyfield® fat-free
         blueberry yogurt
1   cup of fresh blueberries, washed
         and patted dry
1/2   tsp. of dried basil
1   sprig of fresh basil

In a blender, combine the yogurt, blueberries, and dried basil. Blend on high until thick and smooth. Pour into tall glasses and garnish with the fresh basil.

Yield: 1 serving

Nutritional data per serving: Calories, 243; protein, 9 g; carbohydrate, 52 g; dietary fiber, 4 g; total fat, <1 g; saturated fat, 0 g; cholesterol, 0 mg; sodium, 134 mg; vitamin A, 2% of Daily Value; vitamin C, 37%; calcium, 47%; iron, 5%; vitamin E, 7%.

JUST DESSERTS

Chocolate-Walnut Pudding

When I was a little kid, my favorite Easter treat was a chocolate fudge egg surrounded by walnuts. Only one store made it, and it is long since gone. But I still love that chocolate-walnut taste. Here's a quick little dessert that brings back those flavorful memories.

1   box (3.4 oz.) of instant chocolate pudding mix
2   cups of fat-free milk
1   tbsp. of walnut oil
1/4   cup of chopped walnuts
4   walnut halves

In a small bowl, combine the pudding mix, milk, oil, and chopped walnuts. With an electric mixer on low speed, beat for 2 minutes. Spoon into four small custard cups and top each with a walnut half. Refrigerate until ready to serve.

Yield: 4 servings

Nutritional data per serving: Calories, 210; protein, 6 g; carbohydrate, 29 g; dietary fiber, 1 g; total fat, 9 g; saturated fat, 1 g; cholesterol, 2 mg; sodium, 417 mg; vitamin A, 8% of Daily Value; vitamin C, 2%; calcium, 16%; iron, 4%; vitamin B$_2$ (riboflavin), 12%; vitamin D, 12%; folate 4%; omega-3 fatty acids, 104%.

Pink Sunset Parfait

Here's a feast for your eyes as well as your palate—and a great ending for a light supper.

1   cup of fat-free raspberry frozen yogurt
1   cup of mango sorbet
6   oz. of fresh raspberries, washed and dried
6   tsp. of Hershey's® chocolate syrup
2   tbsp. of whipped cream
2   tsp. of finely chopped walnuts

Let the yogurt and sorbet stand for about 5 minutes, or until slightly softened. In each of two parfait glasses, place a spoonful of yogurt, then a spoonful of sorbet, a few raspberries, and 1 teaspoon of the chocolate syrup. Repeat twice, using all the yogurt, sorbet, raspberries, and syrup. Top each parfait with 1 tablespoon of the whipped cream and garnish with 1 teaspoon of the walnuts. Serve with an iced-tea spoon.

Yield: 2 servings

Nutritional data per serving: Calories, 334; protein, 7 g; carbohydrate, 73 g; dietary fiber, 7 g; total fat, 3 g; saturated fat, <1 g; cholesterol, 4 mg; sodium, 79 mg; vitamin A, 22% of Daily Value; vitamin C, 57%; calcium, 20%; iron, 5%; vitamin B$_2$ (riboflavin), 17%; folate, 9%; magnesium, 9%; potassium, 10%; omega-3 fatty acids, 33%.

Mini Banana Split

Nothing speaks to me of utter indulgence like a banana split. But who can take all those calories? Here's a mini version, with all the fabulous flavors packed into one small serving.

1	**finger banana**
$^1/_2$	**cup of fat-free vanilla frozen yogurt**
2	**fresh strawberries, thinly sliced**
2	**tbsp. of fresh pineapple**
1	**tbsp. of Hershey's® chocolate syrup**
1	**tbsp. of toasted chopped walnuts**
1	**tbsp. of whipped cream**

Peel the banana, halve lengthwise, and arrange in a large dessert dish. Scoop the frozen yogurt between the halves. Surround with the strawberries and pineapple, and drizzle the chocolate syrup over everything. Garnish with the walnuts and whipped cream.

Yield: 1 serving

Nutritional data per serving: Calories, 272; protein, 6 g; carbohydrate, 50 g; dietary fiber, 4 g; total fat, 6 g; saturated fat, 1 g; cholesterol, 3 mg; sodium, 61 mg; vitamin A, 1% of Daily Value; vitamin C, 64%; calcium, 33%; iron, 5%; vitamin B_6, 19%; folate, 7%; magnesium, 9%; potassium, 10%; omega-3 fatty acids, 76%.

Blue Moon Fruit Sauce with Frozen Yogurt

I just love Bing cherries, and I usually eat them out of hand. But once in a blue moon, I split them and pit them and serve them to my family and friends over frozen yogurt. My guests are always grateful!

20	**large Bing cherries**
1	**cup of fresh blueberries, washed and patted dry**
1	**cup of fat-free plain yogurt**
2	**tbsp. of seedless black raspberry preserves**
2	**cups of fat-free raspberry frozen yogurt**

Halve the cherries and remove the pits. In a small bowl, combine the cherries and blueberries. In another small bowl, combine the yogurt and preserves. Stir until well mixed and the color is even. Pour over the fruit and stir until well blended. Divide the frozen yogurt among four dessert dishes and spoon one-fourth of the sauce over each.

Yield: 4 servings

Nutritional data per serving: Calories, 183; protein, 7 g; carbohydrate, 38 g; dietary fiber, 2 g; total fat, <1 g; saturated fat, 0 g; cholesterol, 1 mg; sodium, 96 mg; vitamin A, 1% of Daily Value; vitamin C, 13%; calcium, 43%; iron, 2%; potassium, 8%.

Cherry-Chocolate Freeze

Craving chocolate? Here's a healthy indulgence.

1	**cup of fat-free chocolate milk**
1	**cup of frozen pitted dark red cherries (or pitted water-packed canned cherries)**
1	**cup of ice cubes**
2	**tbsp. of unsweetened cocoa powder**

In a blender, combine the milk, cherries, ice, and cocoa. Blend on high until thick and smooth. Pour into a frosty glass and drink with a straw.

Yield: 2 servings

Nutritional data per serving: Calories, 134; protein, 6 g; carbohydrate, 24 g; dietary fiber, 3 g; total fat, 2 g; saturated fat, 1 g; vitamin A, 14% of Daily Value; vitamin C, 4%; calcium, 16%; iron, 16%; vitamin B_2 (riboflavin), 16%; potassium, 16%.

CHAPTER 9

Get Well Soon!

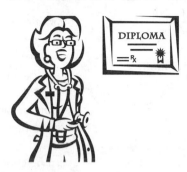

Eating right and getting plenty of exercise are certainly two
of the top ways you can stay happy and healthy. But there
are other factors that can sneak up on you and come into play,
too, which can sabotage all of your good efforts. Stress and lack of
sleep are two such "intruders," and there are plenty more. In this
chapter, I'll share my best secrets on how you can fend them off.

SIDESTEP STRESS

We hear so much about stress these days—and for good reason. As a nation, we're enduring more of it than ever before, and we're learning that ongoing stress can wreck our health. Stress triggers a flood of adrenaline and cortisol, the "fight-or-flight" hormones that quicken your breathing, speed up your heart rate, and tighten up your muscles. That's great when there's a real threat, but in everyday life, unrelieved stress can contribute to accelerated aging, higher blood pressure, foggier memories, bluer moods, and conditions ranging from arthritis to psoriasis. Heck,

the overproduction of cortisol itself may even predispose you to disease because it weakens your immune system. In the short term, stress can cause headaches, digestive problems, eating disorders, and insomnia, and lower your resistance to colds and flu. Need any more reasons to de-stress? I didn't think so. Read on for ways to reduce the stress in your life.

Keep It Under Control

Unfortunately, when under a lot of stress, many folks resort to smoking, drinking, drugs, overeating, self-pity—behaviors that cause *even more* stress to our bodies and minds. Talk about a double whammy! The best "vaccine" against stress is regular exercise, mind-body techniques such as yoga (studies show that a single 50-minute session can lower cortisol levels), and socializing with friends and loved ones. But even seemingly minor, quickie stress busters also offer protection. The idea behind all stress-management tips and techniques is to help you gain a sense of control, because when you feel more in control, you're more immune to future stress. Here are a few easy ways to minimize stress and maximize your sense of control:

Breathe easy. Don't fume when you're in that traffic jam or at the end of a long line at the bank. Instead, take slow, deep breaths and focus on the sensation (called mindful breathing). This easy-to-do technique can lower your heart rate and reduce other harmful effects of stress hormones.

Share a moment with Fido. If you can't sit with the Dalai Lama, being in the room with your golden retriever may be the next best thing. Studies have shown that pets serve as a buffer against acute stress and make you feel less hassled—even more so than being in the presence of a spouse or close friend. One reason: Pets neither judge nor evaluate you.

Commune with nature. As we gardeners know, being outdoors is enjoyable and calming. Now we know why: Researchers believe that biochemical pathways in the brain may respond positively to contact with nature. The interesting part is that you don't even have to be outside! Strolling through a warm, aromatic greenhouse, or simply admiring your neighbor's lawn or the park across the street through the nearest window can do the trick.

Pinch yourself. Once or twice daily, press firmly on the fibrous spot between your thumb and index finger, about an inch from the edge of the web. This acupressure point corresponds to the large intestine, and pinching it may help tone your exhausted adrenals and improve your ability to handle stress.

Play at your desk. Experts say that the major source of stress for adults is workplace pressure, and we may do well to revive certain kindergarten pastimes. Stock your pencil holder with colored pens, for instance, and when you're jotting down notes or thoughts, do it in, say, purple—and keep scribbling/coloring if you have the time and the privacy. Even this little throwback to childhood can help release tension and have a deeply calming effect.

Munch on schisandra. Ongoing stress can wear out your adrenal glands. Schisandra, an herb available at health-food stores, can help perk them up like a jolt of java, but without the jittery side effects. Chew 1 teaspoon of berries

HOME REMEDY

When your blood boils, do your teeth clench tighter than a clamshell? If so, then you're just spreading more tension down into your neck and shoulders. Here's an easy exercise to help you loosen up. Take a deep breath, and drop your jaw. Next, open your mouth and exhale with a long *haaaaaaa* sound. Finally, gently close your lips. Feel the difference? Repeat this exercise throughout the day and soon you'll be able to stop that jaw-busting clench before it starts!

twice daily, sip 2 cups of tea per day, or add 15 to 25 drops of tincture to a glass of water and drink it daily. *Caution:* Don't use schisandra if you're pregnant.

Get Your B's

If your life is in overdrive, it's vital to include fish, milk, beans, peas, whole grains, broccoli, cauliflower, and kale in your diet. These foods all provide a bushel full of pantothenic acid, which is critical for keeping your adrenal glands up to snuff when they may be maxed out. (Not to mention, they're darned good for you, too!) To be on the safe side, supplement daily with a B-complex vitamin that contains 50 milligrams of pantothenic acid.

Think Happy Thoughts

What you tell yourself can absolutely add to your stress level. For instance, the next time you hear yourself saying, "I can't handle this," take a deep, calming breath and swiftly replace that thought with this one: "I am strong, I am in control, and I *am* handling this." Two more ways to calm down:

- Hug someone. Studies show this can help you remain calm during a chaotic day. Just be sure to ask permission first.

- Go ahead, be a crybaby. Believe it or not, having a good cry can reduce your body's levels of stress hormones.

Ease with Teas

Sipping a cup of herbal tea helps you de-stress in two ways. First, you get the calming power of the herbs themselves, and second, you force your body into a relaxing state by sitting down with the warm brew. Some of my favorite ideas for a calming cuppa are:

Black tea. Recent reports indicate that drinking black tea can help speed recovery from stress. It brings cortisol (the stress hormone) levels back to normal, thus minimizing the harmful effects of stress.

Kava. A favorite among herbalists and natural medicine doctors as an antianxiety herb, kava works gently to naturally relax your nervous system and calm you down. While kava has been used safely for centuries, experts say it's not for you if you have liver problems or if you're taking any drugs that could have an effect on your liver. Go the safe route and check with your doctor before trying kava or any other natural remedy.

If you'd like to give kava a try, here's how: Grate 1 to 2 teaspoons of dried kava root into a cup of boiling water. Cover, then let it steep for a good hour. Strain, and then sip up to 2 cups a day. But be forewarned: Kava is mighty bitter-tasting. For most folks, it takes a while to acquire a taste for kava, so you may want to add some honey to your tea.

Passionflower. One of Mother Nature's best tranquilizers, this herb contains alkaloids and flavonoids that deliver sedating effects— making passionflower the perfect herb to rescue you when you're feeling anxious or stressed. In addition, passionflower's natural calming ability comes without the "narcotic" hangover that's commonly associated with prescription tranquilizers, so you can have your tea as a nightcap and still wake up refreshed. The leaf, stem, or vine of passionflower can be used when brewing a tea. Just steep 1 or 2 teaspoons of the dried herb in a cup of boiling water. Wait about 20 minutes, then strain out the herbs before drinking slowly.

Soothe Sense-ibly

Your senses can be some of your most powerful weapons against stress. It's fairly simple to use sight, sound, and smell to tame tension:

- Close your eyes and picture yourself in your favorite relaxing scenario. This is called visualization, and it's a proven technique to reverse the body's stress response.

- A recent study showed that listening to classical or soft and slow music for 30 minutes produced calming effects equivalent to a 10-milligram dose of Valium. So chill out with your favorite calming tunes.

- Researchers reported that a majority of 100 women who took scented baths not only felt more relaxed, but were more relaxed than those who took unscented ones. Another recent study found that the smell of vanilla made folks feel the most relaxed.

Feed Your Calm

Stay away from those traditional "comfort" foods like macaroni and cheese, pizza, French fries, and ice cream in stressful times. They're high in fat and calories and are the worst choices because they'll make you feel lethargic and less able to deal with stress. Here's what you need to eat to beat stress:

- High-fiber, carbohydrate-rich foods like baked sweet potatoes, lentil soup, and sautéed vegetables over rice will cause your brain to produce more serotonin (that feel-good hormone), but won't sap your energy the way a mound of mashed potatoes will.

- Get your daily requirement of calcium (1,000 to 1,500 milligrams, depending on your age) either in supplement form, or through dairy or fortified foods. Calcium will halt the hormones

---

FAST FORMULA

Soothing Soaker

A hot bath is a super stress buster. Make it milky and fragrant, and you're in heaven! When you're tired and irritated, try this simple soother.

2 cups of nonfat dry milk
1 cup of cornstarch
1 tbsp. of your favorite scented oil

Mix up all the ingredients in an old blender. Add ¹/₂ cup of the mixture to your bathwater, sink into the tub, and relax. The remaining mixture can be stored in an airtight container at room temperature until your next stress-induced emergency.

---

that cause stress symptoms, especially during PMS, when levels of these hormones tend to be elevated.

- Include plenty of whole grains, beans, vegetables, nuts, and seeds in your daily diet. They contain magnesium, which you need to combat stress. If you can't fill up on magnesium-rich foods, be sure to take your daily multivitamin.

- Omega-3 fatty acids—the "good" fats found in salmon, sardines, walnuts, and flaxseed—help your nervous system function properly. One of those fats, DHA, is especially helpful in reducing various types of stress. Added benefits of omega-3s are shiny hair, strong nails, and healthy-looking skin. Aim for two 3-ounce servings of fish portions each week. If you're just not fond of fish, and you're not taking blood-thinning medications, take fish-oil capsules instead.

GET YOUR Z'S!

If you're like me and lots of other Americans, there are days when you're running on empty because of a bad night's sleep. Now we all know how much better we feel when we get those z's, but here's the WHY of it all: The proper amount of shut-eye helps us maintain a healthy heart and immune system, keeps stress and weight under control, and enhances physical and mental performance. But before you go to your doctor begging for sleep medication, I'm here to tell you that changing some daytime behaviors and thoughts can often help you take back the night. And it can be more effective than any knockout pill on the market. So if you need a good night's sleep, try some of these tips.

Knock Yourself Out

It should go without saying that physical activity during the day will help you sleep better at night. Exercise reduces stress and induces sleep by depleting stimulating chemicals, such as epinephrine. Exercise also helps you sleep longer and fall asleep faster. Even a brisk walk before dinner can make a big difference in how you sleep at night.

Lull Yourself with Lavender

Lavender has long been used as a sleep aid. Some people spray their sheets and pillowcases with lavender scent; others tuck a dried lavender sachet into their pillowcase. Another way to inhale lavender's calming fragrance is to use a bedside essential-oil diffuser. It mists the room with sweet-smelling, calming lavender, which may help you sleep longer and more soundly. You can buy diffusers from natural products companies and some health-food stores.

Stay Off Stimulants

If you want to get to sleep—and stay asleep—cut out all caffeine after 6 p.m. (make that noon if even a spoonful of cappuccino yogurt revs up your engines). And skip the nightcap; alcohol may make you sleepy, but it will wake you up later. Another piece of sound-sleeping advice: Pass up the late-night news and opt for something more soothing, like listening to classical music.

Get in a Rut

A good one, that is! Start going to bed at the same time every night and getting up at the same time every morning, even on weekends. This will set your sleep clock (circadian rhythms), so your body will know when it's time to go to sleep. How much sleep is enough? The experts say to aim for seven to eight hours.

Work Out Early

Exercise can release tension and help you sleep more soundly, but there is a downside—it will keep you too stimulated if you exercise within three hours of bedtime. Working out five hours before you hit the sack is ideal.

Ouch, That Hurts!

We all assume that as we age, we naturally need less sleep. Well, that's just not true. The real reason older people often sleep less is that they have more medical conditions, like arthritis, that keep them awake. So don't be a stiff-upper-lipper when it comes to pain. To prevent those aches and pains from keeping you up at all hours, talk to your doctor—and then do something about it!

Know Your Type

A morning person goes to sleep relatively early in the evening, wakes up early, and is most effective doing complex tasks in the morning, rather than in the evening. An evening person goes to bed later, gets up later, and is slower coming to full horsepower. He or she does better at complex tasks in the evening, rather than in the morning. If insomnia is a major part of your life, the odds are good that you're fighting your natural sleep type. Just decide which type of person you are and readjust your daily priorities, so that complex tasks are scheduled for the proper time slot. Sleep will soon follow.

Let Darkness Prevail

Your body needs darkness to trigger its sleep cycle. So if you have a big streetlight shining in the window, or if you have to sleep during the day because you're on night shift, close the blinds or pull opaque drapes across your window. That way, the light won't get through.

Soothing Sounds

Make a tape of whatever sounds help your body relax and calm your mind. Then play it just as you turn out the lights.

Get a Live Security Blanket

Many people sleep with their pets, and some say it's like curling up with a security blanket. They know that should anything go wrong during the night while they're asleep, the dog or cat will alert them. This makes them relaxed when they go to bed, and thus primed for sleep.

Time Your Bath

Soaking in a warm bath for 30 minutes raises

FAST FORMULA

Dreamy Dream Maker

If you find yourself unable to get a good night's sleep because something is weighing heavily on your mind, try this helpful herbal nightcap.

1 oz. of passionflower tincture
1 oz. of catnip tincture
1 oz. of hops tincture
1 oz. of skullcap tincture
1 oz. of wood betony tincture

Put all of the tinctures together in a glass container. Cap it with a lid and give it a few shakes to blend. Then take an eyedropper and fill it with the liquid. Put 20 drops of this mix into a glass of water and drink it right before you go to bed. Reseal the bottle and store it in a cool, dry place—maybe in your nightstand!

---

your body temperature, which then drops and makes you drowsy two hours later. The best time for a good, sleep-inducing soak? Two and a half hours before bedtime.

Talk It Out

Talking aloud to yourself at the end of the day, acknowledging your anxieties and concerns, can help you release the emotions that are bothering you so they won't interfere with your sleep. Keeping a bedtime journal can also help. Just jot down your worries before you turn off the light and forget about them.

Pop Some Herbal Valium

Valerian root's active components, called valepotriates, appear to work in a way similar to diazepam (Valium). Its only downsides are that the tea and capsules smell like dirty socks and, as with many substances that relax you, there is a possibility of becoming dependent on it. As long as you're not using any other medications, take valerian root according to package directions.

Savor Evening Oats

Oats have long been used to soothe the nerves and treat insomnia. Adding milk to them further invites drowsiness, since oats are loaded with tryptophan, the amino acid necessary to make the brain chemical serotonin, which controls sleep patterns. If you'd rather sip your oats than eat them, try some oatstraw tea. Purchase the tea and the herbal sedatives dried chamomile, skullcap, and catnip at a health food store. Mix equal parts of each, and steep 1 heaping teaspoon in 1 cup of hot water for 20 minutes.

Hops to It

I'll bet you didn't know that hops—yep, that prime ingredient in beer—is a time-honored sleep-inducing herb. It's used to make "dream pillows" because exposure to air increases its sedative effect. Simply stuff some dried leaves (which you can find at a health-food store) into your pillowcase. Then use the rest to make a tea by steeping 1 to 2 teaspoons in a cup of hot water along with equal parts of lemon balm and valerian root. Studies show that drinking a cup of this concoction 15 minutes before bedtime works directly on the central nervous system and could help you nod off within a half hour or so.

You're Getting Sleepy...

The next time you're lying awake at night, playing a loop of negative thoughts such as "I'll never get to sleep; I'm going to blow my presentation tomorrow," try this positive suggestion instead. Close your eyes, fold your hands over your chest, and say, "Tonight, I will sleep deeply and peacefully, and I will wake up feeling great." Repeat this suggestion 10 times while gently pressing your hands into your chest. This will help anchor the suggestion in your body, so your mind gets the message.

Keep a Cool Head

Try sleeping on an all-natural fiber pillow, or one with a combination of sodium sulfate and ceramic fibers. That will help keep your head cool, thus promoting a sounder sleep.

Catnip for Catnaps

Catnip may turn a lazy feline into a rowdy cat, but it has just the opposite effect on us humans. In fact, long before pharmacists began dispensing powerful chemicals—with all their side effects—to sleep-deprived people, herbalists recommended catnip tea to speed up the journey to dreamland. To make the tea, steep 1 teaspoon of dried catnip in 1 cup of hot water for 10 minutes, then strain and enjoy.

Poppy Power!

Poppies are known for their soporific effects, and the good news is that you don't have to travel to Oz to find them. The common California poppy (*Eschscholzia californica*) is a gentle sleep inducer that can be made into a tea on its own, or added to any of your favorite bedtime herbs. Steep 1 heaping teaspoon in 1 cup of hot water for 15 minutes. Strain, and sip.

A Lube Lullaby

Experts say that warm soles induce sleep, so rub warm, organic sesame oil on the soles of your feet just before bed. Warm woolly socks will also do the trick.

HELP FOR HEADACHES

You overslept. The kids are screaming and fighting for the TV remote. You can't find your purse. And to top it all off, your husband dropped the coffeepot. In the middle of all this craziness, you might notice that your head is starting to throb—and you know from painful experience that within a few minutes, this minor headache could escalate into a major-league skull banger. Stay calm and try these tips to stop the thud, thud, thud.

More Than One

The term *headache* covers a lot of ground, from tension-induced head pain to debilitating migraines. Tension headaches are the most common type, and they're aptly named.

Quick Fix

Talk about a "peppermint patty"! Rubbing peppermint oil—a proven anesthetic—on your forehead may relieve the pain and sensitivity that come with tension headaches. What's more, if you use the oil daily, you may even be able to sidestep future headaches. Simply mix peppermint oil (available at any health-food store) with an equal amount of rubbing alcohol, and apply no more than a couple of drops to your forehead and temples. Wait 15 minutes, then massage the area for 3 minutes. Repeat no more than three times a day.

Whenever you're tense, muscles in your scalp, neck, and shoulders contract and tighten up. Tight muscles have to pull against something, and it's often your head that feels the squeeze.

If you get migraines, your pain is felt as a gradually worsening throbbing on one side of your head or behind your eye that's caused, in part, by blood vessels widening (dilating) and pressing on nerve endings. Nausea and sensitivity to light, sound, and odors are often part of the equation. In addition to migraine pain, sinus headache pain falls into this category, as does the pain of cluster headaches (so called because they usually occur in groups)—a particularly excruciating type of headache that sufferers (mostly men) say feels as though a spike is being driven repeatedly through one eye.

Nearly everyone gets headaches sometimes. It's worth checking with your doctor if you get them all the time or if the pain interferes with your daily activities, but you'll probably be able to manage most headaches on your own. The vast majority of headaches (about 95 percent) are "primary" headaches, which means that they aren't caused by some dangerous underlying illness.

Fight Back

Unfortunately, many medications prescribed for headaches have some serious drawbacks. Corticosteroids, for instance, can cause osteoporosis—dangerous thinning of the bones—and leave you vulnerable to fractures. Other drugs can increase your risk of heart attack and stroke. The good news is that nondrug treatments have proven hugely successful in relieving headaches. Here's how to get started:

Divide and conquer. In this age of highly advanced medicine, we often assume that a therapy has to be just that—highly advanced or technical—in order to be effective, but that's simply not the case when it comes to headache pain. Just keeping blood sugar levels steady by eating multiple meals throughout the day provides relief for half of all people who suffer from migraines.

Watch what you eat. About one-third of all headache sufferers get relief simply by avoiding foods known to trigger headaches. Of the 100 or more troublemakers, the worst offenders include red wine, hot dogs, chocolate, fermented foods such as soy sauce, foods that contain the flavor enhancer monosodium glutamate (MSG), and those that contain the amino acid tyramine, such as aged cheese and preserved meats. But headaches can also be caused by hidden food allergies, and they can be prevented just by eliminating the most common allergenic foods, such as corn, wheat, eggs, soy, peanuts, or milk, from your diet.

Jot it down. To identify your triggers, keep a headache diary. Write down anything that appears to be a trigger, including foods, activities, sleep changes, stressful events, what point you're at in your menstrual cycle, and even the weather. Then try to eliminate as many as you can.

Reach for White Willow

Long before that little Bayer® aspirin bottle became a medicine-cabinet staple, Native American medicine men dispensed the bark of the white willow tree for pain relief. Willow contains salicin, which is similar to the painkilling substance used to make aspirin. But the old-fashioned remedy may be better because it won't upset your stomach the way aspirin can. At the first sign of headache pain, drink a cup of white willow tea or take 3 to 5 milliliters of liquid extract (both are available at health-food stores; to make tea, follow the package directions). Avoid the herb if you're allergic to aspirin, though, and never mix the two or use white willow with alcohol.

Have a Cuppa Chamomile

Relaxing, antispasmodic chamomile can calm migraine-associated queasiness as well as ease the stress associated with tension headaches. Have a cup or two of chamomile tea at the first hint of pain; use two tea bags to maximize its potency and effectiveness. Don't use chamomile, however, if you're allergic to ragweed.

If chamomile doesn't do the trick, valerian, a stronger sedative herb, may be effective. As long as you're not taking any medications, check your health-food store for valerian tincture, then, at the first twinge of pain, add 15 to 30 drops to a cup of water and drink. Just be sure to hold your nose—this herb smells like stinky feet!

Fewer with Feverfew

The herb feverfew should really be renamed "migrainefew." Studies show that taking feverfew in capsule form daily can reduce the frequency and potency of migraines. Just be sure you search the health-food store for standardized capsules that contain parthenolides, the active ingredient of feverfew that appears to affect serotonin levels—and ward off migraines. Follow the label directions.

Medicate with Mocha Java

Caffeine constricts blood vessels, which can ease head pain and even delay or dampen a migraine. If you drink caffeinated beverages regularly, however, your blood vessels will grossly overdilate when the caffeine wears off, triggering the last thing you need—a whopper of a headache! Try weaning yourself off of your daily fix. Then the next time you feel a headache coming on, you can drop by the coffee shop for a cup or two of dark roast.

Sting Sinus Headaches

For headaches triggered by allergies that swell the sinuses and cause blinding pain, nothing works better than stinging nettle tea. This herb contains a compound that's similar to serotonin, the brain chemical that regulates blood vessel dilation. It's most potent in the bulk herb, which you can buy at health-food stores. Add 1 heaping teaspoon to a cup of hot water, steep for 10 to 15 minutes, strain, and sip. You should get relief in anywhere from 5 to 20 minutes.

Forget Ibuprofen

If you're plagued by headaches, you may have already discovered the hard way that popping analgesics doesn't bring relief. Ibuprofen, aspirin, and other nonsteroidal anti-inflammatory drugs (NSAIDs) work by constricting your blood vessels. When their

---

☗OME ☗REMEDY

Whenever I got a headache, my Grandma Putt would give me a cold washcloth to hold at the base of my skull, while I soaked my feet in warm water. According to folk wisdom, this old-time remedy pulls blood out of the swollen blood vessels in the head and moves it toward the feet. And it's always worked for me!

---

effects wear off, however, the vessels typically overdilate, leaving you with even more pain than you had before. Soon, you're taking larger and ever larger doses, but getting less and less relief, and possibly winding up with daily "rebound" headaches. As if that weren't enough, prolonged use of NSAIDs can lead to ulcers and can possibly interfere with the absorption of nutrients, including tryptophan—an amino acid the body uses to make serotonin.

Mind Your Minerals

Magnesium and calcium are the two to pay attention to. Why? Because both tend to be lacking in people who get migraines. When this dynamic mineral duo is combined with riboflavin (a B vitamin shown to crush head pain) and the herb feverfew, it helps ward off severe head pain.

Consider Coenzyme Q10

Next to magnesium (see "Mind Your Minerals" above), this nutrient may be the most promising nondrug headache therapy around. In fact, studies show that people who took CoQ10 daily had 60 percent fewer headaches than when they weren't taking it. Look for supplements at health-food stores and drugstores, and follow the label directions.

Pick Dandelions

This unassuming weed helps the liver metabolize estrogen and may ease migraine pain associated with fluctuating hormone levels. Plus, dandelion is rich in magnesium, which is often lacking in people who experience migraines. Check your health-food store for dandelion capsules, and take 400 to 500 milligrams a day throughout your menstrual cycle. You can also pick some fresh dandelion leaves from a chemical-free lawn and toss them into a salad. If you're taking diuretics or potassium supplements, check with your doctor before using dandelion.

Stick It to Me

Now here's one instance where I won't cringe at getting poked with needles. When researchers at the National Institutes of Health evaluated the benefits of acupuncture (the insertion of hair-thin needles at certain points on the body, supposedly to release blocked energy), relief from chronic headache pain was near the top of the list. Interested in giving it a try? Ask your doctor for a referral to a reputable acupuncturist in your area.

Rub Away a Migraine

A study at the University of Miami School of Medicine Touch Research Institute revealed that when participants had a 30-minute massage twice weekly for five weeks, migraine pain decreased, and the duration of the headaches was shortened by 80 percent. Massage not only feels simply delightful, it also boosts blood flow, removes pain-causing lactic acid from muscles, and promotes the release of natural painkilling substances. A good rubdown also inhibits the release of hormones called catecholamines, which contribute to pain.

Tame Tension

The moment you feel a tension headache coming on, close your eyes and take several deep, cleansing breaths, inhaling deeply through your nose and exhaling through your mouth. As your lungs fill up and deflate, imagine that you've locked your worries—deadlines, concern about a family member's illness, unpaid bills— inside a suitcase tied to a hot-air balloon. Then, in your mind's eye, watch as the balloon lifts your worries up, up, up—and away!

Rewire Your Brain

All those negative, whiny thoughts—"Why me?" "How much longer is this going to last?"—swirling around in your headache-prone head may actually contribute to your pain. In fact, if you recast your self-talk in a more positive light, you may actually rewire your brain chemistry and reduce your pain. So the next time you hear yourself begin an internal moan, repeat the following statement instead: "I have a biological predisposition for headaches, *and* right now, I'm going to focus on things that can help relieve the pain."

Veto Pain with Vitamin C

This vitamin has powerful anti-inflammatory properties, which are important because inflammation plays a role in some tension headaches. You can try taking 1,000 to 2,000 milligrams of vitamin C at the first sign of a headache; if it's going to work, you should feel the benefits within an hour or two.

Lick It with Lemon Balm

Try taming a headache by putting 2 teaspoons of dried lemon balm leaves in a cup of boiling water. Let the mixture steep and cool. Strain the herbs, then sip away.

When to Dial the Doc

Consult your doctor if you have three or more headaches a week, or feel you must take a pain reliever every day. Also, even if it's just a one-time occurrence, dial your doc if you have any of the following, which may indicate an underlying disorder that requires further attention:

- A sharp, abrupt, severe headache

- A headache accompanied by fever, stiffness, rash, mental confusion, seizures, double vision, weakness, numbness, or difficulty speaking

- A headache after a head injury, even if it's a minor fall or bump, and especially if the headache gets worse

- A chronic, progressive headache that worsens after coughing, exertion, straining, or sudden movement

- Onset of new headache pain after age 40

BANISH THE BLUES

We all have times when we pull into ourselves like little box turtles, preferring to be alone with our thoughts or feelings. But if you've been inside your shell for longer than usual, or you're interacting with people with barely contained irritation, you could be depressed. While depression can manifest itself as sadness and despair, it can also show up as irritability and a lack of pleasure in normally pleasurable activities. Even overfocusing at work can be a symptom of depression—a disease that springs from an imbalance in brain chemicals that powerfully affect moods, appetite, and sleeping habits. If you've been paying attention, you know that altering how you feel, what you eat, and how much you sleep is directly related to your physical health. So it's important to learn how to deal with the blues. You should always see your doctor if the doldrums last more than a few days, or head for the emergency room if you have any thoughts whatsoever of suicide. Otherwise, here's some help.

Sad Is Bad for the Heart

Depression has always been linked to heart disease. Johns Hopkins researchers found that depressed people were four times more likely to have a heart attack than those who said they were not depressed. And a study of middle-aged women found that those who had depressive symptoms (sleeping problems, lack of energy, frequent boredom, and crying) and who also felt unsupported by their friends and families had low levels of high-density lipoproteins (HDL), the "good" cholesterol, which is another risk factor for heart disease.

Depression Checklist

Ask your primary physician for a referral to a mental health professional if you've been unable to experience pleasure for two weeks and have any five of the following symptoms:

- A persistently sad, anxious, or empty mood

- Sleeping too little or too much

- Weight loss or gain

- Loss of interest or pleasure in activities you once enjoyed

- Restlessness or irritability

- Difficulty concentrating, remembering, or making decisions

- Fatigue or loss of energy

- Feelings of guilt, hopelessness, or worthlessness

- Obsessive thoughts of death (If the thought of suicide pops into your head even once, head for the emergency room immediately or call an emergency help line.)

Depression can be life-threatening, so if you think you may be depressed, consult your doctor immediately. Ask him or her for a referral to a mental health professional, such as a psychiatrist, psychologist, or licensed clinical social worker, who may recommend that you take an antidepressant medication, such as fluoxetine (Prozac®) or sertraline (Zoloft®). Both of these drugs block the reabsorption of serotonin into the brain, so people who take them always have a constant level of this mood-stabilizing hormone available. You should also be advised to have at least short-term cognitive therapy. Studies show that the two together are much more effective than any other treatment regimen.

Natural Pick-Me-Uppers

For people with moderate or serious depression, the benefits of medication clearly outweigh the side effects (which often include lack of energy, weight gain, and zero libido or sexual function). If your depression is mild, however, you might talk to your doctor about starting with gentler, more natural alternatives, such as those listed below. Just one caveat: If you're already taking prescription antidepressants or have bipolar disorder (also called manic depression), avoid the herbal antidepressants recommended here.

B good. Nearly 80 percent of people with depression are deficient in vitamin B_6. To get B_6 and the rest of the Bs (all of which your body needs to deliver oxygen to the brain, turn blood sugar into energy, and keep feel-good brain chemicals in circulation), doctors suggest popping a B-complex supplement that supplies 20 milligrams of B_6, 500 micrograms of B_{12}, and 400 micrograms of folic acid. Take the supplement with food.

Make strides. When you feel yourself beginning to slip into darkness, don't panic—just act. As quickly as you can, head outside for a brisk

Quick Fix

Studies show that when women spend time with one another, their bodies release a brain chemical called oxytocin that battles the stress associated with depression. Now there's a great reason to make Girls' Night Out a regular happening!

10-minute walk, literally counting your steps in a 1-2, 1-2 military fashion. This simple focusing, almost meditative activity will not only crowd out negative thoughts, it will also encourage your brain to release endorphins—the feel-good brain chemicals that will help lift your mood.

Fish for a lift. Cold-water fish, such as salmon and tuna, are packed with omega-3 essential fatty acids, which help the brain receive serotonin. But they also contain eicosapentaenoic acid (EPA), a component of fish oil that has been shown to help reduce feelings of worthlessness. Since you'd have to eat a boatload of fish to get the antidepressant effects of EPA, your best bet is to eat fish several times a week and take 1 gram (1,000 milligrams) of fish-oil supplements (available at health-food stores) twice a day. Just be sure your supplements contain at least half EPA and half docosahexaenoic acid (DHA). Since fish oil can thin your blood, avoid it if you take aspirin or prescription blood thinners.

Turn to Turkey

Don't wait until the holidays to get your dose of tryptophan, an amino acid that's ultimately converted into serotonin in the body. In one study, when women who were depressed feasted on tryptophan-rich foods, such as turkey, chicken, fish, dairy products, soybeans, nuts, and avocados, their depression eased without the help of medication. One idea: Buy bags of frozen soybeans at the supermarket, pop a bowlful in the microwave to cook, and snack on them (they're crunchy!) throughout the day. Or mash up several avocados to make some yummy, mood-lifting guacamole.

When you're eating turkey or another tryptophan-rich food, pair it with a lower-fat carbohydrate, such as whole-grain bread, brown rice, or mashed potatoes. Carbohydrates trigger the release of insulin, which allows tryptophan to freely enter your brain so that, eventually, your serotonin levels rise.

Get Moving!

A study at Duke University Medical Center revealed that people with major depression who exercised aerobically for 30 minutes three times a week experienced the same relief from depression as people who took antidepressants. There are several reasons for this effect: First, aerobic exercise forces oxygen into your cells, increasing energy production, and second, it signals your brain to release feel-good brain chemicals called endorphins, which boost your mood.

If you do your aerobic exercise outdoors, you may actually boost its antidepressant effect. Exposure to sunlight—even on dim, overcast days—helps boost levels of vitamin D, which then helps the body maintain higher levels of serotonin. In fact, even in a downpour, there is 30 times more light outside than there is indoors.

Rub the Blues Away

Preliminary studies indicate that massage may help reduce symptoms of depression, perhaps by combating a buildup of the stress hormone

---

FAST FORMULA

Take a Whiff

Since fragrance has a mighty powerful effect on our mood, it makes perfect "scents" to find one you love and make it a part of your daily routine. Using essential oils, make your own body lotion, perfume, room freshener, candle, or bath oil. Here's an uplifting air freshener you can try.

1 1/2 oz. of distilled water
1 1/2 oz. of high-proof alcohol (vodka is suitable; rubbing alcohol is not) or
   3 oz. of distilled water
20 drops of lime essential oil
14 drops of bergamot essential oil
4 drops of ylang-ylang essential oil
2 drops of rose essential oil

Combine all the ingredients in a clean 4-oz. spray bottle with a fine-mist setting. (Do not use a bottle that previously held cleaning products or products such as hair spray.) Spray, sniff, and smile!

---

cortisol. To enhance the effect, use some mood-boosting herbal oils, such as bergamot, geranium, jasmine, neroli, or ylang-ylang, which are all available at health-food stores.

Get the Point

A study from the University of Arizona found that three months of twice-weekly acupuncture treatments reduced depression in more than half of the women tested, although researchers aren't sure why. It's possible that insertion of the thread-thin needles stimulates the release of mood-lifting endorphins, or corrects a chemical imbalance involved in depression. Ask your doctor to recommend a reputable practitioner in your area.

Try St. John's Wort

A lot of folks (including me) call St. John's wort the happy herb. Both its flowers and petals have been scientifically proven to contain natural medicines that lift the spirits and lighten up moods. That's why St. John's wort is often regarded as nature's Prozac®—it helps treat mild depression without the risk of addiction or side effects found in prescription medicines. Be patient, though—it may take two to six weeks before you notice a lift in your mood. If you think you may be suffering from depression, be sure to see a doctor before using St. John's wort. In some people, it can cause stomachaches, allergic reactions, and heightened sensitivity to the sun. And do not take St. John's wort with other medications.

Swallow SAM-e

Short for S-adenosylmethionine, this compound helps regulate the breakdown of feel-good hormones and may be a more effective and faster mood booster for people with mild to moderate depression than St. John's wort. You get results with SAM-e in less than a week with no major side effects. Check with your doctor first, then look for quality brands at health-food stores. Follow the package directions, and don't take SAM-e with any other medication.

Stop and Pick the Flowers

Flowers do more than make our world a more beautiful place: Their fragrance, color, and chemical makeup can also lift our mood. Passionflower, lavender, vervain, borage, rosemary, and skullcap, with their beautiful purple and blue flowers, can be just the thing for chasing the blues away. Try making a tea with one of these herbs, or use two or three in combination. Steep 1 teaspoon of either a single dried herb or mixed herbs in 1 cup of boiling water for 10 minutes, then strain. Drink two or three cups per day.

STOP THE SNIFFLES

If you're wondering why modern science hasn't found a cure for the common cold, you're not alone. But consider these numbers: The common cold is actually one of about 200 mild viral infections of the upper respiratory tract. Even if doctors figured out how to cure one of them, what about the other 199? Whichever virus we catch, it creates pesky symptoms, including a runny or stuffy nose, sore throat, laryngitis, teary eyes, sneezing, wheezing, and heavy breathing (not *that* kind!). A cold also blunts our senses of smell and taste, and it can bring on a mild headache and a general feeling of fatigue. With all those symptoms to tackle, no wonder there's no cure! But there *are* some things you can do to make a cold a whole lot less debilitating.

Kick a Cold

Other than curling up in bed, what's the alternative when a nasty cold strikes? Well, you've got to strike back! Until your cold runs its course, here's what you can do to make yourself more comfortable and kick that cold to the curb:

Snooze with booze. Try a hot toddy. There are many variations of it, which apparently originated in Scotland. Start with juice, honey, or tea, and add the liquor of your choice. One version from way back when is a Hot Whiskey Lemonade. Start with 1 cup of boiling water to which you add the fresh-squeezed juice of half a lemon, honey to taste, and a healthy shot of whiskey. Stir, sip, and you'll sleep like a baby.

Take echinacea. Echinacea, or purple coneflower, has a strong reputation as an herbal cold fighter and it's available at most drugstores. Take it according to the package directions at the very first sign of a cold. This immune stimulant battles cold germs after they enter your body. In fact, studies show that it will decrease the length of your cold and cut the severity of your symptoms in half. *Caution:* Echinacea should be avoided by people with autoimmune conditions, such as lupus or rheumatoid arthritis.

Lay off the dairy. When you've got a cold, stick to juices, water, and hot beverages. Avoid milk and milk products, because moo juice promotes mucus formation. If you drink dairy during a cold, you'll not only get a milk mustache, but you'll get more congested, too!

Suck Up Some C

I love to drink gallons of orange and other citrus juices when I have a cold (which is hardly ever anymore). Perhaps it's the vitamin C in the citrus that feels so cleansing, or maybe just the idea that C—even if it's a placebo effect—works for me. While no one has yet proven that vitamin C can cure a cold, some say it acts like interferon, which is a natural body chemical that stops virus growth. It's most effective if you up your C intake at the first sign of a sniffle. Most health professionals agree that vitamin C does have a slight antihistamine affect, so drinking more citrus juice or taking a supplement may help reduce nasal symptoms.

Chicken Soup for the Nose

Why did the chicken cross the road? To get into the soup pot! Nobody knows exactly what chicken soup does—but it sure does help colds. Most doctors believe that the steam from the hot soup promotes drainage and thus makes you feel better. Some believe that neutrophils, the immune cells activated by the cold virus, are slowed down by something in chicken soup. This remedy, which many people know as "Jewish penicillin," has been in use since the 12th century.

Spice Up Your Life

Spicy foods, such as hot peppers and chili con carne, contain capsaicin, a substance that can help reduce nasal and sinus congestion. Try garlic, turmeric, and other pungent spices for a similar effect. Some cold sufferers add these strong spices to chicken soup to promote drainage. Even when you don't have a cold, any hot soup or hot spice will help get your eyes and nose running.

Another good source of heat is gingerroot. The oil in ginger is similar to the capsaicin in peppers. It is slightly irritating, and it thins out mucus. You can clear your head with ginger in several ways: Cut the root into pieces, brew a tea, and then inhale the vapors as you sip; grate it up and toss it into a salad dressing; or chop it up and add it to a stir-fry.

Think Zinc

According to doctors at the Mayo Clinic, there is evidence that zinc may prevent colds; but scientists aren't sure why. They suspect it may keep the cold virus from reproducing, or it may increase the body's own immune response. As with any immune stimulant, overuse can cause problems, so take zinc capsules only as directed. Good food sources of zinc include wheat germ, dried peas and beans, oysters and other seafood, meat, poultry, tofu, and dairy products.

I'll Drink to That!

It's important to drink plenty of fluids when you have a cold to keep your nasal passages hydrated and help clear up congestion. Whether you choose hot or cold versions is up to you. Try these recipes to whet your appetite and put a crimp in your cold symptoms:

- Veto colds with vinegar. Appalachian healers make this remedy from common, household ingredients: Mix a dash of cayenne pepper and a pinch of salt into 1 ounce of apple cider vinegar, and drink it three or four times a day.

- Make a Bloody Mary, with or without the booze. Start with tomato juice, then add some lemon, a celery stalk, and horseradish—and drink it quickly. Tomato juice is full of vitamin C, but it's the horseradish that really does the trick. Its powerful fumes will loosen up mucus congestion, making your cold more bearable.

- Take tea and see. A hot cup of regular tea with honey usually feels great when you have a cold. You can also try other types, such as red pepper tea, which are meant to loosen up the mucus. Lemon and honey, added to weak tea or even plain hot water, will also ease head pain and help break up congestion.

There's the Rub

Using poultices when you have a cold is a good way to make yourself slow down and rest. Make your own chest rub by adding 3 to 4 drops of an essential oil (try eucalyptus, lavender, or thyme) to 1 tablespoon of olive oil. Apply it liberally to your chest, cover with a clean cloth, and settle into a comfy chair with a cozy afghan and a good book.

FAST FORMULA

Keep Vampires (and Colds) Away!

Garlic (*Allium sativum*) has long been used for its potent healing effects, and it doubles as a cold preventative because it keeps other people at a distance! Surprisingly, garlic tea doesn't taste as bad as it sounds. Try it—you may like it!

2 medium cloves of garlic, chopped
2–3 slices of fresh gingerroot
Honey and lemon, to taste
1 cup of water

Simmer the garlic in the water for 10 to 15 minutes. Add the ginger to improve the taste and increase the warming action of the garlic. Add honey and lemon if you'd like. Try to drink 2 to 4 cups per day. *Caution:* People taking blood-thinning medications should steer clear of garlic unless it's approved by their physician.

Peel Me an Onion

Whenever you peel an onion, you cry a river. That's because the chemicals released by an onion are attracted to water. The trick for weepless peeling is to do it at the kitchen sink, so you can turn on the tap and hold the onion close to the water as you peel it. On the other hand, if you want to let those pungent onion fumes help fight your cold, peel a big onion—away from the sink—and hover over it. The fumes will work their way into your mucous membranes and help clear up your congestion.

Keep It Clean

You may think that the common cold is simply a fact of life, expected to hit at some point, no matter what you do. Well, I'm here to tell you that you can take measures to lower your risk and cut down on the number of colds you catch. One of the easiest ways to keep colds at bay is to practice good hygiene habits. Be diligent about the following:

- Wash your hands frequently. Hardy cold viruses can live for hours on doorknobs, faucet handles, books, money—all of the things we touch every day.

- Dispose of the germs. Bacteria and viruses live on cloth towels and sponges for hours, so use paper towels, tissues, and napkins when someone in your house has a cold.

- Disinfect dirty surfaces. Frequently wash places that are constantly touched in the home, such as stair railings, telephones, countertops, and doorknobs. And children's toys are common culprits, too. Wash them in warm, soapy water to kill the bacteria and viruses they collect.

Boost Your Immunity

If your immune system is in tip-top shape, colds will be less likely to catch you. One sure way to beef up your immunity is by maintaining a healthy diet. Increasing your consumption of the following foods will go a long way to keep colds at a distance:

Vitamins A, C, and E. Lots of fruits and veggies will deliver the antioxidant power of these vitamins—just what you need to "A-C-E" colds!

Omega-3 fatty acids. Flax oil and fatty fish (such as salmon, tuna, and mackerel) act as immune boosters by increasing the activity of phagocytes, the white blood cells that eat up bacteria. (Perhaps this is why grandmothers used to insist on a daily dose of that nasty cod liver oil!)

Selenium. This mineral increases natural killer cells that will ferociously attack a cold virus. The best food sources of selenium are tuna, red snapper, lobster, shrimp, whole grains, brown rice, egg yolks, cottage cheese, and chicken (white meat only).

Garlic. It's a powerful immune booster that stimulates the multiplication of infection-fighting white cells, and increases the efficiency of antibody production. The garlic breath that follows may just be worth it!

Get Steamed

If you think you've been exposed to cold germs, steam will kill them on contact if water temperatures are 110°F or more. You can breathe in plain steamy air, or liven things up a bit with herbs, such as eucalyptus, which add a penetrating scent and disinfectant. Put fresh leaves in a bowl, pour boiling water over them, and make a towel tent over your head and the bowl. Lower your face over the bowl (carefully—you can scald yourself if the steam is too hot), and breathe in deeply through your nose. You can also add a few drops of oregano oil to the water. It's nice—a bit like diluted Vicks®—but pricey.

Don't Dry Out

Artificially controlled environments with really dry air, such as offices and airplanes, dry out your nasal membranes and the passages may form tiny cracks that invite viruses. The best defense? Drink plenty of liquids, and use a nasal saline spray often to hydrate those tender membranes.

Drink a Powerful Potion

For an immune-stimulating teatime, combine equal parts of yarrow (*Achillea millefolium*), lemon balm (*Melissa officinalis*), licorice root

(*Glycyrrhiza glabra*), gingerroot *(Zingiber officinale)*, eyebright *(Euphrasia officinalis)*, and rose hips *(Rosa canina)* in a jar with a tight lid. Use 1 heaping teaspoon of the herb mix per cup of boiling water. Drink 2 to 3 cups per day. *Caution:* Licorice root should not be used by people who have high blood pressure or kidney disease.

Quick Fix

It is now widely known among doctors that positive emotions strengthen the immune system by increasing gamma interferon, an immune system hormone that activates other infection-fighting compounds within your body. So the next time you have a cold, rent some funny movies and have yourself a laugh fest that'll chuckle away your cold woes.

Flu: Nothing to Sneeze At

Flu has become a catchall word for any malady, from a bad cold to a stomachache, that hits us in the fall or winter. But influenza is caused by a very specific group of viruses classified as type A, B, or C. These viral strains have been known since the 1930s and 1940s. The worst is type A, which killed 20 million people in a global epidemic in 1918. Type A is also to blame for the 1957 Asian and the 1968 Hong Kong flu epidemics. Type B is also serious, but does not cause such widespread epidemics. Type C is the mildest form, and that is what most of us have had at one time or another.

The flu can hit you quite suddenly with fatigue, muscle pain, headache, fever, runny nose, and/or a sore throat. A dry, hacking cough can follow congestion as the other symptoms

progress. You may feel weak and tired for weeks after the flu has left the building. Follow this advice to both sidestep and handle the flu.

Be Antisocial

The flu is highly contagious. If you happen to be in the same room with an infected person who sneezes or coughs, the airborne bug can literally bombard you with flu viruses. So at the height of flu season, boycott crowded places, such as subways, theaters, and parties, as much as you can. And if at all possible, avoid air travel—spending time on airplanes keeps you in a confined space with recirculated air, which is definitely not a good way to stay flu-free.

Hands Off

The flu is also contagious through indirect transmission. This means that the virus can live for hours on telephones, faucets, or anything that's been touched by infected people who didn't wash their hands. Once the bug enters a particular "community"—such as a school or nursing home—it spreads like a wildfire. So wash your hands frequently throughout the day during the flu season to reduce your chances of contamination. And make sure you wash them every time you return home.

Give It a Shot

Or I should say, *take* a shot. Flu shots aren't just for the very young, very old, and those who have contact with the chronically ill. If you just plain don't want to get the flu, then you need a flu shot. It's best to get it in the fall to give the vaccine time to take effect. In North America, influenza season is from December to March and peaks in February. (It has been known to start before Thanksgiving.) In the tropics, flu thrives year-round. *Caution:* Most doctors agree that those who are allergic to eggs should

189

HOME REMEDY

Garlic *(Allium sativum)* has immune-stimulating and antiviral properties. If you don't mind the odor, you may want to try a garlic foot rub when you're battling a bad cold or the flu. Coat the soles of your feet with olive oil. (Better yet, have someone else do this for you, and enjoy a soothing foot massage!) Slice a clove of garlic in half, and rub the cut end on your well-oiled feet. Put on a pair of clean socks, and go to bed. *Caution:* The oils in garlic can cause burns, so it is imperative that you oil your feet well before applying the garlic to them.

not get a flu shot. If you're in doubt, talk to your doctor before you roll up your sleeve.

Take It Easy

When preventive measures fail, and you're felled by the flu, make yourself as comfortable as you can. Influenza just has to run its course—usually in three to seven days. If you treat the symptoms, you'll at least feel better while your natural antibodies destroy the virus. Take acetaminophen or over-the-counter pain medications to fight the fever and ease the aches and pains while you rest, and drink lots of fluids. (But avoid aspirin and never give it to a child who has the flu. It can bring on a condition called Reye's syndrome, which can be fatal.)

Chamomile Calmer

Chamomile *(Matricaria recutita)* is one of the most versatile herbs—it's an antimicrobial, eases pain, calms the stomach, and induces relaxation. In other words, it's just what you need when the

flu bug strikes. Make a soothing, healing tea with 1 teaspoon of the dried herb per 1 cup of boiling water. Steep, covered, for 10 minutes. Drink 1 cup three times per day. *Caution:* People with ragweed allergies may be sensitive to chamomile.

Clean and Clear

To prevent passing the flu bug by hand-to-hand contact, clean those high-touch household surfaces, such as phones, countertops, and toilet handles. You can disinfect them with a few drops of eucalyptus oil mixed into a pint spray bottle of water. The fumes will also help clear up your stuffy nose as you clean.

When to Dial the Doc

If you have chest pain, wheezing, or difficulty breathing, or are coughing up green or yellow sputum, these can be signs of pneumonia. This means the virus has infected your lungs or compromised your immune system. People over 65 are at serious risk for pneumonia, especially if they have other chronic conditions—such as diabetes, cancer, or heart or lung disease—and if they are in a hospital or nursing home. See your doctor promptly if any of these symptoms arise.

HELP YOURSELF ONLINE

If you've ever attempted to find health information via the Internet, you know that there's a wealth of information out in cyberspace, and believe you me, it's downright overwhelming. The trouble is, anyone with access can post a Web site. So how do you know if you've found reliable information you can trust? Well, I've been doing quite a bit of traveling down the information superhighway, and I've picked up these tips along the way.

Address Smarts

The first thing you need to watch when you go online is *where* you're actually going. Web sites are created by corporations, the government, nonprofits, educational institutions...the list goes on and on. Here's what you need to know when it comes to online health info:

- Beware of Web sites sponsored by manufacturers of pharmaceuticals, supplements, or any product or position. A good general rule is to watch out for site addresses that end in ".com," which tend to be commercial sites; also be wary of any information that's posted anonymously.

- Stay away from sites that tout "miracle cures" or treatments that sound too good to be true. They always are.

- Check when the information was last updated, and who reviews it. Credentials of the reviewers should be provided. If not, move on.

The Top 10

Here's a list of the top 10 Web sites recommended by the American Medical Association and the National Institutes of Health. Log on and check 'em out!

1. Healthfinder. Available in English and Spanish, the U.S. Department of Health and Human Services sponsors this site at **www.healthfinder.org**.

2. Health Information–National Institutes of Health (NIH). The central point of access to all NIH consumer information is **http://health.nih.gov**.

3. Medline. The National Library of Medicine offers this searchable database of over 3,800 medical journals at **www.nlm.nih. gov/databases/freemedl.html**.

4. American Medical Association. The AMA provides consumer health information that has been reviewed by medical experts, with links to other reliable sites, at **www.ama-assn.org**.

5. U.S. Centers for Disease Control and Prevention. Information on diseases, health risks, and prevention guidelines is available at **www.cdc.gov**.

6. U.S. Food and Drug Administration. The latest information on such topics as foods, human and animal drugs, and cosmetics can be found at **www.fda.gov**.

7. Tufts University Nutrition Navigator. Links to nutrition information that has been reviewed by a team of nutrition experts are provided at **www.navigator.tufts.edu**.

8. NIH SeniorHealth. Aging-related health information is easily accessible, and adjustable text size and contrast, as well as audio, are available at **http://nihseniorhealth.gov/**.

9. HealthWeb. A collaborative project of several health sciences libraries, it offers access to evaluated noncommercial, health-related resources at **http://healthweb.org/**.

10. National Women's Health Information Center. A gateway in English and Spanish to the vast array of federal and other women's health information resources is available at **http://www.4woman.gov/**.

CHAPTER 10

A-Head of the Game

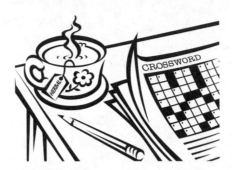

You can't stop the clock on aging. And while every part of your body eventually falls victim to the process, the first signs most often make themselves apparent from the shoulders up. Yep, I'm talking about what's in and on your head: memory, vision, hearing, hair, and teeth. These are the "loss" leaders. But don't panic: The good news is there are things you can do right now to keep your wits (and vision, hearing, hair, and teeth) about you!

BOOST YOUR BRAINPOWER

"**E**xcuse me, I'm having a senior moment." It may seem like a witty way to face the dilemma of forgetfulness, but I know personally that it's also a bit of black humor. Most of us fear losing our minds more than anything else that could conceivably happen with age, so it's reassuring to find out that we can be forgetful for many reasons other than dementia. Memory is all about attention. Just as we clean out our filing cabinets, we do the same thing with our mind's "memory files." Here's how to keep your files from disappearing too soon.

Food for Thought

Once again, nutrition comes to the rescue in matters of the mind. Memory loss is most often attributed to low blood sugar and fatigue. So be sure to eat nutritious, well-balanced meals—especially a good breakfast of protein and complex carbohydrates, such as whole-grain cereals and breads. Other foods that can help keep you as sharp as a tack include:

Grapes. Studies suggest that grapes contain chemical compounds that may help ward off memory loss and improve motor skills. So munch a bunch with lunch!

Tempeh. After menopause, supplies of an important brain chemical called choline dwindle, decreasing the ability of memory cells to communicate with each other. The good news? High-protein foods like soy and tempeh contain choline, so adding them to your diet can help make up for the loss. Enjoy a glass or two of soy milk each day.

Blueberries. Eating $1/2$ cup of blueberries a day may clear the sludge from your memory banks, reports a recent Tufts University study. Blueberries are reported to have the highest antioxidant level of any fruit or vegetable. Eat fresh blueberries when they're in season, and keep bags of frozen blueberries on hand to add to your oatmeal, smoothies, and salads for a brain-boosting treat.

Beans, egg yolks, and cabbage. What do they all have in common? They're rich in lecithin, which produces chemicals that act as messengers for our thoughts and memories. The more messengers the better, so be sure to put these foods on your menu.

HOME REMEDY

If you have trouble focusing—and you have a hankering for chocolate— you're in luck! Chocolate contains phenylethylamine (also known as the "love drug"), which raises blood pressure and blood sugar levels, and methylxanthines, a caffeine relative that increases neurotransmitter activity in the brain to produce more endorphins. What, exactly, does all that mean? Simply that you can get improved mood, energy, and concentration by snacking on a 1.75- ounce bar of dark chocolate (not milk or white) daily. Now *that's* something to cheer about!

Plate It with Pasta

An Italian study recently found that cognitive impairment was less common among elderly people who ate a Mediterranean diet, which includes lots of olive oil—a monounsaturated fat. As their "healthy fat" intake increased, their risk of memory problems declined. So swap saturated, brain-fogging fats such as butter and marbled meats for healthy, monounsaturated fats like olive and canola oils. Use them not only on pasta, but also in salad dressings and hearty soups.

Supplement Your Brain

It may be as simple as popping a pill. Taking soy-extracted isoflavone tablets (55 milligrams) twice daily has been shown to help verbal recall. However, if you have breast cancer or are at risk for it, check with your doctor before using supplements, since isoflavones may have an estrogenic effect on tissues.

Get Extra E

A recent study concluded that taking supplements of vitamins E and C significantly protects against vascular dementia (loss of cognitive function due to atherosclerosis). The study subjects performed better on tests, too. In another study, vitamin E slowed the mental decline of patients with Alzheimer's disease. While your favorite citrus fruit or berry will give you loads of C, vitamin E is harder to come by in foods. So ask your doctor if it's okay to take it as a supplement.

"B" Sharp

If you don't get enough of the B vitamin folate (the natural form of folic acid), your brain could degenerate. Folate, as well as vitamins B_6 and B_{12}, may protect your gray matter by keeping homocysteine levels in check. (Elevated homocysteine is associated with Alzheimer's disease.) So pad your diet with plenty of folate-rich orange juice, broccoli and other cruciferous veggies, avocados, and legumes. Meat, poultry, whole grains, and green leafy vegetables provide vitamin B_6, while vitamin B_{12} is found mostly in meat.

Mind Your Minerals

Studies have shown that deficiencies of iron and zinc can interfere with concentration. You can boost your brainpower by eating a serving of beans a few times a week—they're loaded with both minerals.

We also need magnesium, potassium, and boron, which are important for mental alertness. So give your brain a wake-up call! Millet, dark leafy greens (such as collards, kale, and broccoli), and figs are chock-full of these minerals, so they are your best choices.

Stop the Stress

Chronic stress makes your adrenal glands pump out cortisol, a hormone that—when levels build up—can wreak havoc with your long-term memory, concentration, and decision making. Do all you can to control the stress in your life (see "Sidestep Stress" on page 171)—and consider some counseling if all else fails and you just can't seem to relax.

Bust a Move

If you're serious about getting your exercise, you're more likely to be mentally sharp, too, since physical activity boosts the production of brain chemicals. A study of sedentary people who began taking brisk walks showed that they improved both their mental agility and their concentration. So add a brisk daily walk to your routine. When your brain is well supplied with oxygen, it will remember more—and the rest of you will feel better as well!

Use It or Lose It

Your brain needs exercise, too! Studies of healthy people suggest that ongoing mental stimulation—such as work, continuing education, extensive reading, mentally challenging games, and crossword puzzles—can keep your mind sharp. Scores of laboratory studies link mental activity and the production of protective neurotrophins. Even Alzheimer's disease is less common among the well-educated (although many smart people do get it). The explanation? Mentally active folks may have increased brain reserves, more neurons, and a more complex, cell-to-cell communication system to draw on if some brain cells sustain damage. So take out the chessboard (or learn if you've never played), write in a journal, or design that great gadget you've been thinking about.

Forget Less with Fats

Brain cells are 60 percent fat, which is needed to transmit the impulses that carry thought. In a healthy brain, omega-3 fatty acids predominate; in fact, low levels of omega-3s have been linked to depression and the risk of Alzheimer's disease. How do you get these healthy fatty acids? They're plentiful in oily fish (such as tuna and salmon), walnuts, and flaxseed. To benefit your whole body, add a handful of nuts, a serving of fish, or 2 tablespoons of freshly ground flaxseed to your diet every day.

Choose Brains over Beauty

Consider taking another look at that shy guy who always has his nose buried in a book. A recent study revealed that living with an intellectually stimulating spouse enhances you mentally, too. (Let the boy toys and material girls have each other, so you can make a wiser, more adult choice.)

FAST FORMULA

Brain Brew

Well, I can't promise that you'll suddenly remember everything about Einstein's theory of relativity, or be able to rattle off all of the answers on *Jeopardy*. But you can give your brain a healthy workout by drinking this mind-expanding ginkgo tea every day. One word of caution: People on blood-thinning medication or aspirin should consult their doctors before using ginkgo.

1 tsp. of dried peppermint
1/2 tsp. of dried ginkgo leaves*
1/2 tsp. of dried rosemary
1/2 tsp. of dried gotu kola leaves*
1 cup of boiling water

Mix all of the herbs in a bowl, then scoop a teaspoon of this blend into the water. Let the mixture steep for about 10 minutes. Strain out the herbs, and sip away!

Available in health-food stores

Stay on the Sunny Side

If you're happy with your relationships, you're less likely to develop dementia, according to a study reported in *The Lancet*. Researchers questioned 1,200 people who were at least 75 years old about three aspects of their social lives: whether they lived alone, had friends, and had satisfying relationships with their children. Over the following three years, those older adults with the poorest social networks were 60 percent more likely to develop dementia than those who had only one unsatisfactory area, or who had a rich, extensive social network. So keep your social life lively, and reach out

to people—you'll reduce your stress level *and* stimulate your brain.

Pour on the Protein

Do you have a hard time staying focused on a task? If so, eat a higher-protein, lower-carbohydrate diet—it promotes concentration. While carbohydrates cause your energy levels and focus to soar, then quickly crash, protein helps produce the neurotransmitter dopamine, which sharpens focus. Keep protein-packed munchies, such as string cheese, protein bars, and celery stalks filled with peanut butter, on hand. You'll be surprised at how just a few high-protein morsels can stimulate your concentration.

Remember Ginseng

Ginseng (*Panax ginseng*) is a whole-system tonic that helps you withstand stress, increase endurance, and improve mental performance. To get the most out of it, steep 1 teaspoon of the herb in 1 cup of hot water for 15 minutes. Drink 1 to 2 cups daily for no longer than six weeks at a time. And if you have high blood pressure, check with your doctor first.

SAVE YOUR SIGHT

Seeing is believing, and you'd better believe that without proper care, you won't be seeing nearly as well as you could. Our eyes age right along with the rest of us, and that means macular degeneration, cataracts, and glaucoma are all waiting in the shadows to attack our vision. The best defense is a good offense, so let's shine the light on these eye enemies and learn how you can preserve your peepers.

Have You Seen This Film?

Wise old eyes are wonderful to look into. Yet sometimes, they can seem a little . . . filmy. That "film" is probably a cataract—a clouding of the eye's lens, which reduces or blurs entering light. The biggest causes of cataracts are genes and radiation. If both your parents had cataracts, then it's more likely than not that you'll begin to develop them by middle age. And if your work or your hobbies have meant many years in the sun (and you've not been in the habit of sporting UV-protective sunglasses), then you're at risk, too.

The great news is that cataracts are almost completely curable. Modern laser surgery to remove the cloudy lens and replace it with a clear implant is now safe and effective. But long before surgery, you can do a lot to prevent most cataracts from forming in the first place. Read on for some helpful suggestions.

Go for Antioxidants

Your eyes consume a lot of oxygen because so much light comes through them. But the more oxygen we take in, the more oxidation occurs. Think of a car burning gasoline. The more it burns, the more sludge builds up in the engine. Oxidation creates free radicals in our bodies that muck up the works and need to be removed. Antioxidants come to the rescue by breaking down those oxidation chemicals. Garlic is one of the best antioxidants, but eat a diet that's rich in fresh vegetables and fruits, and you'll also get what you need.

Food Fight

Quercetin, an antioxidant that's essential for eye health, is found in certain foods. Adding these foods to your diet may lower your risk of developing cataracts. Here's the rundown:

Take time for tea. Tea is rich in quercetin. One study showed that drinking several cups of green or black tea a day was associated with lower risk of cataracts. So brew up a pot daily.

Don't hold the onions. The body absorbs twice as much quercetin from onions as it does from tea! And quercetin survives heat, so you can enjoy your onions cooked, as well as raw.

See red. Red wine is another quercetin-rich food. Just be sure to limit your intake to one glass a day (because you don't want to end up "blind drunk").

It's "berry" clear. Bilberry, a close relative of the blueberry, may help prevent cataracts, or at least slow their growth. This shrubby plant is high in bioflavonoids, which are nutrients that enhance the action of vitamin C. Because the lens of the eye naturally contains so much vitamin C, some scientists believe a deficiency can lead to cataracts. You can find bilberry in tincture form in the health-food store; the usual dose is 1 to 2 milliliters twice a day.

Smoke Gets in Your Eyes

Cigarette smoking increases the risk of developing age-related cataracts, and a *Journal of the American Medical Association* article suggests that quitting does reduce the risk of developing them. If you've tried to kick the habit, but so far it's been a losing battle, ask your doctor for help. There are many new and effective ways to help you quit, and the sooner you do it, the better off you'll be.

Shade Those Peepers

Sun exposure triples your risk of cataracts—and it's so easy to avoid! Simply wear a brimmed hat and good sunglasses every time you're out in the sun. And keep in mind that reflected light—from water, snow, or pavement—is often even more damaging than direct sunlight, so wear your shades year-round.

The Eyes *Don't* Have to Have It

You know the old joke: How many people does it take to change a lightbulb? Well, here's a question that's no joke: How often are you changing your lightbulbs and replacing them with higher-wattage bulbs? Why am I asking? Because a major symptom of age-related macular degeneration (AMD) is the need for a brighter light in your reading lamp.

AMD causes blurred vision, which usually begins as difficulty reading fine print. The condition tends to be mild in the early stages, but with the passage of time, it can lead to a severe reduction in vision. This gradual loss of central vision is caused by the degeneration of the macula, which is a tiny bull's-eye point at the center of the retina. By age 65, approximately 15 percent of us will suffer some macular degeneration; by age 75, the prevalence more than doubles to nearly 33 percent. The good news is that even if you come from a family with AMD, you're not likely to develop the disease—if you reduce your other risks. While macular degeneration is a serious disease that needs a doctor's attention, there are many ways to prevent it or catch it in the early—and treatable—stage. The tips below will tell you how.

Oh, Say, Can You See?

See your eye doctor, that is. Get regular eye checkups at least once a year so your doctor can detect any symptoms of AMD, such as the appearance of drusen, which are spots on the retina that are visible during an eye exam. Drusen don't do much damage, but they may cause changes in vision, such as the distortion of straight lines. A telephone pole may appear bent, for example. If you have several relatives who have macular degeneration, begin getting retinal examinations at age 40.

Your Health Is a Clue

It's important for you to be aware of how other medical conditions may affect your vision. For example, hypertension and diabetes increase your risk for macular damage and loss of vision. Hypertension, often related to hardening of the arteries, affects the blood flow throughout your body—including your eyes. Diabetes sometimes leads to diabetic retinopathy, a condition that can interfere with proper metabolism of oxygen in the retina. Talk with your eye doctor as well as your medical doctor about keeping such conditions under control—and AMD at bay.

Sport Some Shades

Wear proper sunglasses and a brimmed hat, and avoid the sun at the peak hours of 10 a.m. to

FAST FORMULA

A Down-Under Chowder

An Australian study found that omega-3 fatty acids may help reduce the risk of macular degeneration. To get more of these "good fats," eat more fish; to get more fish in your diet, try this quick and tasty chowder recipe.

2 white potatoes, cubed
2 large carrots, sliced
1 onion, diced
1 lb. of fish (salmon is one of the highest in omega-3s)
Seafood seasoning (such as Old Bay®)

Place all the ingredients in a pot, and add enough water to cover them, plus 1 inch more. Bring to a boil, then reduce the heat, and simmer until the veggies are cooked and the fish is opaque. See clear to eating it twice a week for maximum results!

2 p.m. Also, make sure your sunglasses provide 100 percent protection from ultraviolet light. Buy the darkest possible lens color to protect your peepers: brown and tan offer the best balance of comfort and protection, with gray and green second best.

Pass the Peppers

Now here's something to sink your teeth into: Bell peppers, especially red ones, pack a powerful punch of lutein and zeaxanthin. A study by the National Eye Institute found that foods rich in lutein and zeaxanthin were associated with reduced risk of macular degeneration. Throw a peck of peppers into stir-fries and salads for healthy eyes in a blink!

Nosh on Nuts

Nuts are loaded with vitamin E, a nutrient that appears to reduce the risk of macular degeneration. Almonds, hazelnuts, and sunflower seeds provide the biggest vitamin E bang for your buck.

Go for the Green

You've already heard me say that eating produce is good for you in all kinds of ways, but now here's yet another reason to munch on your veggies: Kale, spinach, and chard are tops for protecting your eyes. Why? They're loaded with the pigment lutein, which, in the eyes, helps filter out the light implicated in macular degeneration. Lutein supplements are popping up all over the place, but stick to your produce aisle for loading up on lutein, as the long-term effectiveness of lutein supplements has yet to be proven.

Learn to Love Orange

Food, that is. Orange and yellow vegetables and fruits are loaded with beta-carotene, a plant chemical that's converted to vitamin A in the body and used every minute of every day by your eyes. Add a bunch of carrots, squash, cantaloupe, and pumpkin to your menu, along with plenty of greens for healthy vision.

Eggs-ellent Prevention

Lutein and zeaxanthin, the two carotenoids that are critical for preventing age-related macular degeneration, are found in eggs as well as produce. Studies show that your body absorbs them more easily from eggs than from any other food. So scramble to the kitchen and cook yourself some eggs today.

Pair It with Potatoes

To protect your eyes, eat more potatoes. They're high in vitamin C, which is a powerful antioxidant that reduces cell damage from "toxic" molecules in the body.

Brighten Up, Baby!

As its name suggests, eyebright (Euphrasia officinalis) has a long history of traditional use in eye conditions. While this herb may not cure cataracts, a cool compress of eyebright tea can soothe the eyes. To make the tea, drop 1 teaspoon of the herb into 1 cup of boiled water, then refrigerate. When the mixture is cool, soak a clean cloth in the tea, wring it out, and place it over your eyes. Leave the compress in place for 15 to 20 minutes, once or twice a day.

Don't Say Cheese!

If you're having eye problems, avoid those bacon cheeseburgers and other high-fat foods. Just as fat can clog the arteries of your heart, it can also clog those that go to your eyes, reducing the flow of blood and nutrients to your retinas. In fact, studies reveal that many of the same factors that lead to atherosclerosis—smoking, high blood pressure, and high cholesterol levels— also contribute to the development of AMD.

Kick the Habit

Smoking increases your risk of developing macular degeneration by a factor of two to six times! It deprives your retinas of oxygen and constricts your blood vessels, making it more difficult for nutrients to be carried through those vessels to your eyes. Get help today to overcome this addiction.

Drink Ginkgo

What does drinking herbal tea have to do with eye health? Well, we know that increasing the microcirculation of the eyes and enhancing antioxidant activities may help prevent the onset and slow the progression of macular degeneration, and ginkgo and bilberry are two herbs that do just that. So make an infusion of ginkgo (*Ginkgo biloba*) and bilberry (*Vaccinium myrtillus*) by steeping 1 heaping teaspoon of each herb in 1 cup of hot water for 15 minutes. Strain, and drink 2 to 3 cups daily. *Caution:* If you are on blood-thinning medications, do not take ginkgo without checking with your health-care provider first.

Hit the Greens

Do you ski? Sail? Surf? In-line skate? If you're trying to avoid macular degeneration, you might want to trade in your sporting equipment for

---

HOME REMEDY

Milk thistle (*Silybum marianum*) is a powerful antioxidant herb that may help protect vision and eye tissues. For a fast and easy way to reap the benefits of this herb, grind 1 teaspoon of milk thistle seeds (available at health-food stores), and add them to your cereal or a smoothie once a day.

---

a set of golf clubs. Golf, you see, is easier on the eyes. A golf course reflects far less sunlight into your eyes than the ski slopes or the open seas do, and sunlight is so powerful that even reflected rays can damage your unprotected eyes. The bottom line: Always protect your eyes with the proper shades, because even if you think you're not looking at the sun, the sun's rays are still reflecting up at you.

Sneaky Thief of Sight

Because it usually has no warning symptoms, glaucoma is especially dangerous. Ninety percent of the more than 80,000 Americans who are blind as a result of glaucoma did not have to lose their sight. With regular eye examinations, even if you should develop glaucoma, you don't need to join their ranks. If it's caught early enough, glaucoma is highly treatable.

The simplest explanation is that glaucoma is like high blood pressure of the eye. Eye fluid that normally drains away as fast as it is secreted begins to build up—sometimes because of a faulty drainage channel between the back of the cornea and the iris. Drug treatment usually helps reduce the pressure, and laser surgery can open a blocked channel or create a new one, if necessary. Anyone from babies to senior citizens can get glaucoma, but the condition's more common in older folks and those with a family history of glaucoma. According to the Glaucoma Foundation, it's also more common in African-Americans and Asian-Americans. But there are things you can do to keep it in check.

Take This Test

Call your ophthalmologist and schedule a regular eye exam. If you're under 45, being tested every four years is fine. But make an appointment for every two years if you are over 45, are of African descent, have a family history of glaucoma, have diabetes, have had a previous eye injury, or have used cortisone steroid products.

If you have glaucoma, your doctor will probably treat you with eyedrops, pills, surgery, or a combination of methods. Your eyesight's on the line, so it's vital to use your medications correctly. If you change your medication regimen without consulting your doctor, you could develop serious side effects, or even go blind. Here are some other helpful tips to save your sight:

- Refill your prescriptions before they run out, so you don't miss any doses.

- If you are using more than one eyedrop, be sure to wait at least five minutes before instilling the second.

- Never stop your medications just because you have no obvious symptoms.

- Ask your doctor for some hints on how to apply eyedrops properly—it can be tricky.

See with C

Vitamin C is a powerful antioxidant that may help strengthen the vasculature of the eye, which takes in the good stuff and gets rid of the bad. Take 1,000 milligrams of vitamin C with bioflavonoids two to three times daily if you want the healthiest peepers. (And who doesn't?)

Brew Bilberry

Bilberries *(Vaccinium myrtillus)* are high in vitamin C and rich in bioflavonoids, which may help reduce pressure in the eye. Include 1 to 3 cups of bilberry tea as part of your daily fluid intake. Steep 1 teaspoon of the herb in 1 cup of hot water for 15 minutes, then drink to good eye health.

HEAR YE, HEAR YE!

*L*osing our hearing is all too common in our later years. One in every three people over the age of 60—and half of those older than 85—experience it. Of course, it's frustrating and embarrassing, especially when we're trying to talk with friends and family. But did you ever stop to think about how dangerous hearing loss can be? Hearing problems can make it hard to understand and follow a doctor's advice, to respond to warnings, and to hear doorbells and alarms. So listen up and learn the signs, symptoms, and steps you can take to manage this all-too-common condition.

Sound Advice

The two most common causes of hearing loss are age and exposure to loud noise. But you need to see your doctor to rule out other causes, such as a virus or bacteria, heart conditions or stroke, head injuries, tumors, and certain medicines. The National Institutes of Health advises that if you have three or more of the following symptoms, you should see your doctor ASAP to determine why things are not sounding as clear as a bell:

- Trouble hearing when there is distracting noise in the background

- Difficulty following a conversation when two or more people talk at once

- Having to strain to understand when someone else speaks

- Mistaking the normal speech of other people as mumbling

- Misunderstanding what others are saying and responding inappropriately

- Frequently having to ask people to repeat themselves

- Complaints from other folks that the TV volume is too high

- Hearing a ringing or hissing sound frequently

What Can Help?

Depending on what kind of hearing problem you have, some treatments will work better for you than others. If you've got minor hearing loss, some of the tips below should be helpful. If it's more serious than that, you'll need a more serious solution. Either way, consult your doctor, and read on for more advice on getting a better handle on hearing.

Tune In to Technology

I know a lot of folks who would rather struggle to hear than get a hearing aid. They may be reluctant because they've only tried older hearing aids, which were difficult to use and seemed to amplify every sound in the room.

HOME REMEDY

A deficiency of B vitamins can cause tinnitus, which is a ringing or other noise in your ears that you hear when no real sounds are present. If you have tinnitus, taking a B-complex supplement can minimize your symptoms, and possibly even improve the function of the nerves in your ears. Look for a formula that includes thiamine, niacin, and vitamin B_{12}.

But let me tell you, what's out there now is not your grandmother's hearing aid. Newer, digital hearing aids have built-in smarts that allow them to do a better job of figuring out which sounds you want amplified. They are also a heckuva lot smaller than they used to be and practically invisible! Whether it's behind your ear, in your ear, or in your pocket, you'll most likely have to try out a few to find the one that works best for you. It's a complicated process, and if you don't end up with the right aid, it can be frustrating. So get a recommendation from your doctor for an audiologist—who is specially trained to help you through the selection process. Then check out these other innovative aids:

Personal listening systems. They help you hear exactly what you want to hear. You can choose from systems that can make it easier for you to hear someone in a crowded room, or those that are better for personal, one-on-one conversations.

TV listening systems. These allow you to listen to the TV or radio without being distracted by background noise. And they can even be used if you have a hearing aid. Or you can get "direct audio input" hearing aids that plug right in to TVs and stereos.

Telephone amplifying devices. If your hearing aid has a "T" switch, you may be able to get a phone with an amplifying coil (T coil). Putting your hearing aid in the "T" position activates the coil when you pick up the phone. You'll be able to listen at a comfortable volume with less background noise. If you have a mobile phone, then a "loop set" is what you need. A wire loop sits around your neck and connects to the phone. Sound is transmitted directly from the phone to the hearing aid in your ear. Either way, contact your local phone company for details.

Keep It Quiet

Background noise makes it hard to hear people talk, so turn off the TV, radio, or stereo if it doesn't have to be on. When you go to a restaurant, don't sit near the kitchen, which tends to be noisy, if you want to hear your dining companions. And try to avoid sitting near any music playing from a band or from a speaker.

Beef Up

Lean meats are rich in zinc, a mineral that may minimize age-related tinnitus and hearing loss. The recommended intake is 15 milligrams a day, which you can easily get by including lean meats in your diet. Alternate them with shellfish, which is also a good source of zinc. Did I hear someone say "surf and turf"? Yes, please!

Magnify with Magnesium

Low magnesium levels may constrict inner-ear arteries and lead to tinnitus. If you work or play around noisy equipment, ask your doctor about taking 250 milligrams of supplemental magnesium—or just feast regularly on green veggies, whole grains, nuts, and beans, all of which are great sources.

Loud and Clear

It's important to talk to friends and family because they need to know that you're not hearing as well as you used to. The more they know, the more they can help. And make sure that they face you when they talk—their expressions and facial movements can help you understand them better.

When Pain Sounds

Most earaches are not serious and will simply fade away on their own. But if you have ear pain for more than a day or two, you need to see a doctor. If fluid has built up, your doctor may use a small suction device to remove it. For bacterial infections, the standard treatment is an antibiotic, but natural infection fighters, such as the ones that follow, can often do the job just as effectively. These remedies are for adults only, so check with a pediatrician for specifics on how to treat earaches in infants and children.

Since prevention is always the best medicine, here are three time-tested ways to stop earaches before they start:

Douse 'em with vinegar. Anytime you're going to swim in an unchlorinated body of water, such as a lake, a river, or the ocean, take along small bottles of vinegar and rubbing alcohol (a drying agent). After every dip, dry your ears well, then dribble a solution of 2 drops of vinegar and 2 drops of alcohol into each ear.

Bet on boric acid. If you're prone to ear infections, ask your pharmacist to mix up a 3 percent boric acid, 70 percent alcohol solution. The boric acid will acidify the ear canal, discouraging any bacterial or fungal invaders from venturing down that path, while the alcohol will dry it up. Squeeze a few drops into your ears every day to keep them infection-free.

Stop the pops. Painful fullness in your ears during airplane travel is caused by a difference between the air pressure in the middle ear and the atmospheric pressure in the aircraft. If you pick up some pulsatilla extract from your doctor or from a health-food store before your flight, however, you may be able to stop the pops—and the pain. This herb works by reducing inflammation in the eustachian tubes. Mix 10 drops of pulsatilla extract in a glass of water and drink it 20 minutes before your descent. Follow with another dose as soon as you can after landing.

Ease the Ouch

If ear pain happens before you can stop it, try these simple soothers:

- Rub oil behind your ear (where your lymph glands are located), or place a cotton ball saturated with oil inside your ear to soothe the ache and help stimulate the lymph glands into removing the infectious agents. Many folks find that something called sweet oil—a mixture of olive oil and other oils such as lavender, tea tree, chamomile, and hops—works really well. Check your health-food store for sweet oil, or simply make your own by mixing the oils together in equal amounts.

- Get steamed. Eucalyptus is another herbal decongestant that may help ease the pressure in your eustachian tubes and start the drainage of fluid that has been dammed up in the middle ear—especially if you combine it with steam, which also encourages the flow of mucus. Fill a bowl with boiling water, add up to 10 drops of eucalyptus oil (available in health-food stores), and lean over the bowl, but not so close that you could burn your face. Drape a towel over your head and the bowl to capture the steam, then inhale the mist for at least five minutes. You can also place a few drops of eucalyptus oil in your bathwater, but *don't* put it directly into your ears.

- For a natural antibiotic, simply mash a garlic clove with a fork, and saturate it with several drops of olive oil. Let the mash absorb the oil overnight, strain out the garlic, and warm the oil so that it's pleasantly tepid, but not hot. Tilt your head so that your sore ear faces up, and plop 2 or 3 drops of the garlic oil into your ear. Lie down—again, with your sore ear up—and let the oil settle for two or three minutes before you raise your head. Repeat this treatment a few times a day, and your discomfort should disappear within a day or two.

- Sniff some salt water. Dissolve as much table salt as you can in a glass of warm water without the water becoming cloudy. Pour a little of the saltwater into your cupped hand, and sniff the mixture into one nostril, then the other. Repeat several times. This nasal wash acts as a natural decongestant to shrink swollen tissues and unplug your eustachian tubes.

Save the Candles for Romance

If you've ever been tempted to try ear candling, which is an alternative procedure touted to draw out excess earwax or ease earaches, save your money! Here's how it's done: The top of a foot-long cone that's been soaked in beeswax is inserted into your ear while you are lying on your side. Then it's lit and left to burn. The vacuum created by the heat is supposed to draw earwax into the cone and ease your pain, but studies indicate that the only thing that collects in the cone is melted beeswax.

Quick Fix

This old-time remedy soothes an earache—and perhaps stimulates the flow of mucus as well—with warm, moist heat. Simply heat an onion or a potato in the microwave (boiling works, too), then cool it slightly. Put the toasty sphere in a clean cotton sock, and rest your sore ear against it for soothing relief.

203

HAIR TODAY, GONE TOMORROW!

Make no mistake, no one holds on to his or her hair forever. Every day, we shed about 100 of our 100,000 scalp hairs. Whether this loss is replaced with new strands of hair depends on several factors, including hormones, genetics, and age. Like plants in a garden, each hair on your head has its own growing season. Instead of just a few months, however, your hair's growing season lasts about four years. During this period, hair grows about half an inch a month for 46 or so months, then enters a six-week resting phase. At the end of that phase, new hair sprouts from the hair follicle, pushing out the old strand—which ends up in your brush or down a bathroom drain. But as we age, the growth phase gets shorter, the resting phase gets longer, and new hair becomes thinner. That's why I'm offering these tips on how to deal with hair loss. Comb through them—some may be just right for you.

Be Brave and Be Bald

If you no longer have a full head of hair, why not shave off what little is left? After all, bald is sexy. Think of Yul Brynner and Telly Savalas's Kojak. Why, even women can make a statement with their naked pates: Consider pop singers Sinéad O'Connor and Joan Jett. So if you're feeling a bit bold, reach for the razor.

Go for Rogaine®

Rogaine® is a hair treatment that has been approved by the U.S. Food and Drug Administration (FDA) for use by both men and women. Read the directions carefully before you rub it into your scalp. Rogaine® is not for everyone, so ask your doctor if it's safe for you—especially if you have medical conditions that require continuous use of medications.

Pump Up the Volume

Drugstore shelves are literally awash in volumizing shampoos. While these products won't grow more hair, they will plump up your existing hair strands. Use these shampoos daily, then blow-dry or shake out your hair, and it will seem much fuller than it actually is.

Try This Tonic

Elder (*Sambucus canadensis*), nettles (*Urtica dioica*), prickly ash (*Xanthoxylum clava-herculis*), and yarrow (*Achillea millefolium*) are all nutrient-rich herbs that help increase circulation, which is exactly what is needed for healthy hair growth. Steep 1 heaping teaspoon of any of these herbs in 1 pint of hot water. Then let your hair down and drink this beverage warm throughout the day.

Be a Hothead

Here's a mix that may help you keep a full head of hair. Add 1 or 2 drops of red pepper (cayenne) oil to 1 ounce of rosemary oil in a clean, small bottle, then massage your entire scalp with the mixture for at least 20 minutes every day. Afterward, wash your hair with shampoo, to which you've added 5 drops of rosemary oil per ounce of shampoo.

Break an Egg

Old-timers used to swear by this treatment for hair loss. Once or twice a week, beat a raw egg in about 1 tablespoon of olive oil, and massage it into your hair and scalp. Leave it on for a few minutes, then rinse with warm water.

Herbal Hair Repair

Some herbs help stimulate circulation, which may help slow down hair loss. Try any one of these for pate-pleasing results:

Rub it with rosemary. A gentle scalp massage may be just what the doctor ordered to enhance circulation and encourage hair growth. Simply mix 4 to 6 drops of rosemary oil *(Rosmarinus officinalis)* in 1 tablespoon of olive oil, and gently massage the mixture into your scalp. For a deepening effect, cover your hair with a shower cap and wrap a hot, wet towel around your head. Leave it on for 30 minutes or so, then shampoo.

Give your locks lavender. Barbers have long known that massaging the scalp with lavender oil stimulates circulation, bringing both oxygen and nutrients to hair follicles and perhaps stimulating hair growth. To get that barbershop treatment, add 6 drops of lavender oil to $1/2$ cup of warm almond, soy, or sesame oil, all of which easily penetrate the skin. Massage the mixture into your scalp for 20 minutes, then wash it out with shampoo, adding 3 drops of bay oil per ounce of shampoo.

Sage advice. It may be especially, well, sage to use sage to encourage hair growth. Taken internally, this pungent culinary herb helps the body adapt to the hormonal changes that are often at the root of hair loss. To use sage externally to stimulate scalp circulation, steep 2 tablespoons of dried sage leaves (or two sage tea bags) in a cup of hot water for 5 to 10 minutes. Strain, let it cool, then pour the tea over your hair after shampooing. Leave it on for 5 minutes, then rinse. Repeat this treatment

---

FAST FORMULA

Meddle with Nettles

Try this easy-to-make herbal vinegar rinse to help maintain a healthy scalp and encourage hair growth.

1 oz. of nettles
1 cup of apple cider vinegar
1 pint of warm water

Simmer the nettles in the apple cider vinegar for 15 minutes. Strain, and store the vinegar in a cool, dark place. After shampooing, mix $1/4$ cup of the herbal vinegar in the warm water, and use as a rinse. Just remember to wear gloves when handling fresh nettles to avoid their stinging hairs.

---

daily. You can also add a few drops of sage extract to your favorite shampoo.

Kink It Up a Notch

One handy way to disguise thinning hair is to get a perm for fullness. Curls cover more real estate than straight hair does, and gentle mussing also offers some camouflage.

Color Me Full

If your hair color is close to your skin color, your scalp will be less noticeable. So use hair coloring to reduce the see-through scalp look. If you color your hair at home, use only the semipermanent dyes. They are not harsh, but they will plump up your hair shafts so they look thicker. And avoid permanent dyes because they don't wash out, and they create a color line between natural and dyed hair that seems to make thinning hair more obvious.

Herbal Hair Saver

Comb the hair-care aisles of your supermarket or drugstore for herbal hair products that contain camphor and eucalyptus. They'll dilate the blood vessels in your scalp, which will help discourage hair loss.

Pour on the Protein

Because hair is made up of protein, it's especially important to beef up the protein content of your diet. The best way is to drink plenty of milk and eat lots of other protein-rich foods, such as poultry, lean meat, and fish.

Fish for Thicker Hair

Thin, brittle hair may indicate a deficiency of omega-3 essential fatty acids (EFAs), which are found in cold-water fish like salmon, sardines, and herring. To strengthen your hair, you'd need to eat fish two or three times a week. If that's way too fishy for you, supplement your diet with gamma-linolenic acid (GLA), another EFA, by taking either black currant oil or evening primrose oil, which are available at health-food stores. Follow the package directions. After six to eight weeks of taking either supplement, your hair should become shinier, stronger, and, hopefully, thicker.

For Women Only

While vitamins and minerals don't do a thing to jump-start hair growth in men, studies show they may prove helpful for some women. Experts suggest taking a high-potency multivitamin/mineral supplement once a day that contains the B-complex vitamins, 1,000 milligrams of vitamin C, 400 IUs of vitamin E, 15 milligrams of zinc, and 1.5 milligrams of copper. Check with your doctor about taking these supplements, and ask about taking iron, especially if you have hair loss following crash dieting or physical trauma.

For Men Only

Saw palmetto, the herb most noted for shrinking enlarged prostate glands in men, may slow down hair loss for men, too—maybe even as well as prescription androgen blockers. It seems that saw palmetto contains an ingredient that reduces dihydrotestosterone (DHT) levels, which contribute to male-pattern baldness. Check your health-food store for saw palmetto capsules, and take 160 milligrams twice daily.

Lather Up with Licorice

Like saw palmetto, licorice contains a chemical that may prevent testosterone from converting into DHT, which is the chemical that's responsible for baldness and thinning hair in men. To slow hair loss, simply add several drops of licorice tincture or extract to your favorite shampoo.

SAVE THAT SMILE!

Aside from getting the occasional tooth snapped off in the throes of an ice hockey or softball game, most of us lose teeth in more predictable ways: from decay, cavities, and the resulting extractions. As we get older, we are more likely to face these conditions—unless we take preventive measures. Don't worry, it's easy to do...so relax, and smile!

Mom Was Right

You know what they say about pesky people— ignore them and they'll go away. Well, the same can be said for your pearly whites! You've got to take care of them if you want them to stick around. It works just like your mom always said it did: When carbohydrate-rich foods such as candy and soda remain on your teeth, bacteria grow and solidify onto the teeth in a substance called plaque. Eventually, it destroys those teeth—and your smile along with them—unless you brush up on these teeth-saving basics:

Brush more than once. Don't think brushing just once a day will do it for you. Brush twice a day for two or three minutes each time. Although saliva is a natural cleanser, your body doesn't produce much while you're sleeping. So that's when plaque typically does its dirty work. For this reason, it's important to brush in the morning before you eat breakfast to remove any plaque that formed during the night. Then brush again before you go to bed. Plaque takes 16 to 24 hours to develop. If you brush twice a day, you won't accumulate enough plaque to do much damage. Get an electric toothbrush with a pulse timer or beeper to let you know you're brushing long enough.

Be gentle. In other words, don't brush your teeth as though you're trying to scrub shellac off the floor. Hard scrubbing damages your teeth and won't remove any more plaque than gentle brushing. A good rule of thumb is: If your toothbrush bristles are worn down after a month, you're brushing way too hard. Brush gently, but thoroughly.

HOME REMEDY

If you run out of dental floss, dig into your knitting basket. That's right! Pull out some white wool yarn, and use it in place of your normal dental floss. It's thicker than floss, but it will do the job just as well as the commercial stuff—maybe even better!

Buy the right brush. Look for a brush with soft bristles that have rounded ends; if the bristles are hard, they can wear away enamel and damage your gums. Replace the brush every three to four months, advises the American Dental Association. And if the bristles begin to fray, replace it sooner.

Floss the nooks and crannies. There are places your toothbrush cannot reach, and that's why you need to floss. Once-a-day flossing is recommended by experts. Flossing removes plaque from between teeth and under the gum line. And healthy gums mean healthy teeth!

Make Friends with a Hygienist

Every dentist's office has a wonderful person who loves teeth so much she (it always seems to be a she) spends her life getting off every little speck of plaque that you—you naughty person!—didn't get with a toothbrush or floss. This person is a hygienist. Get to know her, see her twice a year, and treat her with gratitude and respect. She just may save your teeth!

Go Green

Green tea contains tooth-loving tannins, which kills decay-causing bacteria and stops them from producing glucan, the sticky substance that helps acid-generating bacteria cling to your teeth. Check your local market for green tea. It's widely available now in tea bags and as loose tea. Drink a cup after every meal. *Caution:* If you have clotting disorders or take heart medications, check with your doctor before drinking green tea.

Kissing Juice

It's been said that kissing helps prevent cavities because saliva cleans the mouth, and kissing produces saliva. How? Well, when you're actively smooching, your mouth is making up to a teaspoon of saliva a minute. (Talk about a wet kiss!) All of which is great unless the person you're puckering up to doesn't take care of his or her teeth as well as you do. That's because cavity-causing bacteria may be transmitted through saliva. So do what you can to make sure your kissing partner brushes up on oral hygiene, too.

Lic' Tooth Decay

Peel a length of licorice root (*Glycyrrhiza glabra*), and chomp on it. Then fray the ends for an instant herbal tooth cleaning. *Caution:* Licorice root should not be used by people with high blood pressure or kidney disease.

No Teeth for Tools!

I know you don't tear off the tops of beer cans with your teeth (at least I hope not!). But that's not the only way to guarantee a broken tooth. If you use your teeth to crack hard nuts, open the lids of pill bottles, loosen knots, or gnaw on candy bars straight from the freezer (as many people do), you're asking for trouble. The top tooth breaker? Ice cubes. So take it easy on your teeth and crunch on some pretzels instead.

Quick Fix

Chamomile tea, a traditional remedy for tooth pain, helps in two ways: It reduces inflammation and has a mild tranquilizing effect. To get the most from chamomile, make a cup of tea, using one tea bag per cup of hot water. Steep the tea for 10 to 20 minutes, let it cool, then swish some around in your mouth for about 30 seconds. Swallow the tea (or spit it out), then repeat until the entire cup is gone. Caution: *Avoid chamomile if you're allergic to ragweed.*

Toothpaste Rx

To try to save a tooth that's suffering from gum disease, pack it with a mixture of powdered myrrh *(Comiphora molmol)* and goldenseal *(Hydrastis canadensis)*. Add enough hydrogen peroxide to the powders to make a paste, and apply around the tooth one to three times daily. When pain is an issue, add a pinch of powdered cloves *(Eugenia caryophyllus)*. Then make a dental appointment, pronto!

CHAPTER 11

Looking Good

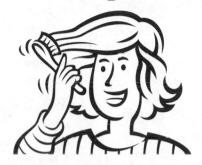

Of course you want to look good. Who doesn't? But maybe you're worried about what's in those beauty aisle products, or are tired of emptying your wallet to buy them. In this chapter, I'll share my favorite beauty and hygiene secrets—using natural ingredients and common household products—so you'll look your best without breaking the bank!

A GAME PLAN FOR GROOMING

Most of us have close encounters of the human kind on a daily basis. To make sure you keep friends and don't make enemies, we'll tackle the most common offenders to personal hygiene here—bad breath, body odor, and dandruff. You'll find my best tips to help you defend yourself.

Bad Breath: Get the Freshest Mouth in Town

Got dinosaur breath? Does your bed partner stuff his or her head under the pillow when you lean over for a good-morning smooch? In either case,

you need help—now! While you're sleeping, your saliva production factory is off-line, too. Busy little bacteria take over, and a few hours later, you wake up with real roadkill breath. A drop in saliva levels allows mouth bacteria to multiply and form plaque. Bad breath may also be a result of poor dental hygiene, poor diet, or a sinus or gum infection. Rarely, it can signal something as serious as kidney failure, liver disease, or diabetes. Ask your doctor about persistent bad breath if you get no relief from the following reliable remedies:

Brush up on your oral hygiene. Are you brushing twice a day with a soft brush? The bedtime brushing is important so plaque doesn't form during the night (while saliva production is off duty). Massage your gums with the brush, too. And before you brush, floss your teeth. Flossing every day helps remove plaque—and bacteria—from between your teeth. And don't forget those twice-a-year visits to your dentist for a good professional cleaning!

Rake your tongue. Most bad breath comes from the wet, boggy areas in the back of your mouth, where bacteria breed a sulfur-smelling plaque on your tongue. So before brushing, reach into your mouth as far as you can go without gagging, and scrape away the plaque. Most pharmacies carry plastic tongue scrapers, or you can save some pennies and simply use your toothbrush.

Fight mouth rage with sage. Put 2 teaspoons of fresh sage leaves (or a teaspoon of dried leaves) in a pint of water on the stove. Bring it to a boil, then turn off the heat and cover the pan with a lid. Let it steep for about 15 minutes. Strain out the herbs, and you now have your very own custom-made mouthwash. Let it cool down before using it; then swish and spit, and say good-bye to bad breath!

Drink lots of water. Keeping yourself well hydrated is a good health practice in general, but it is especially important to help keep bad breath at bay. Drink those eight glasses of water a day to help keep saliva production going strong and to reduce bacteria buildup.

Eat your veggies. Vegetables and fruits are not only valuable sources of vitamins and antioxidants, but they also contain chlorophyll, a natural deodorant that sweetens your breath. So eat five to nine servings a day for a healthy body and healthy breath, too.

Pucker up. Sour foods, like pickles and lemons, will jump-start the flow of saliva,

---

> **FAST FORMULA**
>
> ## Native Spice Mix
>
> Here's a Native American cleansing and refreshing mixture that clears up bad breath while brightening your teeth; it also makes a fine gargle and mouthwash. You can use this tooth powder daily, or alternate it with a commercial brand.
>
> 1 tbsp. of baking soda
> $^1/_2$ tsp. of sea salt or kosher salt
> $^1/_2$ tsp. of powdered allspice
> $^1/_2$ tsp. of ground sage
>
> Combine the ingredients in a small dish. Sprinkle the mixture onto your toothbrush and brush, or stir 1 teaspoon into 1 cup of warm water and gargle.

which helps to flush away any nasty halitosis bacteria that are in your mouth.

Make It Myrrh-velous

To keep your breath kissably fresh, try this mouth mix: Stir 1 teaspoon of tincture of myrrh *(Commiphora molmol)*, which you can find at a health-food store, in $^1/_4$ cup of water and use it as a mouthwash. Then get ready to pucker up!

Take It from Eve

An apple a day not only will keep the doctor away, but it will also keep bad breath at bay! In fact, an apple is a great remedy for garlic breath. In a healthy mouth, garlic odor usually goes away after a while, but you'll speed up the process if you dilute the pungent aroma with an apple, and then brush your teeth.

Chew on It

Some Native American traditions call for using

spearmint or bergamot leaves as a quick and easy digestive aid and breath freshener. Try it for yourself by slowly chewing on a leaf or two. Or try this other portable breath freshener: Carry a sandwich bag or pouch of mint or parsley leaves; chewing on them periodically throughout the day will give you the freshest mouth in town.

Go for the Burn

Fight fire with fire—kill dragon breath with cayenne's firepower! Cayenne not only kills germs, but also leaves your breath feeling spicy fresh. Just dilute 5 to 10 drops each of cayenne tincture and myrrh tincture (both are available in health-food stores) in half a glass of warm water, and use it as a mouth rinse to burn bad breath away.

Get Seedy Relief

Chewing fennel *(Foeniculum vulgare)* or dill seeds *(Anethum graveolens)* after meals will not only help freshen your breath, but it'll be a boon to your digestive tract, too!

Lose the Stink!

Aren't you glad we're not living back when people only bathed once a week—or less—and masked their body odor with heavy perfumes, powdered wigs, and lots of rarely washed clothes? I sure am. Whee-ew! Our bodies need to sweat to regulate temperature, but perspiration's not the problem—in fact, your sweat is composed of nearly odorless water. The odor comes from the presence of bacteria and fungi in the sweaty areas. These busy little stinkers particularly like to get between your toes, into your armpits, and on your private parts. And they can leave your clothes smelling less than sweet as well. Here are some tips for keeping the odors away:

Gobble up the garnish. Some body odor is caused by what you eat. Those all-too-familiar smells of garlic and onions can come right through your pores. But there's no need to boycott these favorites: Just neutralize their potent aromas by eating parsley and other green leafy vegetables that contain chlorophyll (a natural deodorant) along with the stinky stuff. That's the origin of the parsley-as-garnish tradition. If you keep it up, you'll begin to notice a distinct difference in just a few days.

Zap the stink with zinc. A deficiency of the mineral zinc in your diet can leave you smelling a little pungent. Make sure you get it in a multivitamin, or in foods such as seafood, oatmeal, meat, pumpkin seeds, and eggs.

Sip some sage. Sage tea can help curb sweat gland activity and may be especially helpful when your perspiration is stress induced. Simply steep 2 teaspoons of dried sage in 1 cup of boiling water for 10 minutes, then sip it in small doses—but only during tense situations. Regular ingestion of sage may cause dizziness, hot flashes, and other problems. *Caution:* Don't drink sage if you're pregnant or nursing.

Can the caffeine. Coffee and tea increase the activity of the apocrine sweat glands. So if you have a body odor problem, eliminate these offenders for a week or so and see if you don't smell sweeter.

Get Your 'Phyll

Chlorophyll, that is! As I mentioned earlier (see "Lose the Stink!" at left), this odor eater is found in parsley and green veggies. Well, alfalfa sprouts contain a generous amount of chlorophyll, too. If you're not too crazy about the idea of eating lots of sprouts, you can get all the benefits by drinking up to 3 cups of alfalfa tea daily or by taking alfalfa tablets.

Balance Your Bacteria

Maintaining a good diet can go a long way toward solving the BO problem. That's because a high-fat, high-sugar, low-fiber diet can upset the balance of bacteria in your intestines, throwing a monkey wrench into your digestion and ultimately, provoking odor.

Give Stinky Feet the Boot!

If foot odor is your particular bugaboo, then the next time you buy deodorant, look for one of these natural odor neutralizers: sage *(Salvia officinalis)*, tea tree *(Melaleuca alternifolia)*, and green clay. Sprinkle one of them in your shoes, and you'll soon say *sayonara* to foot odor.

Flower Powder

Or rather, powdered flowers, which can help absorb odors. Mix together equal parts of the powdered flowers of calendula *(Calendula officinalis)* and lavender *(Lavandula officinalis)*, and add them to an equal part of slippery elm *(Ulmus fulva)* powder. Dust under your arms once or twice daily and body odor will take a powder.

Clean from the Inside Out

What's your largest body organ? Nope, not your heart or your lungs. It's your skin! Not only does it protect what's inside of you, but skin is also an important player in the elimination of toxins from your body.

So what does all this biology have to do with BO? Well, body odor can sometimes be the result of sluggish or poor elimination. So to get things cleaned from the inside out, make a tea from these gentle cleansing herbs:

Calendula *(Calendula officinalis)*

Cleavers *(Galium aparine)*

Peppermint *(Mentha x piperita)*

Red clover *(Trifolium pratense)*

Yarrow *(Achillea millefolium)*

Combine equal parts of the herbs, and store in a container with a tight lid. Add 1 heaping tablespoon of the herb mix to 1 quart of warm water. Steep for 15 minutes. Drink throughout the day for a good internal cleansing.

A Little Dab Will Do Ya!

Splashing some rubbing alcohol under your arms may help to reduce the bacteria population that's found a home there. For a persistent odor problem, try using alcohol in place of deodorant—just don't do this after shaving or if you have any nicks or cuts in your skin. That would sting like heck!

Go for the Gold

Natives of the U.S. Southwest and Mexico have long used calendula flowers as skin fresheners because of their mild, pleasing fragrances and skin-soothing minerals. A cream made from these flowers absorbs well into the skin, especially during summer's heat. To make your own soothing salve, combine 1 ounce of dried, crushed calendula petals with glycerin or beeswax, distilled water, and some dried mint or bergamot. Simmer in the top of a double boiler for about three hours to create a fine emulsion. Then pour it into a clean bowl, and whip it with a hand beater or electric mixer until it cools and sets.

You may also want to try making another Native American recipe: Mix crushed calendula leaves with cornstarch for a refreshing body talc.

Shake Those Flakes for Good

Many people shed a dandruff flake or two every now and then, especially in winter, when scalps tend to dry out. More serious dandruff, however, results when tiny oil glands at the base of the hair roots run amok. The scalp's skin normally replaces itself once a month; but if you have dandruff, somehow this shedding process gets accelerated. Hair becomes greasy, and those telltale crusty, yellowish flakes sprinkle your shoulders. Chances are, they're not your favorite fashion accessories.

Another type of dandruff occurs when the scalp's sebaceous glands become plugged. Hair loses its gloss, and the dandruff flakes are dry and grayish. Because more men than women have dandruff, doctors suspect that the male hormone testosterone may have something to do with it. Other factors that can give you a case of the flakes include family history, food allergies, excessive sweating, alkaline soaps, and yeast infections. And although no one knows exactly what causes dandruff, stress does provoke it. See a doctor if you are losing hair, your scalp seems inflamed, or you have itching, scaly skin on other parts of your body as well, which may indicate a more serious problem such as psoriasis. Otherwise, there's a lot you can do to control dandruff. Read on for my advice on your best options.

Shampoo Savvy

A good, dandruff-fighting shampoo reduces scaling of the scalp and allows medication to penetrate. Look for shampoos that list tar or salicylic acid among their ingredients. Although there are many over-the-counter dandruff shampoos, the U.S. Food and Drug Administration (FDA) has approved only five active ingredients as safe and effective against dandruff: coal tar, pyrithione zinc, salicylic acid, selenium sulfide, and sulfur. Stick to one of these for fighting flakes.

Once you find a good shampoo, use it daily. Washing your hair every day will break up larger flakes of dandruff, making them less noticeable. It'll also prevent the buildup of hair spray, gels, and other hair preparations—some of which can look a lot like flakes as they wear off your hair. Massage the shampoo into your scalp, and let it sit there for three to five minutes—longer if your dandruff is severe. Make sure you rinse thoroughly to get all of the shampoo out.

Lemon Squeeze

After shampooing, rinse your hair with lemon juice or—if you can stand the smell—vinegar. Dilute each with enough water (say, 2 ounces of lemon juice or vinegar to 1 quart of water), so you don't feel a burning sensation on your scalp. This hair treatment is popular with many folks because it leaves hair shiny and squeaky clean. Rinsing with or dabbing these weak acids right onto your scalp helps remove dandruff flakes, too.

Get to the Roots

Native American healers use the roots of the yucca plant, pounded and whipped with water, to treat dandruff. Yucca roots contain soapy substances called saponins. Don't feel like whipping and pounding? No problem. You can pick up a ready-made yucca root shampoo at your local health-food store.

Hang Up Your Hair Dryer

Whenever you can, let your hair dry naturally, rather than blowing it dry. When you must have extra volume for a special occasion, be sure to use a lower heat setting. That hot wind really dries out the scalp, making you more vulnerable to developing dandruff.

⏳ *Quick Fix*

It flavors beer—that's what most of us know about hops. Yet the wild hops plant is found all over the world, and Native Americans use it as a cure for dandruff (among other things). But you don't need to comb the forests and fields in search of hops—just rinse your hair with beer, or add a good squirt of the suds to your regular shampoo.

Dandruff-B-Gone

The B vitamins, particularly biotin, are essential to having a healthy scalp. And a healthy scalp could mean flake-free hair. So make sure your multivitamin contains biotin, or find a B-complex vitamin that contains 300 micrograms of biotin, and take it every day.

Herbs for Your Head

Enlist these herbal helpers in your fight against dandruff (use once or twice a week):

Get steamy. Steaming your scalp with nutritive herbs is a deep-cleansing treatment that fights dandruff. Mix together equal parts of dried or fresh rosemary, nettle, and peppermint leaves. Add 2 tablespoons of dried herb mix ($^1/_2$ cup fresh) to 2 cups of hot water and steep, covered, for 10 minutes. Strain the infusion, cool slightly, and apply it carefully to your scalp. Cover your hair with a shower cap and wrap your head in a hot, wet towel. Sit and relax for 30 minutes, then finish with the thyme rinse below.

Take a thyme out. Try this routine—dab some thyme oil diluted with olive oil (4 drops of thyme oil per teaspoon of olive oil) on your scalp one hour before washing your hair. Then, after shampooing, it's thyme for an antidandruff rinse. To make the rinse, boil a handful of dry thyme leaves in 1 quart of water, strain, and cool.

Styling Sense

While it's important to choose the right shampoos and rinses to fight dandruff, it's equally crucial to style your hair properly. Use a natural-bristle brush to brush your hair from the scalp outward with steady, firm strokes. This action carries excess oil away from your scalp, where it can cause dandruff, to the hair strands, where it gives your hair a nice, healthy shine.

When you're perfecting your hairdo, use only nonoily gels and mousses. Greasy hair fixatives can make a dandruff problem worse.

HEALTHY HAIR AND SKIN

Have you noticed all the natural and herbal products that are showing up in shampoos, lotions, and facial cleansers? Manufacturers are finally getting wise to what some of us have known for years: The best routes to healthy hair and skin can be through the gate to your garden, the freeway to your fridge, and the path to your pantry.

No More Bad Hair Days

We all want healthy, shiny hair, but the number of hair-care products out there is enough to make your head spin. Read the labels and you'll think you need a graduate degree in chemistry to figure out what's inside! Fortunately, there are a number of ways to manage your locks naturally, without that fancy degree. Here's what to do to maintain your crowning glory:

Count on bunny food. Carrots can help absorb excess hair oil without drying out your scalp. To put them to work for you, chop up three raw carrots, and then puree them in a blender. Apply this mix to your scalp, leave it on for 15 minutes, then hop along to rinse it off with cool water.

Say holy guacamole! What's the cure for dry hair? How about a ripe (overripe is even better) avocado that's been skinned and mashed. Apply the puree to your hair, leave it on for 15 minutes, and then rinse it out with cool water for luscious locks.

Change the oil. Herbal experts say that a 500-milligram capsule of black currant oil, taken twice a day, is the surest cure for dry hair. But you need to be patient; it takes six to eight weeks to see the difference. Once your hair is in better condition, you can cut the daily dosage in half.

Scramble for moisture. Eggs are rich in protein, and therefore, they make an excellent conditioning pack for hair. Beat an egg until it's light yellow, and then apply it to your hair. Leave it on for 10 to 15 minutes, then rinse thoroughly, using cool to tepid water.

Drink to Healthy Hair

Like the condition of your fingernails, hair health is a reflection of internal health. So make it a practice to drink nutritive teas that are rich in minerals to optimize your skin and hair health. Any or all of the following herbs taken daily will do the trick: nettles *(Urtica dioica)*, oatstraw *(Avena sativa)*, horsetail *(Equisetum arvense)*, and red clover *(Trifolium pratense)*. Steep 1 heaping teaspoon of any one of these herbs in 1 cup of hot water, and drink 1 to 2 cups daily. *Caution:* Be sure to wear gloves when handling fresh nettles so you don't get stung.

Get L.A. Locks

For deep conditioning that fights heat, smog, and fog, mash 1/2 cup of fresh avocado with 1/4 cup of mayonnaise—the real mayo with eggs and oil in it. Apply to your scalp first, massaging well, then comb it out to the ends of your hair. Cover with a shower cap and wrap a hot, wet towel around your head. Leave on for 30 minutes or longer and you'll be ready for Hollywood!

S'more Conditioning

Marshmallow (no, not the kind that floats in your cocoa) is a great natural moisturizer for dry hair. Put 2 teaspoons of dried marshmallow root (available at health-food stores) into 1 cup of boiling water, and steep for about 15 minutes. Strain out the herb and let the solution cool in the refrigerator before using it to rinse your hair.

Soften Up Your Birthday Suit

Skin that feels itchy and dry, and looks dull, is just no fun to live in. Dry skin, medically known as xeroderma, can result from cold weather, frequent bathing, sun exposure, or chemicals that leach the natural oils from your skin. *Note:* If your skin is dry, itchy, and flaking, it could be an allergy or infection, or a systemic condition that needs your doctor's attention. If not, all you need to do is replenish the moisture—inside and out—for a healthy all-over glow. Here's how to get the moisture back into your birthday suit so you can get comfy in your skin:

Go for fats. Dry skin, especially in the winter, can be the result of too little of the right kind of fats in your diet. Our skin is where water and oil meet, and both are essential to good skin health. So make sure your diet includes one or more servings a day of omega-3 fats found in cold-water fish (salmon, mackerel, sardines), nuts (almonds, walnuts, pecans), and seeds (sesame, flax, sunflower).

Massage in moisture. Are you so rushed that you barely have time to apply a moisturizer after a shower when your body is damp? Well, I hate to tell you this, but you really need to give yourself a few extra minutes each day for a postshower mini massage. Take your time and rub a moisturizer all over your body. The massage will stimulate blood flow to your skin, which helps the moisturizer be even more effective.

Keep your rain barrel full. You need lots of water to keep all parts of your body working well, including your skin. It's really quite simple: The more water you drink, the more water you will make available to pump up and out to your epidermis. So don't be stingy with the H_2O—drink at least 8 to 10 glasses a day—and carry a water bottle with you whenever you're exercising or are out in the heat.

Honey, Pass the Milk!

A milk and honey massage is one way to start your day off on the right foot. Simply mix equal parts of honey and milk and, starting at your feet, massage the lotion into your thirsty skin. This is kind of messy, so it's best done in the shower, where you can simply rinse off when you're finished. Then use a towel to gently pat dry.

FAST FORMULA

Extinguish That Itch!

When added to a bath, this mix will relieve itching and restore the proper pH to your skin.

1 cup of apple cider vinegar
1 cup of barley flour
1 tubful of warm water

Add the apple cider vinegar and barley flour to a tepid bath. Don't worry, the vinegar smell will dissipate quickly, and you'll soon be luxuriating in the silky, soothing solution.

Soak Away Psoriasis

To soften scaly areas of skin on your hands and feet caused by psoriasis, sprinkle 1 cup of Epsom salts in your bathwater and soak for a spell. After patting the itchy areas dry, rub them gently with some warm peanut oil, and top the oil with a paste made of baking soda and castor oil. Then put on some white cotton gloves and socks, and get into bed. In a few nights, your scales should disappear.

Breakfast Beauty

I remember walking into the kitchen one day to find my Grandma Putt sitting at the breakfast table with mashed strawberries on her face. She called it her "beauty regimen." But strawberries are just one of several breakfast foods you can use to give yourself a facial. Try any one (or a mixture) of the following: chamomile tea, oatmeal, pureed fresh strawberries, sunflower oil, wheat germ oil. Leave it on your skin for about 15 minutes, then rinse off with cold water. You'll be glowing all day!

A-Peeling Skin Care

For a great facial cleanser, try this tangy recipe. First, grind lemon peels in a blender or coffee grinder, then mix about 1 tablespoon of the ground peels with enough plain yogurt to make a paste. Wash your face with the mixture, rinse with cool water, and pat dry. If your skin is on the dry side, substitute vegetable oil for the yogurt.

Don't Let Your Bubbles Burst

If you're like me, you really look forward to a nice, long soak in the tub. It's so relaxing and soothing that you never want to get out—especially if you have some music or a good book with you. Well, I've learned this lesson: Don't overstay your welcome. A bubble bath and even some bath oils can dry out your skin if you soak for too long.

Banish Breakouts

Pimples are a pain in the fanny no matter how old you are. As teens, we could cover the angry bumps—those on our foreheads, anyway—with a fringe of bangs. Adult acne, though, which typically crops up on the chin, isn't so easily hidden. And it's possibly even more vexing than the teenage variety because it's so unexpected—and so totally unfair.

When we get pimples as adults, they tend to appear anytime we're stressed out. For women, breakouts often occur right before their periods, during pregnancy, and in the years just prior to menopause. Not coincidentally, these are all times when hormones are raging, pumping out excess oil that can clog pores, trapping dead skin cells there. Then bacteria can multiply like fish behind a dam. The result is an infected, inflamed pore, better known as a pimple. If the blockage is really deep, it can create lumps (cysts) beneath the skin surface, which are the most severe form of acne.

While some breakouts require heavy-duty prescription treatment, the occasional pesky pimple outbreak usually doesn't require any medication—prescription or over-the-counter. It doesn't even call for wearing bangs. What it does need are just a few of these milder zit-zapping tricks that you can whip up in a flash.

On-the-Spot Relief

It sounds like a tabloid headline—Whipped Egg White Shrinks Pores!—but it's true. Simply dab a bit of whipped egg white on each pimple, let it dry, and rinse off. Then cover with a flesh-colored acne lotion—*not* regular makeup.

Stop Popping

I know it's oh-so-tempting to squeeze, but curb the urge—it's counterproductive. When you press on a zit, you can inadvertently push pus and bacteria farther into the pore, causing deeper, more serious inflammation. Instead, apply a warm washcloth to it several times daily. This will coax the bacteria to the surface, so the blemish can burst naturally.

No Digging Allowed!

Don't even think of excavating blemishes with a mechanical or electric pore extractor. Pore extractors can force bacteria deep into the skin tissues, causing deep-rooted inflammation and infection. The result: acne so angry that it may leave scars that only lasers can remove.

Cleanse with Calendula

Many folks just assume that if their skin is oily and prone to pimples, they should be scrubbing it like crazy. Not true! The key to keeping outbreaks under control is to wash with a gentle touch. Using your fingers, not a washcloth, cleanse with warm water and a mild herbal soap such as calendula (which you can find

217

at health-food stores). The herb is a mild, but potent natural astringent that will gently strip your skin of oils. Finish with a splash of cold water to close the pores.

A Cup to Clear It Up

Traditional herbal blood purifiers are said to clear the skin of blemishes and spots. To try one, mix together equal parts of the dried root of burdock *(Arctium lappa),* yellow dock *(Rumex crispus),* and dandelion *(Taraxacum officinalis).* Bring 1 cup of water to a boil, and use it to steep 1 tablespoon of the dried root mixture for 20 minutes. Strain, and drink. Honey and lemon may be added to taste. *Caution:* Dandelion greens are rich in potassium and should not be taken with potassium tablets. Consult your health-care provider if you have concerns.

Value These Vitamins

Several vitamins are known to help skin stay in the clear. Here's a rundown:

- B vitamins—particularly B_6. These help regulate those pesky hormones that set the stage for adult acne, especially breakouts triggered by hormonal changes during menopause and menstruation.

- Vitamins A, C, and E. Collectively referred to as antioxidants, these vitamins protect your body from oxygen-related free radicals that damage skin cells and promote inflammation, which can lead to blocked pores. Make sure your daily multivitamin/mineral tablet provides all three so you get a little extra breathing room for your skin.

- Zinc. This mineral helps your oil-producing glands work properly. To benefit from this supplement, take 15 milligrams of zinc along with 1 milligram of copper once a day with food to help absorption.

Nature's Skin Soldiers

While vitamins create healthy skin from the inside out, herbs have been used for centuries to clear skin on the surface. These mixes will combat acne and keep your dermis trouble-free:

Try tea tree oil. This herbal oil, which you can find at health-food stores, battles acne just as well as medicines like Clearasil® do, but with much less skin irritation. The only drawback: It works more slowly, has an unpleasant odor, and may sting a bit. Dilute the oil with water before applying it to your skin, and don't use it more than twice daily.

Grab some goldenseal. If you've got acne, don't leave your health-food store without picking up powdered goldenseal root—a mild, but effective disinfectant. Add $1/2$ teaspoon to 12 drops of tea tree oil, and dab the resulting paste onto your blemishes. Rinse after about 20 minutes. Apply the paste twice a day, and your pimples will vanish.

Take vitex. Also known as chasteberry, this herb (which you can find in tablet form at health-food stores) is a mild antiandrogen that may also help regulate progesterone levels and squelch premenstrual breakouts. The recommended dose is 40 milligrams a day, but talk to your doctor before taking it— especially if you're on prescription hormone drugs of any kind.

Just Say Clay

French women often use clay as a cleansing mask because it soaks up excess oil and sloughs off dead skin cells without irritation. So take a hint from this culture synonymous with classic beauty and pick up some green clay at your local health-food store. Then add a little water to 1 teaspoon of clay, and mix a few drops of lavender oil into the paste. The oil's antibacterial and anti-inflammatory properties will help your acne heal faster, and its lovely aroma will help to lower your stress level. Leave the mask on for 15 minutes, rinse off, and say *au revoir* to oily skin!

Get Your EFAs

Taking 2 tablespoons of flaxseed oil or evening primrose oil daily could make up for a deficiency in your diet of essential fatty acids (EFAs). Both oils are excellent sources of gamma-linolenic acid (GLA), a type of EFA that spurs production of an anti-inflammatory prostaglandin known to promote healing. That means it'll help clear things up a lot quicker. Check your local health-food store for both oils.

Wine Away

Here's a skin-care solution that even teetotalers will love. You can control breakouts by dabbing a little wine on your skin. Do it once or twice a day after washing your face. Use white wine for fair skin, and red wine for darker complexions. Cheers!

BEAUTY ON A BUDGET

Before you run off and spend every last dime on those high-priced creams, gels, and scrums that crowd the department store shelves, try some of my old-time skin-care and antiaging techniques. They'll not only keep your skin looking beautiful, but they'll save you a bundle of money, too! Best of all, just about everything you need is probably already in your cabinets, cupboards, and fridge.

Double-Duty Beauty

What's more of a bargain than a two-for-one deal? Nothing, in my book! Here's a little secret: Some common household items can play a dual role, giving you more "bang for your beauty buck." Here are some of my favorites:

Baby yourself. Baby oil makes a great eye makeup remover. It's gentle enough for even sensitive eyes, yet tough enough to remove waterproof makeup. Add baby oil to your bathwater, soak, pat yourself dry, and moisturize. Just be careful not to slip in the tub. In places where your skin is extremely dry, such as your feet, rub on some additional oil. Then wear socks to bed so you won't get your sheets all greasy.

Fix flat hair. No need for pricey mousses and gels! Just rub some shaving cream into the

---

FAST FORMULA

Skin Smoothie

This delectable drink will discourage blemishes and delight your taste buds. These ingredients are packed with alpha hydroxy acids, which help unclog pores by dissolving the "glue" that holds dead skin cells together.

1 tsp. of sugar (glycolic acid)
A few tablespoons of milk (lactic acid)
5 grapes (tartaric acid)
1 kiwi, peeled and sliced (citric acid)
1 apple, peeled, cored, and sliced
   (malic acid)

Combine all of the ingredients in a blender and puree. Apply a little of the mixture to each blemish, leave it on for 10 minutes, and rinse with warm water. As an added bonus, you can slurp up any leftovers!

roots of your locks. It'll give your hair plenty of texture and lift.

Shave and soothe. Whether it's for your face or your legs, witch hazel makes a super-soothing alternative to commercial aftershaves. Just mix 1 part witch hazel and 1 part apple cider vinegar in a bowl, and slap it on after shaving to soothe your skin.

Bag it. Black tea's astringent nature makes it an excellent remedy for baggy eyes. Simply wet two black tea bags, and place one over each eye while you rest for 20 minutes or so.

Steal from your fridge. Baking soda keeps your fridge odor-free, so why not you? Use it as a dusting powder or body rub, or sprinkle a handful in your bathwater.

Get a lift. Saggy skin can get some uplifting help from a mixture of 1 teaspoon of green tea leaves in $1/2$ cup of witch hazel. Gently dab it onto your face and neck with a cotton pad. There's no need to rinse.

Make your own toothpaste. A few drops of hydrogen peroxide added to baking soda makes a great whitening toothpaste. Just don't expect it to taste good while you brush; the reward comes afterward, when your teeth will shine like the sun.

Oatmeal, Anyone?

Treat yourself to a whole-body oatmeal mask. Make a big pot of the cereal, cool it slightly to a tolerably warm temperature, and slather it on from head to toe. Leave it on for 20 minutes or until dry, and rinse it off. Better yet, soak it off in a tubful of warm water. For ease of removal, lightly oil your skin before applying the oatmeal.

Say Hello to Jell-O®

Unclog pores with this easy, peel-off facial mask. Mix $1^1/2$ tablespoons of unflavored gelatin with $1/2$ cup of raspberry fruit juice in a microwave-safe container, then nuke it until the gelatin is completely dissolved. Put the mixture in the fridge until it's almost set (about 20 to 25 minutes), then spread it on your face, let it dry, and peel it off.

Cucumber Toner

To tighten your pores, mix 3 tablespoons of coarsely chopped cucumber, 1 cup of witch hazel, and the juice of one lemon in a jar with a lid. Set the mix aside for two days, then strain out the cucumber, and pour the liquid into a bottle. Keep it in the refrigerator, and dab it on with a cotton ball whenever the need arises.

A Is for Antiaging

You can't stop Father Time, but getting plenty of vitamin A can help keep your skin looking younger, longer. Vitamin A is one of a group of substances known as retinoids that are vital for skin repair and renewal (they're also the main ingredients in many antiaging prescription drugs, such as Retin-A®). To get nearly the same protection without the high cost of drugs, just fill your plate with vitamin A–rich foods, such as cantaloupe, carrots, and apricots.

Go Bananas

It's all monkeyshines for your skin and hair with these tropical treatments:

- To revive dull skin, mash a banana and add 1 tablespoon of honey to it. Cover your face with the mixture, let it sit for 15 minutes, then rinse with warm water and pat dry.

- To make your hair shine, mash half a ripe banana and half a ripe avocado in a bowl. Add 1 tablespoon of extra-virgin olive oil and 3 drops of lemon oil. Mix together and work it into your hair. Cover with a shower cap, wait 60 minutes, then shampoo as usual.

- To make your skin glow, puree one banana and one avocado in a blender. Apply the mixture to your skin, and leave it on for at least 20 minutes. Rinse with warm water and pat dry.

Bathe in Buttermilk

Lots of fancy, high-priced skin-care products boast of containing exfoliating alpha hydroxy acids (AHAs). But you don't have to break the bank to get AHAs. Since they come from lactic and citric acid, you can find these skin-smoothing acids at your grocery store—in buttermilk. For ages, women have enjoyed lolling in buttermilk baths, because of buttermilk's high lactic-acid content. To fill a tub, though, you'd need your own cow. But you can affordably bathe your face and/or hands in buttermilk once or twice a day.

Potatoes for Your Peepers

Most puffiness under the eyes is due to a buildup of fluid in that area. One culprit is eating foods with too much salt. Just like the old trick of putting a potato in a pot of too-salty soup to soak up all that sodium, the same can work for your peepers. Make a potato-patty compress by grating a raw potato and wrapping it in clean cheesecloth or gauze. Place it over your eyes for 20 minutes while resting. A simpler method is to

thinly slice a raw potato, and lay the potato slices directly on your skin.

Berry White Teeth

Get a whiter, brighter smile with strawberries. Believe it or not, fresh strawberry juice is said to whiten teeth over time. Try it for yourself: Paint the juice on your teeth, and leave it in place for five minutes. Follow up with a rinse made of a pinch of baking soda in warm water for a 'berry' bright smile.

Freckle Rx

If you'd like to lighten the look of your freckles and age spots (also called "liver spots"), reach for the enzyme activity of horseradish and yogurt. Combine 1 tablespoon of grated horseradish and $1^1/_4$ cups of plain yogurt, and refrigerate the mix. Dab the yogurt mixture on spots daily until the desired results are achieved. Follow each application with a drop of vitamin E oil or wheat-germ oil to moisturize and smooth your skin.

Lighten Up with Lemon

Help fade age spots with this "lemon-aid." Mix equal parts of lemon juice and water, apply a little to each spot, and leave it on for five minutes before rinsing. Repeat three times a week, and the brown spots may fade to taupe. Use more lemon juice and less water as your skin gets used to the preparation. The goal? To eventually apply the juice "straight up."

A Fading Formula

To get rid of those unwelcome age spots, mix 1 teaspoon of vinegar, 1 teaspoon of lemon juice, 1 teaspoon of grated horseradish, and 3 drops of rosemary oil. Dab the spots with a cotton ball soaked in the mixture. Don't be put off by the strong odor—it really works!

Grow a Beauty(full) Garden

Why spend your hard-earned dollars buying pricey potions and lotions, when you could have some of the best beauty secrets growing in your own backyard? If you don't already have these veggies, flowers, and herbs gracing your garden, here's several great reasons to start digging!

Make your own massage oil. Put a handful of rose petals into a 1-pint glass jar. Add a sprinkling each of dried calendula (leaves or flowers), chamomile, comfrey, and lavender. Then fill the jar nearly to the top with vegetable oil. Twist the lid on tight. Stash the jar in a warm place, such as near your stove. Every morning, give the jar a vigorous up-and-at-'em shake. Do this for a couple of weeks, then open the jar, and strain out the herbs, using a fine-mesh sieve. Finally, add a few drops of lavender essential oil. You now have your very own massage oil to rub into your dry skin each day.

Send those bags packing. To deflate those pesky pouches that seem to plague your under-eye areas, place a 1-inch thick slice of chilled cucumber over each eye, lie down, and relax for 15 or 20 minutes.

Blondes have more...marigolds? Herbal rinses add sheen—and a little color—to the hair shaft, while relieving scalp irritations. Traditional herbs include rosemary and sage for dark hair, chamomile and marigold for blondes, and cloves for auburn or red hair. Make a strong tea using 4 tablespoons of herb to 1 quart of boiling water. Steep for 15 minutes, and add ¼ cup of apple cider vinegar to restore the scalp's proper pH. Use the resulting mix as a final rinse after shampooing your hair and you're guaranteed to turn heads!

Mind your elderflowers. These flowers *(Sambucus canadensis),* known for keeping the complexion clear and free of blemishes, have their origins in folk medicine and are still used today in many commercial skin creams. Make your own elderflower water by steeping 1 ounce of fresh elderflowers in 1 pint of distilled water overnight. Strain, and use it as a wash following your daily cleansing regimen. If it's refrigerated, the solution will keep for four to five days.

Deflate Puffy Eyes

A cold compress made with fennel tea can reduce the swelling around puffy eyes. Just pour 1 cup of boiling water over 2 teaspoons of fennel seeds. Cover, and allow the brew to steep for 10 minutes before storing it in the refrigerator overnight. In the morning, strain out the seeds, and your eye-pleasing medicine is ready! To use, dip a paper towel into the fennel tea. Find a quiet place to lie down, shut your eyes, and put the moistened paper towel over them. In 10 minutes or so, your eyes will sparkle and look refreshed.

Warts Away

If dandelions are growing in your lawn, get out there and pick yourself a wart cure. Herbalists say you should apply the sap from the flower stem to your wart three times a day for as long as it takes for the wart to disappear.

SOOTHE SKIN DISTRESS

If you're plagued by unsightly skin conditions—anything from an annoying rash to psoriasis to rosacea—you know how embarrassing, uncomfortable, and even painful they can be. Well, you don't have to put a bag over your head or hide inside your house until the skin crisis has passed. Instead, try some of these down-home remedies that are sure to get out the red, ditch the itch, and end the discomfort.

HOME REMEDY

For almost-instant pain and itch relief, take a clean spray bottle, fill it with water, and drop two aspirin tablets in it to dissolve. Then spritz your rash. If you'd like, you can add a drop of glycerin to the mix to reduce skin redness and swelling.

Don't Be Rash

If you haven't had a rash since your diaper days, consider yourself extremely lucky. Those red bumps are itchy and unsightly. And pinning down the culprit behind a rash isn't always so easy when you consider the dozens of suspects you come into contact with daily. The list goes on and on, including detergents; cat dander; nickel in rings, earrings, and zippers; latex and rubber in protective gloves, balloons, and waistbands; hair, shoe, and clothing dye; and the worst offender—fragrances, which are found in everything from detergents to lotions. If you're susceptible, any one of these offenders can leave a rash (sometimes with raised, angry welts) at the point of contact.

You can also get a blotchy rash in response to stress and an itchy, hivelike rash with bumps the size of quarters from taking penicillin, certain pain relievers, and other medications or from

eating nuts, chocolate, shellfish, strawberries, or foods that contain additives or preservatives. In some cases, a rash can be a symptom of a fungal infection, toxic shock syndrome, or an underlying disease such as lupus, psoriasis, or meningitis. Finally, there are the rashes that fall into the "heaven only knows" category. Whatever the cause, here are some simple solutions to help you battle the bumps.

Play Detective

No matter how annoying your rash is, resist running pell-mell to the medicine chest in search of hydrocortisone cream. Instead, spend some time trying to ID your suspects, so you can avoid them (and the need for any kind of cream) in the future. For instance, if you think your rash may be related to something you're eating, keep a food diary for a week, then see your doctor for a skin test to confirm any suspects you come up with. In the meantime, check out the following rash remedies. They can provide relief even if you haven't a clue yet about what's getting under your skin:

Feel your oats. Forget the fancy aromatherapy bubbles and sink into a cool, slimy colloidal oatmeal bath for anywhere from 5 to 30 minutes. When this finely ground grain (available at health-food stores) hits the tub, the water turns milky and coats your irritated skin, moisturizing it and reducing the itch. You can also mix colloidal oatmeal with a bit of water to form a paste, and apply it directly to the rash.

Season, don't scratch. For a rash of unknown origin, simply chew a fresh oregano leaf (a strong antiseptic), spit it into your hand, and slather it on your rash. If you prefer a less primitive method of application, use a few drops of oregano oil, which is available at health-food stores.

Soothe it. A good Rx for any itchy rash is to mix up a paste with 3 parts baking soda and 1 part water or witch hazel (an astringent), then dab it directly onto your skin. Or simply scoop some gel from an aloe leaf, mix it with a drop of peppermint oil (which also relieves pain), and smear it on the affected area.

Add fat. If you've erupted in a red, bumpy rash on your forearms and thighs, it could be a telltale sign that you're lacking essential fatty acids—the kind found in fish, flaxseed, and evening primrose oils—which help keep skin lubricated, supple, and smooth. Take 1 teaspoon or 500 milligrams of flaxseed oil, evening primrose oil, or fish oil (all of which you can find at health-food stores) three times a day. You can also apply evening primrose oil directly to your rash. If it's progressed to the point where the skin is cracking, you should see healing within a week or two. *Caution:* People who take aspirin or prescription blood thinners should not take flaxseed oil or fish oil.

A Gem of a Remedy

If you've been bushwhacked by poison ivy and live in the eastern United States, look for another plant—jewelweed—to treat it. Simply squeeze the juice from the stem, and apply it to the affected area. The jewelweed can help keep the irritating urushiol oil in poison ivy from binding to your skin and spreading. If you don't happen upon any jewelweed growing in your neighborhood, a few drops of jewelweed extract, which you can find at health-food stores, will work, too. To keep a reserve handy, mix a few

drops of the extract with water and freeze the solution as ice cubes to use on any itchy spots that might crop up.

Beat Bikini Bumps

To keep your bikini line from looking like a minefield of razor bumps and infected hair follicles the next time you shave, use shaving gel. Leave it on for a few minutes, then shave using a wet razor—this technique will allow more water to soften the hair for a closer shave and less chance of ingrown hairs. Afterward, smooth on a cream with alpha hydroxy acids (AHAs), which can reduce ingrown hairs and minimize the bumps. Follow this up with a vitamin C–based cream to reduce redness.

When to Dial the Doc

A rash accompanied by wheezing, dizziness, or fever (or any other symptom, really) is potentially very serious. You could be having a life-threatening allergic reaction caused by inflammatory histamines released by your body's mast cells, so don't wait—seek medical help immediately!

Give Psoriasis a Pause

An old friend of mine had psoriasis that flared so badly when he got nervous or stressed that he wore long sleeves to camouflage the silvery scales that appeared on his elbows, even if it was 90 degrees in the shade. Unfortunately, scientists still aren't entirely sure what causes psoriasis. They can tell us only that this autoimmune (and probably hereditary) condition involves overexcited T cells, or immune cells, that trigger an overgrowth of skin cells. Like widgets spewing from a revved-up conveyer belt, the dead skin cells pile up in scaly plaques on the knees, elbows, scalp, and other areas instead of being shed.

Nutritionally oriented doctors believe this psoriatic pileup stems from allergies, nutritional deficiencies, too much animal fat in the diet, or a buildup of toxins in the liver. But most doctors agree that hyped-up emotions and other forms of stress set the plaque attack in motion, as can dry air, cigarette smoking, and too much or too little sun exposure. Fortunately, there are a number of safe, natural methods that help tame T cells and put the brakes on the rapid overgrowth of skin cells. Here's what you need to know:

- Relief starts with consuming more veggies and fewer dairy foods and meats (animal fat spurs inflammation and toxic waste buildup). Also drink at least eight glasses of water a day to flush out toxins.

- In one study, aloe gel helped improve itchy lesions in more than 80 percent of participants with psoriasis. For the best results, coat your lesions with aloe gel (either scooped straight from the plant, or purchased at a health-food store) three times a day for one month.

- A bathtub with a water-agitation attachment or a whirlpool tub will help soak off dead skin and relieve the itching. To soften really thick lesions, add 1 to 2 pounds (one to two boxes) of baking soda to the water.

Dunk in the Dead Sea

Actually, in Dead Sea *salts*. According to research from the Dead Sea Mor Clinic in Ein-Bokek, Israel, soaking in a special blend of salts scooped from the Dead Sea clears 90 percent of psoriatic lesions in a majority of patients. You can buy the salts on the Internet. Soak for at least 45 minutes three times a week in a warm, salty bath for best results.

Kitchen Cabinet Cures

Relief from psoriasis is right at hand. Just take a look in your kitchen and bathroom cabinets for these common household products that'll work like magic:

Douse with cider. To take the sting out of irritated lesions, splash a little apple cider vinegar on scaly areas, and leave it on for 1 minute or so before rinsing.

Rub it in. Bathe your plaques twice daily, pat them dry, and immediately rub in layer after layer of petroleum jelly or vitamin E oil. Within a week, at least 80 percent of your problem will disappear.

Peanuts, anyone? To soften hand or foot lesions, soak in a bath laced with Epsom salts, pat your itchy areas dry, and massage them with warm peanut oil. Then cover the

Quick Fix

Counterintuitive though it may be, if you apply an over-the-counter cream containing capsaicin—the ingredient that gives chili peppers their bite—to your lesions, your skin will be less irritated. That's because capsaicin helps tamp down chemicals that transmit pain and itching. You'll find capsaicin creams at most drugstores. Be sure to wash your hands well after using the cream, and don't get it near your eyes, or apply it to broken skin.

oil with a paste made from baking soda and castor oil, don white cotton gloves or socks, and hop into bed. Your scales should soon melt away.

Don't Worry, Be Happy!

Studies show that worrywarts with psoriasis heal more slowly during UV light therapy (a common treatment for psoriasis) than their more carefree colleagues. The next time you're bathing in light, try listening to stress-reduction tapes that feature meditation and visualization. If you visualize smooth, scale-free skin while inhaling deeply through your nose, your lesions could clear up three times faster than if you don't.

Sunbathe Sensibly

If you have mild psoriasis, and you can get a half hour of natural sunlight daily (slathering unaffected areas with sunscreen) at least three days a week, your lesions may start to heal within six weeks. But do your sunning outdoors, not in a tanning booth.

Got Milk?

Thistle, that is. Milk thistle helps the liver eliminate leukotrienes, which are responsible for inflammation and the deregulation of skin cell growth. The suggested dose is 120 to 175 milligrams of standardized extract in capsule form or $1/2$ teaspoon of liquid extract twice daily. Check health-food stores for milk thistle combined with other liver tonics (such as burdock, yellow dock, red clover, or sarsaparilla) in tea, capsule, or liquid form, then follow the label directions.

Strike Oil

People with psoriasis tend to have low levels of omega-3 essential fatty acids, which help to squelch inflammation-causing arachidonic acid. To rebalance your acids, limit animal fats in your diet and take 4 to 6 grams (4,000 to 6,000 milligrams) of fish oil daily in capsule form, divided into three doses. That's a lot of fish oil, so you need to get your doctor's okay first, especially if you take aspirin or prescription blood thinners.

Rosacea: Stop Seeing Red

Do you blush rather easily? Maybe it happens when you hear a bawdy joke, drink hot coffee, eat spicy nachos, sip Bordeaux, exercise strenuously, or simply come in from the frosty air. Well, your quick-to-turn-crimson cheeks may put you at risk for rosacea, an inflammatory skin condition involving the blood vessels of the face. Rosacea affects 13 million adults, most of them fair-skinned women between the ages of 30 and 60.

Doctors believe that people with rosacea have either "twitchy," reactive blood vessels, a chronic bacterial infection caused by microscopic skin mites, and/or an ulcer-type infection that affects the blood vessels. Any one

Quick Fix

If you've got rosacea, try to avoid the midday sun and stay in air-conditioning on humid summer days. You should also take steps to keep cold air off of your face in winter. The more you cover up when you're chilled (which makes the blood vessels overconstrict to conserve heat), the less your vessels will dilate as they throw off heat when you come inside.

of these can precipitate leakage of blood from the vessels, triggering low-grade inflammation that may gradually progress from blushlike episodes to permanent ruddiness marked by red, spidery, "broken" blood vessels and, in some cases, tiny, red, pus-filled pimples. Depending on its cause, rosacea is usually treated with topical antibiotics to squelch the infection and subsequent inflammation, sulfur agents such as permethrins (Elimite®) to kill the skin mites, or an antifungal gel. But there are steps you can take to keep the blush at bay.

Think Ahead

There's no need to make a mad dash for the drugstore—especially if your rosacea is mild or occasional. Surveys conducted by the National Rosacea Society indicate that simply avoiding triggers helps curb 96 percent of flare-ups. They also suggest that the best way to begin is by limiting the big three vessel dilators: sun, red wine, and heat in all its forms, from spicy or piping-hot foods to steamy showers. Here are a few other things you can do:

Sidestep the sting. Steer clear of things that sting, such as products containing ethyl alcohol, witch hazel, menthol, peppermint, eucalyptus oil, or clove oil. Where there's stinging, redness usually follows.

Baby it. Treating your skin like a baby's is vital—no harsh or scented soaps or rough washcloths allowed!

Pop a pre-meal pill. Take an antihistamine two hours before you partake of a food that typically turns you red as a beet. It could prevent the release of inflammatory histamines in skin cells that color your cheeks. Common histamine-prompting foods include red wine, beer, vermouth, cheese, soy sauce, vinegar (watch out for those salad dressings), processed meats, eggplant, nuts, chocolate, shellfish, papaya, pineapple, and strawberries.

Switch spices. By simply trading spices when you cook—using cumin mixed with oregano instead of red pepper or paprika, for example—you can minimize flushing without sacrificing flavor.

Beat the Blush

If you follow the above advice, you may be able to keep flushing flare-ups to a minimum—without even a modicum of medication. Then when redness flares, here's how to strike back:

- Hold the cream. If you've been smearing an over-the-counter corticosteroid cream on your facial "rash," cease and desist! Topical steroids make rosacea worse. In fact, studies show that stopping their use (and, in the research, taking an antibiotic) could help clear up your flushing problem.

- Slick on silymarin. You can use cover-up lotions to try to camouflage your redness, but studies show that preparations containing silymarin and vitamin E can actually help reduce redness—even if you have long-standing rosacea. Silymarin is a component of milk thistle that may help squelch free radical–generated inflammation, and vitamin E is an antioxidant that may reduce swelling. If you use such a preparation when your face is merely pink, it could prevent the rosacea from progressing to the red stage. Look for silymarin-based preparations such as Rosacure® on the Internet.

- Tone up. All of the dilation that occurs when you flush can leave your blood vessels flabby and less likely to constrict the way they should, dermatologists say. Taking vitamin C along with bioflavonoids to help tone the blood vessels is a good idea. As long as you don't have kidney or stomach problems, check your local drugstore or health-food store for combination formulas, then take 500 milligrams three times a day.

- Rub it in. Try using herbal creams, such as horse chestnut cream, which improves the tone of vein walls and is used to help shrink varicose veins, or rose wax cream (both of which are available at health-food stores). Applying either cream twice a day may help to minimize rosacea.

- Reduce inflammation. Grapeseed extract is an excellent natural anti-inflammatory that also shores up collagen. Take 50 milligrams in capsule form three times a day. Look for it at your local health-food store.

Breathe Deeply

Surely you've heard the advice to "slow down and take a deep breath" when you're stressed or nervous. Well, according to a survey of National Rosacea Society members, it also applies to halting the crimson tide. When you're feeling overwhelmed, inhale and count to 10, then exhale for 10 more counts. Repeat this exercise several times, and you'll be less likely to flush.

Try Hypnosis

A step beyond deep, measured breathing, hypnosis teaches guided imagery and progressive muscle relaxation techniques to help you actually prevent your blood vessels from dilating. Are you getting very…intrigued? Ask your dermatologist about hypnosis and for a referral to a trained clinician in your area.

HOME REMEDY

Say good-bye to rosacea redness with aloe vera. Its anti-inflammatory and antibacterial properties may go a long way toward relieving your redness when it flares up. Apply pure aloe vera gel to your skin twice a day to reduce symptoms. You can buy the gel at any health-food store, or slice open a leaf from the plant growing in your kitchen.

CHAPTER 12

Stay Safe

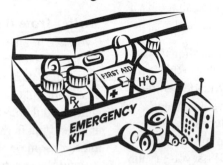

For many of us, "stay safe" took on a new meaning after 9/11 and Hurricane Katrina. Gone are the days when it simply meant taking care of ourselves and our loved ones in the event of broken bones, burns, or blackouts; we now need to know how to proceed in times of graver danger. In this chapter, I'm going to share everything I've learned to treat all of life's emergencies—no matter how big or how small they are.

HOME, SAFE HOME

From a fire to an act of terrorism, our home, sweet home can unfortunately become the scene of a disaster in a matter of seconds. We'd all feel a whole lot better—and do a better job of staying safe—if we had the keys to prevention and preparation in our back pockets. Here's a brief rundown on what you should do in case of a household emergency.

Get Ready!

Are you prepared for the unthinkable? According to the Department of Homeland Security, there are three basic "gets" to staying safe during a disaster, whether it's brought on by Mother Nature or it's man-made. They are:

1. Get prepared. When readying for a possible emergency situation, the first thing you need to do is create an emergency supply kit. Remember the basics of survival: fresh water, food, clean air, and warmth. Any well-stocked supply kit can take care of this and more. (See the Home Remedy box on page 231 for a list of recommended items that every basic emergency kit should contain.)

2. Get a plan. Your family may not all be together in one place when disaster strikes, so plan in advance how you'll reach one another and get back together. Also remember to choose an out-of-town contact. In the event that local telephone service

is down, an emergency contact person outside your area can be a big help in communicating with your family. Just make sure everyone has the emergency contact number and a way to make the call (coins, a cell phone, or a prepaid phone card).

3. Get informed. Do you live in earthquake-prone California? Tornado Alley in the Midwest? Or how about Hurricane Central down South? If so, there are some major differences between these types of emergencies that will determine what kind of action you need to take. What you should do during a hurricane is not necessarily what you'd do in the middle of an earthquake, for instance. By thinking ahead and having a sound game plan in place, you'll be in a much better position to deal with disaster and reunite with your family and loved ones—safely—during an emergency. To prepare yourself, simply follow the three-step strategy in "Disaster Smarts" below.

Disaster Smarts

As the Boy Scouts always remind us, it's important to "be prepared." Before disaster strikes, follow this procedure:

Step 1. Find out what kinds of disasters, both natural and man-made, are most likely to occur in your area. Talk to your neighbors and local emergency personnel (police and fire), and visit your local library for disaster information.

Step 2. Learn how you will be notified in the event of an emergency. The methods vary widely from community to community, ranging from a special siren to telephone calls to special broadcasts by emergency radio and TV.

Step 3. Find out what emergency plans, if any, are already in place at work, day care, and school. If no plans exist, consider volunteering to help create one.

Shelter from the Storm

If you live in an area where flooding isn't likely, then a "safe room" in your home might be your best refuge during a powerful storm. Specially designed and tested to withstand battering winds and flying debris, these types of rooms are best built in the basement, garage, or an interior room on the first floor, as long as it's structurally isolated from the main house and securely anchored to the foundation of your home. It can even serve double-duty as a bathroom or closet! The Federal Emergency Management Agency has ready-to-use plans for homeowners to build such a shelter in an existing house or in a new house. Check it out at **www.fema.gov/library**.

Be Fire Ready

Did you know that here in the United States, one home fire is reported to a fire department every $1^1/_2$ minutes, and someone dies in a home fire every $2^1/_2$ hours? It's true, so don't let it happen to you! Follow these 10 precautions to prevent everything you love from going up in smoke:

1. Install and regularly check smoke detectors. Make sure that there's a smoke detector on every level of your home (even the basement) and that they are all working properly. Test them every month, and replace the batteries once a year, or whenever a detector "chirps" to signal that its battery is weak.

2. Sit down with your family and map out an escape plan from every room in your house.

Make sure that everyone knows where at least two unobstructed exits are from every room. (Elevators don't count!) Then pick a place to meet outside after your escape that's far enough away from the fire, yet easily accessible. And be sure to hold a family fire drill at least twice each year, so everyone gets the plan down pat.

HOME REMEDY

Here's a rundown of what every home emergency kit should contain. Put these items in several plastic storage containers with tight lids (don't use one large container, or it will be too heavy to pick up and move), and keep them in an easily accessible place.

- **Water—a three-day supply for drinking and sanitation (1 gallon per person per day)**
- **Food—at least a three-day supply of nonperishable food**
- **One blanket or sleeping bag for each person**
- **Flashlight with extra batteries**
- **Battery-powered radio with extra batteries**
- **First aid kit**
- **Whistle—to signal for help**
- **Dust mask—to filter out any contaminated air**
- **Moist towelettes and garbage bags for personal sanitation**
- **Crescent wrench or large pliers to turn off utilities**
- **Local map**
- **Can opener for any canned food**

For a list of other items to consider adding to your kit like pet food and important documents, visit the Department of Homeland Security's Web site at www.ready.gov/america.

---

3. Never leave anything cooking unattended. And when you're cooking, wear clothes with short, rolled-up, or tight-fitting sleeves. Turn pot handles inward on the stove, so you don't bump them and children won't grab them. And look around—is there anything combustible near the stovetop? If so, move it at least 3 feet away. (This goes for outdoor grills and barbecues, too!) If grease happens to catch fire in a pan, don't throw water on it. Instead, slide a lid over the pan to smother the flames, and then turn off the heat.

4. Keep all portable space heaters at least 3 feet from anything that's combustible or can burn. Make sure that children and pets don't have access to the heaters, and never leave any type of heater on when you leave home or go to bed.

5. Have a qualified serviceperson inspect your home's chimneys, fireplaces, woodstoves, coal stoves, and central furnace once a year. If they need cleaning or any kind of repairs, don't put it off. The cost of a cleaning or repair is far cheaper than repairing your house after a fire!

6. Replace any electrical cords that are cracked or frayed, and never, ever run any cords under carpets or rugs. Don't overload your electrical outlets or extension cords, either. And don't even *think* about tampering with your fuse box or using improper-size fuses! If an electrical appliance smokes or has an unusual smell, unplug it immediately, then have it serviced before using it again.

7. Keep candles away from all combustible materials. It goes without saying that children should never be left unattended in a room with lit candles, and obviously, you should never leave candles burning without an adult in the room. Keep candles, matches, and lighters out of the reach of children. And don't ever display lighted candles in windows or near exits where a wayward draft could send flames soaring.

8. Don't smoke! As if there aren't already enough reasons to kick this bad habit, careless smoking—like smoking in bed or when you're drowsy—is the leading cause of fire deaths in North America. If you've got smokers in your house, give them large, deep non-tip ashtrays and soak the butts in water before dumping them into the trash. Then, before going to bed or leaving home after someone has been smoking, check under and around all cushions and upholstered furniture for any smoldering cigarettes or ashes.

9. Stop, drop, and roll—and stay low! You learned this in grade school, but it bears repeating: If your clothes catch fire, whatever you do, don't run. Stop where you are, drop to the ground, cover your face with your hands, and roll over and over to smother the flames. And remember: During a fire, smoke and poisonous gases rise with the heat, so stay low because the air is cleaner near the floor. If you run into smoke while you are escaping from a fire, immediately find an alternate escape route.

10. Have at least one working fire extinguisher for every level in your home—and another one in the kitchen. Be sure you, and all of your family members, know how to properly use the extinguishers. If you're unsure, call your local fire department and ask for training in how to use them.

Guard Against Gas Leaks

It's no wonder that gas leaks are often referred to as "the hidden hazard" and "the silent killer." You can't see or hear gas leaking, and often, you won't smell it, either. There are two kinds of gas that pose the greatest threat to home safety if they're emitted: natural gas and carbon monoxide. The tips below will help you guard against the danger.

Natural Gas Disaster Plan

Though they're a rare occurrence, natural gas leaks are a real hazard because they substantially increase the risk of fire and/or explosion. Natural gas is colorless and odorless, and is most often used for cooking and home heating. A leak would be tough to "sniff out" if gas companies didn't add a "rotten egg" or sulfur smell to the fuel for easier detection. The only trouble is, many folks, especially seniors, have a diminished sense of smell. That's why it's crucial to have a natural gas detector in your home. You can find one at your local hardware store or home center. Here's what to do if that alarm sounds—or if you smell natural gas or suspect a leak:

- Get out of the house immediately, leaving the doors and windows open, if possible.

- Don't smoke or light any matches in or anywhere near the house.

- Call your gas company or 9-1-1 from a neighbor's phone. Do NOT make the call from your home—it can also cause a spark.

- Do not turn any lights off or on (even a flashlight) or operate any electrical appliance

During a power outage, your fridge and freezer will stay cold 24 hours longer if they're full. So plan ahead and stock up if you're expecting bad weather.

because it could cause a spark that could ignite a fire.

- Do not go back into your home until it has been inspected by a gas company or other official who has made any repairs and deemed it safe to return.

Improve the Odds

To help prevent a natural gas leak in the first place, make sure all of your gas appliances are properly installed and vented, kept clean, and are in good working order. Have a qualified heating contractor inspect your furnace or boiler annually. A properly tuned furnace may not only save your life, but it'll also save you energy and help avoid costly repairs.

Steer Clear of Carbon Monoxide

Anytime a fuel such as gas, oil, kerosene, wood, or charcoal is burned, carbon monoxide (CO) is produced. That makes cars, fireplaces, kerosene heaters, gas ranges, and oil- and gas-fired furnaces the most common producers of this deadly gas. You can't see or smell carbon monoxide, but at high levels in an improperly vented area, it can kill a person in minutes. It's so dangerous because it attaches itself to blood 210 times faster than the oxygen your blood needs! CO detectors are affordable, widely available in stores, and easy to install. If you don't already have some in your home, pick up a couple today.

CO Safety Drill

If your CO detector sounds its alarm, follow these steps right now:

Step 1. Check to see if anyone in your household is experiencing symptoms of CO poisoning—headaches, dizziness, mental confusion, nausea, or shortness of breath. If they are, get them out of the house, and seek medical attention immediately.

Step 2. If everyone is feeling OK, open all the windows and doors to air out your house. Then turn off all potential sources of CO: your oil or gas furnace, gas water heater, gas range and oven, gas dryer, gas or kerosene space heaters, and any vehicle or small engine.

Step 3. Get a qualified service technician to inspect all of your home's fuel-burning appliances and chimneys to make sure that they are operating properly. Also have the technician verify that nothing is blocking any fumes from being vented out of the house.

Don't Get Lazy

Merely buying a CO detector shouldn't lull you into a false sense of security. Preventing CO from becoming a problem in your home in the first place is still very important. Use this checklist to safeguard against this silent killer:

- At the beginning of every heating season, have all of your fuel-burning appliances inspected by a service professional. Make sure all flues and chimneys are cleaned out and in good working condition.

- Buy appliances that vent directly to the outside, whenever possible. If you must use an unvented gas or kerosene space heater, follow the manufacturer's directions and cautions to the letter. When you're using them, be sure to keep the door to the room open, and even crack open a window for extra ventilation. And do not ever sleep in any room with an unvented gas or kerosene heater.

- Don't let your car idle in the garage, even if the outside garage door is open. CO fumes can build very quickly and create a deadly situation if you're not careful.

- There are some things you should never, ever do, and here are two of them: Never use a gas oven to heat your home, and never use a charcoal grill indoors—even in a fireplace.

- Never use any gas-powered engines, such as mowers, blowers, trimmers, or generators, in enclosed spaces. Adequate ventilation is always a must.

Clear It Away

To reduce the chance of fire in your home, be sure to keep these products away from furnaces, water heaters, ranges, or other gas appliances: paint stripper, fabric or water softener, bleach, adhesives, or salt for melting ice. The chlorine or fluorine in these items can cause the metal in appliances to weaken and corrode, which makes it much more likely that they'll fail and burst into flames.

FIRST AID KNOW-HOW

It's a rare soul who can go through life without needing a bit of first aid once in a while. A new pair of shoes brings on a blister, a pot holder wears thin, a shave gets too close, or a mosquito makes a meal of you. Never fear, though, 'cause ol' Jer' is here. I'll show you how to handle almost any minor mishap or malady using some all-natural remedies and a little good old-fashioned common sense.

Blisters: Avoid the Friction

Blisters are the pits. Whether they're caused by a tight shoe, a hand tool, burns, bug bites, infections, or poison ivy, they're a real royal pain in the you-know-what. So learn how to protect yourself from getting those fluid-filled sacs in the first place.

Shop with fat feet. It's a fact: Your feet are bigger toward the end of the day. So the best time to shop for new shoes is while they're at their largest. Or shop one hour after working out, when your feet are still a bit swollen. That way, your new shoes will be big enough and won't be blistering your toes after you've been walking around all morning long.

Lace up right. When putting on running or other sports shoes, be sure to lace them up properly, so your foot is held firmly in place. Otherwise, your foot will rub against the inside of the shoe and create a painful blister.

Be sport specific. If you play basketball in shoes designed for running, they won't pivot with your feet and may rub and cause blisters. So get the shoes to fit the sport.

Practice safe socks. Throw away all those worn-out and laundry-stiffened socks. Wear soft, cushioned socks with no ridges or seams to rub against your foot inside your shoe.

Lose the shoes. Some athletes, especially runners, like to toughen up their feet by going barefoot as often as possible. If you're game, try running barefoot on the beach, or in a grassy field for 10 to 15 minutes after a workout.

Reduce friction. Try this two-part friction fighter: First, apply a commercial, friction-reducing gel, such as Hydropel®, to your feet. Then wear silk or fine-cotton sock liners under your regular socks to further reduce friction. You can find sock liners at sports apparel stores.

Soak up the soggy. Blisters on your feet are most likely to develop if your feet are too sweaty. If your socks are often soggy after working out, the origin of your blister problem may be sweaty skin. Try sprinkling a little cornstarch into your socks before you put them on, and dust some between your toes, too.

An Ounce of Prevention

Before a blister appears, you'll usually notice a hot spot—a red, tender area on your skin. Acting quickly at this stage may prevent a blister from forming. If you've had a burn, for example,

---

HOME REMEDY

Did you know that many plants and trees contain compounds called tannins, which can strengthen your skin? To stop blisters before they start, soak your hands or feet in a strong, tannin-rich infusion of black tea, oak bark, or pine twigs.

To make the infusion, simply soak a handful of the tea, bark, or twigs in a basin of boiling water. When the water cools, strain the infusion, and then soak your hands or feet for 10 to 15 minutes. *Caution:* People with diabetes should talk to their doctors before soaking their feet in any solution.

---

quickly apply ice to the area, and keep it there for about 20 minutes. If the hot spot is caused by friction, cushion the area with moleskin, gauze, or another type of padding.

Protect Your Hands

It's a good idea to always wear gloves whenever you work with household or construction tools. Likewise, you should always wear gardening gloves when you're raking or pruning. Here are a few more of my hand-saving tips:

Loosen your grip. A golf club, squash racket, or tennis racket is a blister machine. To minimize the damage, loosen your fingers, and change your grip as often as you can while playing.

Play with gloves. When you play softball or other sports that require a bat, racket, or club of some kind, wear gloves like the pros do. And if your favorite pastime is sailing the high seas, remember: You can also get some pretty bad blisters from sailing without gloves. Oh, how those lines burn when you're coming about in a heavy wind!

Toughen up. Before you dive "hands-first" into that home building project or any other activity that could be a shock to your soft hands, get them ready. Rub denatured alcohol on them three times a day for several weeks before beginning any manual labor.

Bye-Bye Blisters!

Most blisters will go away on their own, usually within a few days to a week. But that doesn't mean you can ignore them in the meantime. Blisters can easily become infected—and when that happens, watch out because they hurt like the dickens! The persistence of blisters, along with swelling, inflammation, or bleeding can be a sign of infection, so you should see a doctor immediately. Also, see your doctor if a blister is accompanied by a fever or other symptoms of infection. Otherwise, once you've got 'em, here's what you can do to speed up the healing process:

Pop it only if it's painful. You should break a blister only if it is very large or painful; otherwise, you'll risk infection. To pop a blister properly, sterilize a needle with a match, and then pierce the blister gently. Let it drain, and keep it bandaged for three or four days until it heals.

Get comfrey. Ointments containing comfrey root *(Symphytum officinale)* are speedy healers. For open, inflamed blisters, add a pinch of powdered goldenseal *(Hydrastis canadensis)* or echinacea *(Echinacea* spp.) to the ointments to prevent infection and soothe irritated tissues.

Wash away the germs. The best way to keep infection-causing germs out of blisters is to clean them (and the surrounding skin) once or twice a day. Wash the area well with soap and water, then dry it thoroughly. You need to keep it dry because too much moisture will soften the blister and make it more likely to break open before it's ready to.

No worries with "wort." The herb St. John's wort *(Hypericum perforatum)* is great for killing germs and easing pain. Use an alcohol-based tincture (available at health-food stores) to moisten a square of gauze, then apply it to the blister after you've thoroughly washed it.

Lay on some yarrow. Big blisters sometimes take a long time to heal. You can speed things along by applying yarrow *(Achillea millefolium),* an herb that naturally (and safely) draws out the fluid and helps dry it up. Whether you're using fresh or dried yarrow,

chop or crumble it up as finely as you can, then add enough water to make a paste. Apply the paste to the blister, and cover it with an adhesive or gauze bandage. Replace the dressing once a day, until the blister is gone.

Count on clover. Red clover oil is a great choice for healing blisters. You can put the oil directly on the sore, then cover it with a bandage to promote healing. Repeat the treatment once a day, until the blister's gone. The oil is available in most health-food stores, but be sure the product you buy is made for topical use. What you don't want is an essential oil, which is too concentrated to apply directly to your skin.

Let it breathe. Even though it's good to protect a blister with a bandage, let it come up for some fresh air for at least 20 minutes a day. A little air circulation will help protect the area from infection-causing bacteria, which thrive in dark, moist places.

Take comfort in calendula. To reduce blister tenderness and help speed healing, apply a salve that contains the herb calendula *(Calendula officinalis)* along with skin-protecting vitamins A and E. You can apply the salve once a day. Or you can buy dried calendula, crumble it between your fingers, and add just enough water to make a paste. Cover the blister with the paste and leave it on for 20 minutes or so, then rinse it off.

Bug Bites: Ditch the Itch

Whether it's mosquitoes circling your head looking for a late-night snack, fleas making the long jump from your pet to you, or flies nipping at your nose at the beach, insects are here to bug us. Fighting off these stinging, sucking, and biting creatures can be a pain in the you-know-what. With a few dangerous exceptions (the black

FAST
FORMULA

A Spicy Solution

If you're worried about a blister becoming infected, you can reduce that risk with two of the strongest antiseptic herbs that are probably in your kitchen right now—rosemary and thyme. Try this brew on your next blister:

1 tbsp. of dried rosemary
1 tbsp. of dried thyme
1 cup of hot water

Add each herb to the hot water, and steep for about 10 minutes. Let the liquid cool to room temperature, pour some on a cloth, and hold it against your blister for about 20 minutes. You can repeat the treatment once or twice a day, until the blister is gone.

widow spider comes to mind), most bites and stings are only minor nuisances. But you should see a doctor as soon as possible if you get bad hives or other serious reactions. Otherwise, keep reading to learn how to win the battle of the bugs.

Make Yourself Repellent

Natural bug repellents are effective only if you use them frequently and there are not a lot of mosquitoes around. Some doctors think that the best kind of repellents contain neem, lemongrass, or citronella oil. If you plan to use a repellent that contains any of these, first test an area of your skin to make sure it doesn't irritate you. Then spray or dab it directly onto your skin, following the package directions. Studies show that neem oil (from an Indian tree) provides significant protection from malaria-carrying mosquitoes for up to 12 hours; another study

found that lemongrass and citronella oils are both highly effective against most species of mosquitoes.

Squish Some Sassafras

Sassafras (Sassafras albidum), or "green twig," as the Algonquin Indians named it, is said to have insecticidal properties. Native Americans make a repellent by crushing fresh sassafras leaves with a charcoal tablet (not a briquette from the barbecue!), or a small piece of charred wood from the fireplace. Then they mix it with 1 or 2 tablespoons of vegetable oil. The resulting mixture is called sassafras squish topical insect repellent. Dab it onto exposed skin, then rub it in gently. Reapply frequently.

Dress for Success

Cover up your juicy body from dusk to dawn when mosquitoes are most voracious—or stay indoors. If you're outside, wear dark or neutral-colored long pants and long sleeves; save the short-shorts for daytime. Avoid bright jewelry, too, since stinging insects are attracted to colors.

Don't Smell Like a Rose

Or any other flower for that matter. Bees will hover if they like your perfume. The same goes for scented hair sprays and makeup. So leave all the smelly stuff off when you're going to be outside, where the bugs are.

Foil the Little Buggers

Some mosquitoes don't travel far from where they hatch in water, so it's important to eliminate possible breeding sites near your house. Check out this list:

● Get rid of standing water in buckets, old tires, and storm gutters, where mosquitoes lay eggs and larvae hatch.

- Change the water in birdbaths and wading pools often.

- Keep swimming pools clean with chlorine.

- Don't overwater your garden, leaving a lot of stagnant puddles standing around.

Bug Bite Rx

It's easy—start by washing any bite thoroughly with soap and water as soon as possible. Apply ice to decrease swelling and reduce the spread of venom, and elevate the bitten area. Watch for any spreading of redness, which could indicate an infection—and the need for a doctor's attention.

If you need to pull out a stinger, do it carefully. Stinging insects, such as hornets, bees, wasps, and yellow jackets, don't transmit disease, but they do inject venom, which can cause a severe and life-threatening allergic reaction in some folks (called anaphylaxis). If you have trouble breathing after being stung, or if you've received multiple stings, dial your community's emergency number—usually 9-1-1—and breathe deeply and slowly to keep yourself calm until help arrives. If you get stung, don't squeeze your flesh to get the stinger out because you'll only force the venom farther in. But if you aren't experiencing a medical crisis, go ahead and pull out or scrape off the stinger with your fingernail or a pair of tweezers held flat against the skin. Some folks say that rubbing a bar of soap or an ice cube over the area will draw out the stinger. Even a coin or a credit card edge can come in handy. Then clean the area with plenty of soap and water.

Spit and Polish

This is not the most pleasant solution to avoiding bugs, but Southwestern Native Americans commonly chewed tobacco, and then applied the moistened juice to their skin. This kept bees away (and probably everyone else, too!). A "chaw" remedy is plantain (*Plantago* spp.), favored by the Shoshoni of the Northwestern Plains. They chewed plantain to make a paste that they then applied as a compress on the bitten area.

Quick Fix

Baked hazelnuts contain an oil that Native Americans have used for a variety of things, including getting rid of mosquitoes. The next time you're at your local health-food store, look for natural insect repellents that list hazelnut oil as a main ingredient. Apply it, and then watch those skeeters scurry!

Keep Your Shoes On

Bees can be hard to see because they hover just above the ground, gathering food from clover and low-to-the-ground flowers. So don't go barefooting across that gorgeous green grass in bee season—you could step on a bee and get seriously stung. And don't pick the flowers—at least not without checking them for bees first. Angry bees may not appreciate your cutting into their food supply.

Get Shot, Then Fly

No, I don't mean get hit by a bullet! Instead, be sure to get the right immunizations from your doctor before you travel to areas where disease-carrying insects are common. Then, if you do develop flulike symptoms after a bite, get medical attention right away.

Fight Fire Ants

It's a fact of life: Fire ants are on the march

throughout the South. They inflict multiple stings around their original bite, which, if you are sensitive, can cause anaphylaxis—a potentially fatal reaction. Want to be on the safe side? If you live in fire ant country, get desensitized with allergy shots right away.

Ease the Itch

Bug bites (and even stings, after the pain goes away) can itch like the dickens. But you don't have to suffer. Try some of these soothing scratch attackers:

Pack a sage poultice. You can make a great bug bite poultice using sage and vinegar. Just run a rolling pin over a handful of freshly picked sage leaves, bruising them along the way. Put the leaves in a pan, cover them with cider vinegar, and simmer the mix on low until the leaves soften. Drain off the vinegar, carefully wrap the leaves in a washcloth, and place the pack on stings and swellings for instant relief.

Put a sock in it! Oatmeal baths provide a soothing remedy for itching skin. Place 1 cup of oats in a sock, and hang it from the faucet while running a bath. While soaking, squeeze the sock, and let the milky water cascade over your bites. Very hot water can sometimes exacerbate the itch, so it's best to do your soaking in warm water only.

Freeze the bite. Applying ice to a bug bite can freeze a painful insect sting in its tracks. Ice also soothes the itchiness of mosquito bites. Simply wrap some ice cubes in a washcloth or small towel to make a cold pack, then hold it against the affected area for about 20 minutes. Remove it for at least 20 minutes, then continue applying it this way until you're feeling better.

A little dab'll do ya. Ammonia is the main ingredient in those over-the-counter anti-itch sticks for mosquito bites, so why not save a few bucks? Just put a little household ammonia on a cotton ball or swab, and apply it to the bite before you've scratched it. But be forewarned: If your skin is broken at all from scratching, you'll be doing the "Oooo, Ow, Oooo, Ow, It Stings!" dance in a hurry.

Make a venom vacuum. The next time you get a bite or sting, mix a little baking soda with water, and smear a generous layer of the paste on the spot. It helps pull venom out of the skin. Don't have baking soda? Then apply a dab of mud. Soil almost always contains a little clay, which helps draw out the venom to reduce the pain and swelling.

Prepare to repair. To help your skin repair itself after a bug bite, be sure to get plenty of vitamins C and E, two nutrients that are critical for skin health. You'll get enough of both—along with other important vitamins and minerals your body needs—just by taking a daily multivitamin.

Take Ticks to Task

Little ticks are capable of making big trouble. Lyme disease has been on the rise since the 1960s, when suburbs began expanding into deer territory. According to the Centers for Disease Control and Prevention (CDC), it's now the leading pest-borne illness. A tiny deer tick, the size of the period at the end of this sentence, causes flulike symptoms and joint pain. If it's caught early, Lyme disease can be treated with antibiotics. When it's left untreated, however, it can cause severe illness. Rocky Mountain spotted fever, which causes a measleslike rash that spreads from the arms and legs to the palms and soles of the feet, is carried by a half dozen

Itch Relief

To zap that itch, make a strong infusion of this hardworking herbal combo.

Equal parts of chickweed (*Stellaria media*), balm of gilead (*Populus gileadensis*), and peppermint (*Mentha x piperita*)
1 cup of boiling water
¼ cup of distilled witch hazel

Place 1 heaping teaspoon of the herbal mixture in the water, and steep, covered, for 15 minutes. Add the witch hazel, chill, and place the mix in a spray bottle. Mist it onto your skin for soothing relief.

varieties of ticks. It hits children hardest and must be treated quickly with antibiotics. Unless you want to spend the summer months hiding in the living room, learn how to protect yourself from ticks and the diseases they carry:

Take the tick off. If a tick has attached itself to you, grasp it firmly with fine-point tweezers, and pull straight up—not at an angle—or the head might break off and stay embedded in your skin. The tick will still be alive, so seal it in a vial or wrap it in tape before disposing of it. Be sure to wash the area well. If you think you have contracted a disease from a bite (if headache, fever, muscle ache, or skin rash develops), see a doctor immediately. And take the tick with you, if you still have it.

Get slick. If the tick has already bitten you, cover it with some oil—olive oil, motor oil, suntan oil—any kind of oil will do. That'll loosen its grip on you, making it easier to remove with tweezers.

Cover up out in the country. Ticks will cling to your legs when you walk through the grass, and they'll drop from the leaves of overhead trees. If you're walking in the woods or grasslands, tuck your pant legs inside of your socks or boots to keep the ticks off of your legs. Then be sure to look for tiny hitchhikers on the outsides of your socks when you get home. And wear a hat and a long-sleeved shirt whenever you're in tick territory.

Dress in white. Ticks are just tiny black spots, so you'll have a hard time finding them on dark clothing. If you wear white and light colors, the ticks will be easier to find.

Douse with DEET. Before you venture into tick-infested areas, spray your clothes with an insect repellent that contains DEET. Read the labels to make sure that the bug spray you select targets ticks, and follow all directions to the letter.

Time Your Traipse

When you're hiking on trails in the woods, stay in the center of the trail. That way, you'll avoid brushing against trees and shrubs and will be less likely to attract ticks. And keep track of time. Check yourself every hour or so to see if any ticks have begun homesteading on your body. Then do a full-body search when you get home, and remove any ticks right away.

The Royal Treatment

Pennyroyal (*Mentha pulegium*) is an herb that has been used since Roman times to keep fleas away. The good news is that ticks find it obnoxious, too, because pennyroyal contains pulegone, a heavy-duty insect repellent. To use pennyroyal, just pick a bunch of leaves, and rub them on your skin and clothing. Or, you can pick up a bottle of pennyroyal essential oil at a health-food store. Rub a few drops on the tops of your shoes and on your socks (rubbing the oil directly on your skin can irritate it), and those tiny terrors will head for the hills!

Burns: Beat the Heat

We all have a lot of heat in our lives—and I don't just mean the dog days of summer. I'm thinking about the dry heat from barbecues and ovens, moist heat from boiling pots of pasta and whistling teakettles, and electrical heat from space heaters and hair dryers. It's no wonder, then, that many of us get singed from time to time. Read on for my tips on how to help cool the burn.

Keep Current

Accidental burns often happen at home or at work. So keep an easy-to-use, first aid handbook nearby, where you can locate it in a hurry. Emergency medical treatment is constantly changing, so make sure your emergency information is up to date. Whatever you do, toss out that medical handbook you inherited from the Roosevelt era, and get a new one.

A Matter of Degrees

I recently seared my fingers on a spoon that was marooned in sputtering oil while I was stir-frying. In a flash, the burn stung and turned redder than a chili pepper. Experts classify burns like mine— the type that affect only the top layer of skin, or epidermis—as first-degree burns. A second-degree burn penetrates to the second layer of skin, the dermis, to cause blistering. When all the layers of the skin are destroyed, this horror is known as a third-degree burn. Fire, prolonged exposure to hot substances, and electrical burns are the most common causes of third-degree burns—and safety is the best prevention.

For third-degree burns, or if a burn is from a fire or chemical, if it's on your face, or if a child is the victim, get medical help immediately. For more minor burns, however, you don't need a medical degree to put out the fire, prevent infection, and reduce the chance of winding up with an ugly scar. Here's what you should do.

Cool It

First, you need to put out the flames, wash off the chemicals, or break contact with whatever is causing the burn. Then immerse the burn in cool water. If you can't hold the burned area under a running faucet, cover it very lightly with a cloth soaked with cool water. Or pour on any handy cold liquid, such as iced tea or soda. By immediately cooling a heat or chemical burn and continuing to immerse it in cool water for at least 30 minutes, you can reduce its size and depth. Just one caveat: Be sure the water is cool, not icy cold. Ice sends blood away from the area, and as it returns, it creates throbbing pain.

Cover Up

After cooling down a first- or second-degree burn with water, apply a nonfluffy sterile or clean bandage to the area. Do not use a cotton or fluffy towel because it might leave pieces of lint on the burned area, which will only increase the risk of infection.

Forget the Butter!

Putting butter or any oily substance on a burn is the worst thing you can possibly do. After heat singes your skin, it continues to cook the tissues, so you want to try to cool the burn immediately. For that to happen, the heat has to be able to escape. Butter doesn't allow it to escape, so keep the butter where it belongs—on your bread!

Keep It Clean, Please

After the initial cooling and cover-up of a first- or second-degree burn, it's time to keep the area clean to guard against infection. You'll also want to hasten the recovery of the injured skin and soothe that burning feeling. Any one of these topical home remedies will do the job very nicely:

Aloe. To encourage healing and guard against infection, you can't do much better than the thick juice inside the leaves of the aloe plant. Aloe vera is called the "burn plant" because it inhibits the action of a pain-producing peptide, and it helps healing and skin growth. If you buy aloe in the form of a cream or processed gel, make sure it contains at least 70 percent aloe. Another alternative is to keep an aloe plant nearby. To use, simply break off a leaf, split it open, and rub the soothing juice over the burn.

Calendula (*Calendula officinalis*). This herb is an anti-inflammatory, astringent (cleanser), and antiseptic (germ killer) all rolled into one. Plus, it helps repair tissue and prevent scarring. Ground petals combined with sunflower seed oil or corn oil can be rubbed on minor burns and other skin irritations. To make a wash, steep 1 heaping tablespoon of fresh calendula flowers in 1 cup of hot water until the water cools. Strain, then pour over the burn for soothing relief.

Plantain (*Plantago* spp.). If the blisters on the burn area burst, dab the burn with water and apply plantain to it. This antibacterial Native American plant contains the healing agent allantoin and is sometimes called "nature's Bactine®" because it's good for healing all kinds of wounds. Brew a tea (you can find packaged plantain tea at a health-food store), let it cool, and apply the liquid to your burn.

St. John's wort (*Hypericum perforatum*). You may know this herb for its reputation as a treatment for minor depression, but it also helps heal minor burns quickly and with minimal scarring. Apply the extract directly to the burn several times a day for healing relief.

Sweet oil. Ever since French perfume chemist René-Maurice Gattefossé healed his burned hand by plunging it in a vat of lavender oil, this scented herb has been used to guard against infection and prevent scarring. Apply several drops of oil (available at health-food stores) directly to your burn throughout the day. Quite simply, it makes perfect "scents"!

This Spud's for You!

Believe it or not, you can actually soothe a minor burn by rubbing it gently with the freshly cut surface of a raw potato. The enzymes in the potato help reduce pain and swelling.

Spice It Up

You love oregano on sizzling hot pizza, and your sizzling skin will love it, too. Essential oil of oregano contains vitamins A and C, as well as the minerals calcium, phosphorus, iron, and magnesium. When rubbed on the skin, it aids in healing minor burns.

Healing from the Inside Out

Supporting the inside of your body with healing agents can help speed recovery of the burn on the outside. To jump-start your "inside job," try any one of these fabulous food remedies and super supplements:

- You should eat five or six servings of antioxidant-rich foods daily to help your skin heal after a burn. You need antioxidants to battle the harmful effects of free radicals, which are oxygen molecules that are produced as a result of burns. They can cause additional damage to skin cells, so bombard

FAST FORMULA

Soothing Cedar

Take a tip from Native American healers who make this burn-soothing salve from dried white cedar (*Chamaecyparis thyoides*) leaves, which are loaded with minerals that calm irritated skin and burns.

1 bunch of dried white cedar leaves
1 pint plus $^1/_2$ cup of oil (olive, almond, or sesame)
2 oz. of grated beeswax
$^1/_2$ oz. of cocoa butter
1 tbsp. of raw honey
3 or 4 drops of vitamin E oil

Chop and place the cedar leaves in a clean glass jar. Cover the herbs with $^1/_2$ cup of the oil. Let the jar sit in a warm oven at 100°F for 12 hours. Then heat 1 pint of oil over very low heat, adding in the beeswax, cocoa butter, and honey. Remove from the heat when melted, and combine thoroughly. Add several drops of vitamin E oil. Keep the mixture in the fridge for freshness.

them by eating whole grains—one of the best sources of antioxidants.

- Snack on pumpkin seeds. They pack a lot of crunch and even more zinc, which helps wounds heal. So munch a bunch!

- If your burn is serious, your body's supply of vitamin E may be diminished. To replenish your stores, take 400 IU daily until the burn heals. Then when the wound is starting to heal, break open a vitamin E capsule, and apply the contents directly to the burn twice daily to help fight cell damage.

- As long as you don't have kidney or stomach problems, take 1,000 milligrams of vitamin C a day by mouth to reduce cell damage as you heal. This vitamin is a super topical healer as well! Just stir 2 tablespoons of powdered vitamin C into $^1/_2$ cup of aloe juice, then apply the mixture directly to the burn.

Season Your Singe

Did you ever accidentally brush against your piping hot grill and singe your finger? If so, then just mash up some of the raw garlic or onion you may have next to the grill, and apply it directly to the burn. This simple homemade poultice will cool the area, act as an antiseptic, and help ease the pain.

Cuts and Scrapes: Save Your Skin

Most of the cuts and scrapes we get in the course of our busy lives are caused by the smallest things: trimming gnarly tree branches, say, or moving a little too fast with the paring knife. These small wounds, however, can deliver a surprising amount of pain, and the risk of infection is very real.

When you get a cut or scrape, your body almost immediately goes into action. It secretes a host of chemical compounds, including gluelike substances that stop the bleeding and seal the cut. Obviously, you need to see a doctor if you're bleeding a lot or have a deep puncture wound. In most cases, though, all you need is some simple first aid.

Run for Water

Hold your wound under running water, or pour cool water over it from a cup. Using mild soap—the brand you normally use when you bathe should be just fine—and a soft washcloth, thoroughly clean the edges of the wound and the surrounding area, being careful not to let any soap stray into the open skin. If dirt is embedded in the wound, dip some tweezers in rubbing alcohol, then pick out the particles. Better yet, use a very soft, clean nailbrush to remove any tiny, deeply embedded bits of debris.

Put On the Pressure

Once the wound is clean, press a clean cloth or tissue on it for 15 minutes (about how long it takes to stanch the flow of blood), especially if the cut is on your scalp, hand, or foot, where blood vessels are close to the surface. If blood seeps through the cloth, add another layer, and reapply the pressure gently, but firmly. If the cut is on your arm or leg, raise the limb above the level of your heart to help slow the bleeding. *Note:* If your cut bleeds in spurts or blood drenches the bandage after 10 minutes of firm, direct pressure, go to the emergency room immediately.

Stay Covered

Once the injury is clean, cover it with an adhesive bandage—one that's snug enough to keep out the dirt, but not so tight that it prevents circulation. But you're not done yet. Even if you wash and cover a wound promptly, bacteria can get inside while it's healing. To prevent infection, it's important to change an adhesive bandage every day. Wash the wound with soap and running water, dry the area with a clean towel, and apply a fresh bandage. Most cuts don't require any more attention than that. Experts advise staying away from hydrogen peroxide because it can actually damage your skin tissue.

Cream the Pain

One of the quickest ways to ease the pain of abrasions is to apply a thick coat of triple antibiotic ointment to them. The cool cream feels good going on, it protects the wound from infection, and it can even help prevent scars.

Quick Fix

Yarrow (Achillea millefolium) is my favorite herb for healing minor wounds. It's easily found, and it acts as both an astringent to stem the flow of blood and an anti-inflammatory to calm the pain. To use it, simply rinse some fresh yarrow leaves, chew them into a paste, and spit out the mashed poultice directly onto your wound. The fresher the leaves, the more quickly the bleeding will stop.

Call on Herbal Healers

Some of the most effective remedies for cuts and scrapes come direct from Mother Nature. By planting such healing herbs as calendula, rosemary, and comfrey, you can grow your very own "first aid garden." If you haven't got the space or place to plant an herb garden, never fear…the extract form of your favorite natural remedy is as close as the nearest health-food store. Put these helpers on your shopping list:

Calendula. It fights a broad range of bugs, including bacteria and fungi, so use calendula as a poultice to clean out any lingering debris. To prepare a poultice, saturate a piece of sterile gauze or cloth with calendula extract, place the soaked material on your injury, and leave it there for about an hour to help soften the skin and make any debris easier to remove. Afterward, pour a drop or two of extract directly onto the wound to keep it germ-free and to reduce the chance of scarring.

Cloves. The next time you cut yourself, raid your spice rack for whole cloves, which contain the chemical eugenol—an excellent antiseptic and painkiller. Crush the cloves into a powder, then sprinkle it directly onto your wound to speed up the healing process.

Comfrey. The leaves and roots of the comfrey *(Symphytum officinale)* plant contain the healing agent allantoin, which stimulates healthy tissue growth, speeding healing and reducing scar formation. You can find comfrey cream at a health-food store, or you can crush fresh, clean leaves to apply to your wound as needed. Since comfrey encourages scab formation, use it only on shallow cuts that you've thoroughly cleaned. Otherwise, you may inadvertently seal in some germs.

Echinacea. If you have a severe laceration or puncture wound, this natural immune booster will help bring white blood cells to the area to fight infection. Take two capsules three times a day for one week. *Caution:* Don't use echinacea if you have an autoimmune disease such as lupus, rheumatoid arthritis, or multiple sclerosis, or if you're pregnant or nursing.

Gotu kola. This versatile Indian herb contains no fewer than three compounds that stimulate collagen, the connective tissue that forms the basis for skin repair and scar reduction. In fact, studies say that gotu kola can help prevent keloid scars—those big, bulging, ugly scars. Simply pour a drop or two of extract directly onto the wound daily as it heals.

Honey. When undiluted honey was applied to infected wounds in a recent study, they healed twice as fast as wounds that were treated with antiseptics. The thick honey covers the wound and may serve as an antibacterial to keep infection at bay. Plus, honey appears to reduce swelling and pain. Just be sure to thoroughly wash your cut, use pasteurized honey (which won't contain bacteria of its own), and watch for signs of infection, such as red streaks around the wound, a fever, or increased tenderness.

Rosemary. To reduce the risk of infection, wash the wound with rosemary extract, which is available at health-food stores. This aromatic herb is a mild antiseptic that appears to penetrate the skin. It may allow the wound to dry out better than antibiotic creams and ointments, which can smother the skin and may seal in germs.

Vitamins C and E. To help your skin repair itself, be sure to get plenty of vitamins C and E, which, as we've mentioned, are two nutrients that are critical for skin health. You'll get enough of both—along with other important vitamins and minerals—just by taking a daily multivitamin.

When to Dial the Doc

Head to the hospital or call your doctor immediately if you are wounded and:

- Blood gushes from the wound in spurts, which may mean you've nicked an artery.

- You're unable to stem the flow of blood after 10 minutes.

- The wound is on your face or lips, where scarring is most likely.

- The wound resulted from a puncture. You may need a tetanus shot if you've been punctured by a rusty object and it's been more than 10 years since your last shot.

- You can't get the edges of the wound to stay together (no matter how small it is). You may need stitches.

- You see red streaks around the wound or develop a fever, both of which may indicate that an infection has developed.

Turn Up the Heat

When I was just a small boy and I got a cut, my Grandma Putt would take me by the arm and walk me into the kitchen. After washing that cut really well, she'd sprinkle just a teensy bit of cayenne pepper onto it. No, she wasn't being mean. And no, it didn't sting—not too much, anyway. What it did do, she told me, was stop the bleeding and close up the cut faster. Of course, don't try this on a huge cut—for one of those, you'll want to get right to the doctor.

Poison Ivy: Soothe Your Skin

I once got a nasty case of poison ivy from a gardening glove I had worn a whole year earlier, while clearing out some poison ivy vines. I've also gotten it from my neighbor's cat, who, in rubbing up against my ankles, brought the oil from the plant to me on his coat. But these are both pretty odd ways to get poison ivy. More often than not, most people simply stumble into the toxic plant because they don't recognize it, forgetting the old adage: "Leaves of three, let it be!"

If you've been exposed to poison ivy, you'll see a rash (first red patches, then blisters) in about two days. It will be miserably itchy by about the fifth day; then the symptoms will begin to fade. The rash is usually completely gone in 7 to 10 days. If the rash lasts more than two weeks, or shows signs of infection (pus oozing from the blisters), have it checked by your doctor. It may not be poison ivy after all, and it may be something more serious. Also, have your doctor examine the rash if you get it near your eyes. Otherwise, the following tips should bring you some relief:

Pop an antihistamine. An over-the-counter antihistamine, such as Benadryl®, will reduce that itch. Simply follow the package directions.

Bathe in baking soda. Dump $1/2$ cup of baking soda into your bathwater, and soak for a good, long while. Ahhh…relief!

Make a grindelia compress. A compress soaked in a strong infusion of grindelia (*Grindelia camporum*), which is available at natural-health stores, can relieve itching and reduce inflammation. Steep 2 heaping teaspoons of grindelia in 1 cup of hot water for 15 minutes. Strain, and let cool. Apply to the affected area, continuing to wet the compress as it dries out. Leave it on for an hour at a time, if you can. It's also available as a tincture and a spray.

Soothe with salve. After you pat yourself dry, apply calamine lotion or zinc oxide ointment to the area. This treatment should help put those itchy nerve endings into a coma.

Patch your patches. Place sterile gauze patches over any blisters. This will keep your skin clean and help absorb any fluid that drains from the blisters.

In Up to Your…

Yikes! Are you standing knee-deep in poison ivy? If you catch yourself in the act, here's how to minimize your exposure:

- Hit the showers—immediately! Poison ivy penetrates the skin within 20 minutes. So if you're near home, head for the shower, and use plenty of strong soap and cool water (which closes your pores) to shut out some of the ivy toxin.

- Always carry a small container of liquid soap and some bottled water in your backpack or picnic basket. In case of a poison ivy encounter, you can use it to wash off your skin no matter how far you are from home.

- A poison ivy product called Zanfel™ is said to remove the toxins from your skin in less than a minute. It's pricey, but if you're seriously affected by poison ivy, it may be worth purchasing. Keep the cream in your backpack when you're hiking, and head for the nearest stream—or even a puddle—so you can wash away the toxins as soon as possible.

- Gardeners and hikers alike swear by the power of jewelweed *(Impatiens capensis)* to clear up poison ivy. Look for this plant, which is a wild type of impatiens, wherever poison ivy grows, because they're usually found side by side (isn't Mother Nature thoughtful?). You'll recognize jewelweed by its bright yellow or orange flowers. Folk healers suggest you squeeze the juice from the stems or leaves, then swab it onto your skin.

- Creams containing calendula *(Calendula officinalis)* or chickweed *(Stellaria media)* may ease the itching and discomfort of poison ivy. You can find products containing both of these herbs at your local health-food store.

- Vitamin C may help reduce your reaction to poison ivy. Once you've been exposed, take 1,000 milligrams of vitamin C every two hours, up to 6,000 milligrams per day. The side effect of taking too much vitamin C is loose stools. Should this occur, simply lower the dose by 1,000 to 2,000 milligrams. Keep this regimen up for three to four days. *Caution:* Anyone who has kidney disease should avoid vitamin C supplements.

Splinter Removal: A Thorny Issue

You don't have to be a carpenter to have a close encounter of the splintery kind. The danged things are everywhere—on worn windowsills, old garden tools, and Grandma's end table, to name just a few

---

> **FAST FORMULA**
>
> ## Kitchen-Counter Itcher Ditcher
>
> **If you've got the poison ivy itch, relief is as close as your kitchen. Comb your cupboards and make a paste using one of the following combinations:**
>
> **Water and cornstarch**
> **Water and oatmeal**
> **Water and baking soda**
> **Water and Epsom salts**
> **Witch hazel and baking soda**
>
> **Apply the paste to the rash, and you'll soon say good-bye to the itchies!**

---

possibilities. And it's amazing how much a teeny-weeny, hardly-nothin'-at-all sliver of somethin' can hurt. Well, there's a good reason why they hurt so much. It's because your fingertips, the usual places you get splinters, are filled with sensitive nerve endings. That's what makes them so deft at knitting or putting puzzles together, but it's also what makes them sting like the dickens when a sliver of wood gets under your skin. To get rid of the little troublemaker:

Loosen your flesh. Yep, that's what I said. If the splinter's under the skin, but not deeply embedded, you can ease it out by first loosening the skin around it with a sterile needle. Then use the needle to try to ease the splinter out.

Tweeze it out. Sterilize metal tweezers by holding them over an open flame, then have at it. If the splinter is sticking out of the skin, tug it out gently, making sure to pull it out in the same direction that it went in. This will reduce the chances that it will break off in your skin.

Let it bleed. Once you're done removing the splinter, squeeze the wound so that blood will wash out the germs.

Ease 'Em Out

If you don't feel up to splinter surgery, an herbal poultice can do the job for you. Plantain (*Plantago* spp.) is one of the best herbs to use, and you can buy it fresh or dried at many health-food stores. Chop or grind the herb and add enough water to make a paste, then slather it over the splinter. Cover it with a bandage, and replace the poultice daily until the splinter comes out. Here are two other splinter easers you may want to try:

- The powerful salicylic acids in wart removers can also help you get rid of a splinter. The superficial layers of skin break down and become soft from contact with the acid. Use wart remover disks because they have a higher salicylic acid content than liquid wart removers do.

- Marshmallow ointment (available at health-food stores) can coax a stubborn splinter to the surface of your skin. Dab some ointment on the site, bandage it, and leave it alone for a few hours. When you remove the bandage, the

splinter will have inched close enough to the surface for you to easily pluck it out with a pair of sterilized tweezers.

What Splinter?

If the splinter is lodged close to the surface of the skin, and the area isn't bleeding or painful, it's okay to just ignore it. Your body will generally work it out of there on its own. Keep an eye on it, though, to be sure it isn't digging any deeper into the skin or getting infected.

Clean Like Crazy

Once the splinter's been removed, be sure to keep the skin around the injury clean. Wash the area gently with soap and water once or twice a day, and cover the area with a bandage if it's likely to get dirty. Check the injury site for signs of infection—redness, pus, swelling, and so on. You can treat a minor infection with some triple antibiotic ointment, but you should see a doctor if it doesn't clear up in a day or two.

Herbal Rinse

Wash a deep splinter wound with the following herbal infusion: Combine equal parts of calendula (*Calendula officinalis*), echinacea (*Echinacea* spp.), and comfrey (*Symphytum officinale*). Steep 1 heaping tablespoon of the mixture in 1 pint of hot water for 20 minutes. Strain out the herbs, then wash the wound in the infusion.

When the wound is dry, dust it with goldenseal (*Hydrastis canadensis*) powder to prevent infection and soothe skin irritation.

Splinter S.O.S.

If a splinter breaks off inside of your skin, if it is very deeply embedded, or if the wound becomes infected, seek medical help immediately. You may need a tetanus shot.

HOME REMEDY

Strange as it may seem, you can coax a stubborn splinter out with a potato. Use a potato poultice, or in the case of a finger or toe, simply carve or hollow out a piece potato for a custom fit. Tape or bandage the spud in place overnight, and you'll be able to easily pluck out the splinter the next day!

Sunburn: Watch Out for Ol' Sol

Yes, we all love a bright, sunny day. But it's also important to know the "dark" side of our solar friend. Too much of it—and you get burned! If you're fair-skinned like me, we have less of the skin pigment melanin that helps block UV penetration, and are more likely to burn. And we're more likely to incur skin damage down the road. Both long-term sun exposure and sunburn cause skin cell damage, which—over time—can lead to the development of skin cancer. Severe sunburn also increases your risk of developing melanoma. In fact, five incidents of sunburn while you are young can double your risk of getting this deadly disease later in life. But if you follow my advice, you won't get fried.

Start with a Screen

Did you get burned even though you slathered on gobs and gobs of sunscreen? If so, then it's possible that you used the wrong product. Most sunscreens protect against UVA and UVB, the sun's two types of burning rays, but they don't necessarily give all the protection you need. To choose the best protection:

- Buy only products that contain oxybenzone, titanium dioxide, mexoryl, zinc oxide, or Parsol® 1789 (also called avobenzone). They provide optimal protection against both types of harmful rays.

- Choose a sunscreen with a sun protection factor (SPF) of 30 or higher.

- Use a waterproof brand if you'll be swimming, or you perspire heavily.

- Apply it at least 20 minutes before going outside—it takes that long for the protective ingredients to "kick in."

- Reapply sunscreen every two hours, no matter what it says on the label.

Rely on Vitamins

If you're a sun worshipper, vitamin C is the one nutrient that you need the most. For one thing, your body uses it to build healthy skin that's at least somewhat resistant to the sun's burning rays. Vitamin C is also an antioxidant that blocks the damaging effects of free radicals, which are harmful oxygen molecules that are produced in profusion when the sun toasts the skin. Finally, vitamin C helps repair sunburn damage.

Another sun lover's nutrient is vitamin E, which, like vitamin C, is a protective antioxidant that helps prevent, or at least minimize, skin damage. Take 800 IU daily when you're nursing a nasty sunburn. You can also apply vitamin E cream or oil directly to the burned areas. They'll heal more quickly, and you'll be less likely to have permanent scars.

Go Green

When green tea is applied topically, it may help prevent sunburn and skin cancer, according to one report. If you're already burned, it may help stave off cellular damage. So brew a pot, let it cool, then pour it into a spray bottle. Spritz it on your burn daily, and the green may help stop the red!

Don't Get Burned!

While you know how important it is to always wear sunscreen when you're out in the sun, there are a few other things you need to be mindful of:

Beware of bergamot. Wearing cosmetics that contain citrus oils, such as bergamot, can predispose you to sunburn. So read the labels carefully before you buy or apply!

Mind your meds. If you're going to be exposed to the sun for any period of time, be extra careful if you take such drugs as antihistamines, antibiotics, birth control pills, antidepressants, and even St. John's wort. All are considered to be "photosensitizing" substances that will increase your risk of getting burned. So slather on the sunblock!

Boycott the Blaze

The sun is most damaging when it's at its highest peak, when the force of the UV rays is 10 times stronger (at noon) than it is three hours earlier or later. Try to avoid exposure between the hours of 11 a.m. and 1 p.m., when the sun is directly overhead. And remember, the sun is up there 365 days a year. Although we may not always feel it or see it, it's still emitting those dangerous rays. So get into the habit of wearing sunscreen with at least an SPF 15 every day, rain or shine, all year long. It's the best protection under the sun!

Slurp Spaghetti Sauce

Tomatoes are chock-full of lycopene, a substance that can stop free-radical damage to cells caused by overexposure to the sun. Eating these scarlet veggies cooked with oil—like your favorite spaghetti sauce—has been shown to help protect the skin from sun damage and redness. And the oil helps our bodies better absorb the lycopene.

Sunburn Alert

It almost goes without saying that severe burns—whether you get them in the kitchen or on the beach at Acapulco—always need to be treated by a doctor. If your skin blisters or develops open sores, or if you feel dizzy or nauseated, see a doctor immediately. Severe sunburn can also cause chills or fever, which is an early sign that you may be going into shock. Of course, most sunburns aren't this serious. For your normal, run-of-the-mill sunburn, there are steps you can take to ease the pain.

Skin Soothers

If you stayed out in the sun a bit too long, you're looking for a remedy anywhere you can get it. Start in your kitchen to get some soothing relief by using these everyday products as follows:

Get milk! Whole milk dabbed on sunburn for 15 minutes every two to four hours can be ultra-soothing. It's the fat content that does the trick, but don't try it until the heat has gone out of the burn, or you'll feel as though you've jumped into a fire.

Bag it. Black tea contains tannins that help change the skin's protein structure and calm burning. Put several tea bags in your bath and soak your pain away. Or place brewed tea in a spray bottle, chill, and mist it on your skin as you feel the heat. Strawberry leaves and witch hazel, both of which are rich in tannins, are also effective.

Try vinegar. Apple cider vinegar is another great source of tannins and an old-time remedy that can soothe larger sunburned areas. Simply add 1 cup of apple cider vinegar to your bathwater, and soak for 15 minutes or so.

Take comfort in comfrey. The herb comfrey (*Symphytum officinale*)—a staple in Native American medicine kits—contains allantoin, which boosts tissue growth and promotes healing. Soak a clean cloth in cooled comfrey tea (which you can buy at health-food stores), and use it as a compress on your sunburn for 15 minutes twice daily.

Be cool as a cucumber. You can soothe the burn by placing chilled slices of cucumber on your simmering skin. A dab of cold yogurt or a splash of vinegar will do the job, too.

Take a Bath

Cool water is a refreshing treat for sunburned skin. As soon as you can, soak a washcloth, wring it out, and apply it to the burned area, or better yet, lounge in a cool bath or shower. Apart from providing nearly instant relief, cool water helps hydrate the skin and prevents it from drying out. Another option? Fill your tub with cool to lukewarm water, and add some baking soda or oatmeal to it. Soak long enough for your skin to feel soothed.

Munch on Antioxidants

To help your skin heal itself and to protect against free-radical damage that can cause skin cancer, include five to six servings of antioxidant-rich foods in your daily diet. Berries of all types are tops, followed by citrus, mango, papaya, dark leafy greens, broccoli, Brussels sprouts, nuts and seeds, whole grains, and legumes.

Ease the Itch

Whatever you do, don't scratch when your sun-damaged skin starts to get itchy. Scratching will only make your skin hurt more and encourage infection. So hands off! Instead, try cold compresses to ease any itching as your skin heals. Calamine lotion works well, too.

Deal with the Peel

When your damaged skin peels or the blisters break, gently remove as much of the dried fragments as you can. Then apply an antiseptic ointment or hydrocortisone cream to the skin below to help with the healing.

FAST FORMULA

Capsule Cure

For mild sunburn, mix your own soothing oil using these ingredients.

6 capsules of vitamin A
6 capsules of vitamin E
1¼ cups of flaxseed oil

Mix the contents of the capsules with the oil, and apply frequently to the burned areas. You can also add this combination to ¼ cup of aloe juice and smooth it over your skin for another slick way to soothe that burn.

This Enzyme Is Fine

An enzyme called photolyase, which is made from ocean algae and added to some sunburn products, is said to be the magic elixir for a painful sunburn. Photolyase helps reverse some of the critical DNA damage that's caused by soaking up too much ultraviolet light. In fact, studies have shown that photolyase reduced redness and DNA damage by as much as 45 percent. Look for the enzyme in the ingredients list of sunburn products.

Let the Soap Slide

For the first day or two after getting burned, don't use any soap on the painful areas. Why not? Because soap dries out the skin and can make the pain worse. Of course, you may have to use soap if the area is dirtier than usual. But it's better to have a little irritation than to risk a nasty infection.

Drink Up

Sunburn removes part of your body's natural

moisture barrier, so you'll need to drink plenty of water to compensate for this loss. Drinking water also helps your body repair the burn and keeps your immune system in good shape to repel any bacteria that invade through the damaged skin. So drink as much water as you can hold—anywhere from four to eight glasses a day, depending on your size and how active you are.

Wallow in Aloe

The aloe plant may have been put on Earth just to help heal sunburned skin. Aloe thrives in any container, in any room, in any part of the country. If you get burned, simply break off a leaf, squeeze out the gel, and apply a generous amount. You can also slit a leaf lengthwise and tape the open area against your skin.

Pop an Analgesic

When you're suffering with sunburn, you not only need something to soothe your sensitive skin, but you also need to dull the pain. So take an analgesic. While aspirin, ibuprofen, and other pain relievers won't help heal your sunburned skin, they are very effective at reducing pain while your skin is recovering.

More Moisture

To ease the heat of sunburned skin, slather on a moisturizer. These miracles of modern science pump healing fluids back into the skin and create a temporary cooling sensation. Just make sure your moisturizer is fragrance-free, or your skin may be irritated by an allergic reaction that can make the sunburn worse.

Spritz This Fix

Lavender is an antiseptic, cooling herb that can relieve burning skin and protect against secondary infections. To fix this mix, fill an 8-ounce spray bottle with cold water and add 6 drops of lavender oil. Shake well, then spray on the sunburned area.

Get Gotu Kola

Now what the heck is gotu kola? It's an Indian herb that is known to fight infection and speed healing. The recommended dose is 200 milligrams twice a day. You'll find this wonder herb at health-food stores.

PART THREE

THE JOY OF GARDENING

CHAPTER 13

Go for the Green

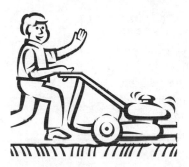

What's more American than apple pie? A lush, green, toe-ticklin'
lawn—that's what! Well, friends, whether you're starting a
brand-new lawn, reviving one that's seen better days, or simply
want to put a little more pep into your old home ground, you've
come to the right place. In this chapter, I'll show you how to
turn any plain old yard into a regular field of dreams.

TENDER LOVIN' LAWN CARE

Just like any other plant, turf grass
requires certain care to help it grow
strong and healthy, and to enable
it to fend off trouble from wicked weeds,
dastardly diseases, and pesky pests. So
here's the lowdown on turf-grass TLC.

Breakfast Time

When the first balmy breezes float through the
air in spring, your lawn (like everything else in
nature) wakes up rarin' to grow. That's the time
to get it up off its grass with this four-step launch
routine:

Step 1. As soon as your grass starts rubbing
the sleep out of its eyes, give it this wake-up

treat: For every 2,500 square feet of lawn area, mix 50 pounds each of pelletized gypsum and pelletized lime, 5 pounds of bonemeal, and 2 pounds of Epsom salts in a wheelbarrow. Apply the mixture to your lawn with a broadcast spreader. This will help aerate the turf, while giving it something to munch on until you start your regular feeding program. Then immediately serve up a good, healthy dose of my Get-Up-and-Grow Tonic (at right).

Step 2. No more than two weeks later, give your lawn its first solid meal of the season. Add 3 pounds of Epsom salts to a bag of your favorite dry, organic lawn food (enough for 2,500 square feet). I use a 20–5–10 mix. Be sure to mix the salts in well. Apply half of this mixture at *half* the rate recommended on the fertilizer label, with your spreader set on the medium setting, moving from north to south in parallel rows across your yard. Set the other half of the mixture aside where you can get at it easily— you're going to need it soon.

Step 3. It's snack time! No more than two days after you spread the fertilizer/Epsom salts mixture, mix 1 can of beer and 1 cup of dishwashing liquid in a 20 gallon hose-end sprayer, filling the balance of the jar with ammonia. (*Note:* When adding dishwashing liquid, do not use detergent or any product that contains antibacterial agents.) Then overspray your lawn to the point of runoff. Apply this bracing beverage before noon—the earlier in the morning, the better.

Step 4. One week later, haul out the second half of the dry lawn food/Epsom salts mixture from step 2 above, and pour it into your spreader. This time, apply it in rows moving from east to west. This "checkerboard" maneuver will guarantee that every square inch of turf gets

---

FAST FORMULA	**Get-Up-and-Grow Tonic**

After giving your lawn its wake-up treat (see Step 1 in "Breakfast Time" on page 253), overspray it with this tonic to kick it into high gear.

1 cup of baby shampoo
1 cup of ammonia
1 cup of regular cola (not diet)
4 tbsp. of instant tea granules

Mix these ingredients in a 20 gallon hose-end sprayer, and apply to the point of runoff. This tonic will get all that good stuff working to help your grass off to a super start—so get ready for the most terrific turf in town!

---

fed, and you won't have any light green lines in your lawn that mark the spots you missed.

Note: If you use a synthetic, slow-release lawn food instead of an organic one, spread the Epsom salts on your lawn first, and *then* apply the fertilizer. The reason is that synthetic fertilizers contain an ingredient that slows down the normal, lightning-like speed of the chemicals they're made from—and that makes them turn into a gooey mess when they're mixed with Epsom salts.

Summer Picnics

Once you've given your lawn its hearty spring breakfast, it's time to begin a series of regular, but light meals that will carry it through to the first cold days of fall. (After all, not even turf grass wants to eat big, heavy meals when the weather's so hot you could grill a steak on the sidewalk!)

Still, heat or no heat, those grass plants need sustenance, and for my money, the best way to provide it is with my All-Season Green-Up Tonic (see page 256). It delivers a light, refreshing combo of nutrients that give your little green plants the growing power they need without filling them up and slowing them down. Serve up this tonic every three weeks right through the first hard frost, and your lawn will romp like a pup through the dog days of summer!

If the heat gets you down so much that you'd rather not fuss with mixing up tonics, you can substitute a good liquid lawn food or fish emulsion. Whatever you use, just remember to keep it "lite."

Gettin' On Toward Bedtime

For your final fall feeding, repeat the spring routine (see "Breakfast Time" on page 253), only this time, use a 10–10–10 dry, organic fertilizer instead of the 20–5–10 version you used earlier. Once again, mix 3 pounds of Epsom salts into a bag of food (enough for 2,500 square feet), and apply half of the mixture at half the recommended rate, moving from north to south across your lawn. One week later, spread the remaining food/Epsom salts, going from east to west. (And again, if you use a synthetic, slow-release fertilizer, spread the salts first, and *then* the food.) Then within two days after your second feeding, serve up a season's-end drink of my Last Supper Tonic, which is described below.

Last, But Not Least

Finish up your turf's bedtime ritual just before winter sets in by applying what I somewhat irreverently call my Last Supper Tonic. This soothing beverage is the equivalent of a bedtime cup of cocoa for your lawn. Immediately after the last fall feeding, mix the ingredients in a big bucket, pour the solution into a 20 gallon hose-end sprayer, and apply it to the grass to the point of runoff. It'll soften up the dry fertilizer, so your grass's roots can absorb the nutrients all winter long. As for the ingredients, you'll need $^1/_2$ can of beer and $^1/_2$ cup of each of these common liquids:

- Ammonia
- Apple juice
- A sports drink that contains electrolytes
- Baby shampoo
- Fish emulsion
- Regular cola (not diet)
- Urine

Drink Up

Every living thing on earth needs water to survive, and turf grass is no exception. But too much moisture can lead to all kinds of problems, ranging from thatch buildup to root rot. To stay in peak form, most types of grass need roughly 1 inch of water each week during the growing season. That's about 62 gallons for every 100 square feet of lawn—and that's a *lot* of H_2O! If you're like most of the folks that I hear from these days, you're finding that Mother Nature is providing less of that supply than she used to— and as a result, you're watching your water bills climb higher every year. Well, don't fret: You can curb your lawn's drinking habits and still keep it healthy, happy, and handsome.

A Grass-Roots Movement

The road to a water-thrifty lawn starts with a strong, healthy—and deep—root system. Although most of a grass plant's roots grow in the top 6 to 8 inches of soil, many of them will dive a whole lot deeper if you give them a chance. And just how do you do that? Well, for starters, you do it by filling your soil with plenty of organic matter, thereby providing the kind of loose, healthy, teeming-with-life surroundings that roots love best. Some more ways you can coax those underground parts to take the downward plunge include:

Bide your time. On the first hot day of spring, it's tempting to give your lawn its first nice, cool drink of the season. Don't do it! If you start watering too early, you'll encourage the roots to stay in the top few inches of soil. But if you wait until the soil has dried out some, the roots will scurry down to deeper, damper territory. And the moisture they'll find at those levels will sustain them later on, when the weather turns hot.

Get it down. When you water your lawn, always make sure the H_2O seeps down to the full depth of the roots. Shallow watering actually does more harm than good because it encourages the roots to stay in the soil's upper reaches—making for weak grass with a thirst that just won't quit.

Deliver dribs and drabs. When it's time to serve drinks, give your grass about $1/4$ inch of water, wait 10 minutes, then give it another $1/4$ inch. Continue this water-then-wait approach until you've moistened the soil all the way down to the bottom of the roots.

Hit the deck. Or rather, raise it. One of the easiest ways to encourage long grass roots is to set your mower deck higher. That's because like most other plants, the height of the grass blade is directly related to the length of its underpinnings. The reason is that the upper part of the plant produces carbohydrates, which make roots grow longer and longer. If you routinely give your lawn a crew cut, you'll deprive the roots of needed nourishment, and they'll stay short.

Water Wisdom

There's really no great skill involved in knowing when to water your lawn. When your turf is thirsty, it'll speak up loud and clear—in sign language, of course. Here are three signs that translate into "Give me a drink!"

1. The grass turns from a healthy green color to a dull, grayish blue, and the blades curl up or fold in along the edges.

2. The soil changes. Heavy soil hardens into a solid block; lighter soils turn tan-colored and crumbly.

| FAST FORMULA | **All-Season Green-Up Tonic** |

This sensational solution will give your lawn the nourishment it needs to sail through the summer's heat—and supercharge the rest of your green scene all season long.

1 can of beer
1 cup of ammonia
$1/2$ cup of dishwashing liquid*
$1/2$ cup of liquid lawn food
$1/2$ cup of molasses or corn syrup

Mix all of these ingredients together in a large bucket, and pour the mixture into a 20 gallon hose-end sprayer. Then spray your lawn (and every other green, growing thing in your yard) to the point of runoff every three weeks throughout the growing season.

Do not use detergent or any product that contains antibacterial agents.

3. When you walk across your lawn, the grass doesn't spring back to life. Instead, your footprints remain in the grass for a long time—often for several hours.

See for Yourself

The key to keeping your lawn green and healthy is to water it just *before* it starts showing any symptoms. And, believe it or not, you can learn to read your lawn's mind. How on earth can you do that? Simple—just get a shovel and dig up a block of turf. Then grab a fistful of soil from the turf block. If you feel moisture, it's not time to water yet. Keep sampling the sod this way throughout the summer until you get a good sense of how long it takes the soil to dry out. And be sure to take samples from different parts of your yard, because moisture vanishes at different speeds, depending on many factors. The most common of them are:

Slope. Soil at the top of a hill can be bone dry when the ground at the bottom is still damp. As for the soil along the way down—how it's holding up will vary depending on the steepness of the incline.

Sunlight. It practically goes without saying that the more sunlight there is, the faster the soil will dry out.

Wind. Wide open spaces will lose moisture much more quickly than areas on the leeward side of a fence or wall.

Is It Time?

I've got a simple—and foolproof—way to tell whether it's time to water your lawn: Just push a long screwdriver into the ground. If you have to struggle to get the tool 6 inches or so into the soil, then it's time to give that turf some liquid refreshment!

The Kindest Cut of All

On the face of it, cutting your grass seems about as simple and straightforward as a yard chore can get: You just crank up the ol' mower, and off you go. But in reality, mowing is *the* most important part of lawn care. Your timing, your technique, and even the equipment you use can spell the difference between a beautiful, healthy, trouble-free lawn, and one that gives you nothing but grief—and could even go belly-up. I know: It seems impossible that something as simple as taking a little off the top can affect the health of your turf. So let me briefly explain mowing from two points of view.

Unnatural Acts

The most important thing to remember about mowing is that your lawn doesn't like it one bit. If that grass had its druthers, it would go through life doing what Mother Nature intended: growing straight up, maturing, and setting seed for the next generation. Turf grasses can tolerate mowing simply because they are what scientists call "basal-growing" plants, meaning they grow from a point in the crown, close to the soil line. When you cut off the tips (which are actually the oldest parts of the plant), new growth shoots up from the crown. But the fact remains that having growing tissue suddenly whacked off takes its toll on the plants in several ways:

- It reduces the plants' ability to snag carbon, oxygen, and hydrogen from the air and, with the help of the sun's energy, turn them into food. The result: less nourishment for the grass—both above- and belowground.

- The height of the grass blades is directly related to the depth and vigor of the roots. The shorter you cut the blades, the shorter and weaker the roots will be. And grass without a strong root system not only has a constant

Quick Fix

Are you sick and tired of scraping grass clippings off of your mower blades? Well, stop scraping! Instead, before you crank up the engine, just coat the underside of your mower with any of these lubricants:

- *Cooking oil spray*
- *Household oil spray, such as WD-40®*
- *Liquid car wax*

thirst, but also is a sitting duck for pests and diseases. In fact, if you remove more than 40 percent of the top growth at any one time, the roots simply stop growing.

- It creates openings that work like a wide-open barn door. Moisture inside the plant goes out and, given half a chance, diseases come marching in.

- Cutting the grass too short (as a lot of folks tend to do) lets in the sunshine, which both dries out the soil and helps weed seeds to germinate.

Having Said That...

the fact that cutting grass isn't *natural* doesn't mean it's *bad*. In fact, if you go at it the right way, you'll actually produce turf that's thicker, stronger, and more resistant to weeds and drought. That's because when a grass plant is cut, it responds in the same way many garden plants do when you prune them: In an effort to reproduce itself, it sends out side shoots—a process known in lawn circles as "tillering." Furthermore, when you mow, you let in light that lets those baby shoots grow and develop into a lush carpet of toe-ticklin' turf.

What's "the Right Way"?

To ensure that your grass bounces back like a champ every time you cut it, simply remember these four words: Mow high, mow sharp. As for the first part of that rule, never cut more than one-third of the height of the grass at any one time. "Mow sharp" simply means that you need to keep a razor edge on your mower blade. That way, it'll slice cleanly through the grass, leaving as little wiggle room as possible for escaping moisture and invading germs.

High Is Good, But Higher Isn't Better

Having delivered my mow-high lecture, I must tell you that it *is* possible to let your grass get too high. Turf grasses that grow much over 3 inches tall tend to get thin and stringy; they don't form that nice, uniform look that we love in our lawns. Overly tall grass also tends to fall over, and gets all matted up in wet weather. Then it may take a long time to dry out, and in the meantime, fungal diseases can set in.

SHAPE IT UP

Have you just bought a house with a yard that's seen better days? Or maybe your old home ground is starting to lose its youthful good looks. (After all, lawns *are* like people, and after a certain age, it doesn't take much to start that downhill slide!) Unfortunately, you can't simply roll up your grass and send it off to a fancy spa for a few weeks. But with my timely tips, you *can* nurse your lawn back to its lush, luxurious self and bring a healthy glow to its cheeks, er, blades.

Dispatch Thatch!

Of all the woes that can befall a lawn, thatch just might be the nastiest. Not only does it keep water, air, and nutrients from reaching the grass roots, but it also provides a dandy home for hordes of bad-guy bugs and dastardly diseases. Well, here's my foolproof plan for sending thatch to the Great Beyond—and keeping it there.

Just What *Is* Thatch, Anyway?

Contrary to what a lot of folks think, thatch is *not* a thick blanket of old grass clippings. Rather, it's a tightly woven layer of stems, roots, and crowns—both living and dead—that forms between the grass blades and the soil line. These plant parts are high in *lignin*, a type of organic material that breaks down more slowly than most. But in a healthy lawn, it *does* break down. (Grass clippings, on the other hand, are made up mostly of cellulose, which decomposes in a flash.)

A little thatch is actually a good thing. A layer of half an inch or so cushions the turf, guards against soil compaction, and helps conserve moisture in the soil. The trouble starts when the stack of stuff builds up beyond that level.

How'd It Get in *My* Lawn?

Before you attack the thatch that's in your lawn, it helps to know what caused it to get out of hand in the first place. That way, you'll be better able to keep it under control later. Any, or (more likely) a combination, of these factors can lead to big-time thatch trouble:

Frequent, shallow watering. It encourages both roots and organic debris to concentrate near the soil surface.

Infrequent, too-high mowing. Whether you rake up the clippings or not, this practice

contributes to thatch. I must confess that I don't entirely understand the reason, but research has confirmed it time after time.

Overfeeding, especially with potent chemical fertilizers. It makes for overly lush growth, which in turn leads to thicker thatch. In particular, supplying more nitrogen than your grass needs will quickly lead to trouble.

Herbicides, fungicides, and pesticides. All of these potent weapons kill the soil-dwelling critters (including droves of earthworms and billions of beneficial bacteria and other microscopic organisms) that break down organic material and prevent thatch buildup.

Improper soil pH. It prevents grass from absorbing the nutrients it needs, and can also discourage the presence of earthworms, which help keep the soil loose and healthy. To find out whether this is a problem in your lawn, send a soil sample to a testing lab. The experts there can tell you the pH level and, if it's out of whack, how to amend it. (Believe it or not, turf grasses differ in their pH preferences, so enclose a note with your package saying what kind of grass you're growing.)

Heavy clay soil—and any type of soil that's become compacted. Both lack openings through which air, water, nutrients, and decomposing organisms can travel. That, in turn, means that grass roots migrate to the surface in search of sustenance, and the underground breakdown squad dies off. The result: big-time thatch in double-quick time!

Take It Off!

With dethatching, as with most lawn chores, you can choose between two modes of operation: manual and mechanical. These are the tools in question:

A thatching rake. This looks much like a normal rake, except that instead of tines, it has knifelike, double-ended blades. You can buy one at a large garden center or hardware store, and you use it in the same way you'd use a garden rake. There's just one difference: Raking up thatch with this tool is a whole lot tougher than raking bare soil! Unless you have a teeny-tiny lawn, take my advice and go the mechanical route.

A dethatcher. This is a machine that cuts through the thatch and yanks it out of the ground. It does the job with a fraction of the effort required with a thatching rake. Most equipment-rental yards rent these machines. Bear in mind, though, that dethatchers are big, heavy mamas, and they can be mighty tricky to handle. If you've never used one before, have the folks at the rental place walk you through the procedure, and follow their instructions *to the letter*. And if you're not accustomed to working with power equipment of any kind, do yourself a favor and turn the task over to someone who is.

No matter who does the "driving," it's important to get the right dethatcher for your grass. There are two kinds. One has vertically rotating, steel blades; it's just the ticket for thick grasses such as Bermuda and zoysia. For finer-bladed types, such as fescue and Kentucky bluegrass, use a wire-tined model. (If you're not sure which machine you need, ask the folks at the rental yard.)

Boy, That's Hard!

All kinds of things can make soil harden up and become what professional lawn and garden tenders call "compacted." And when that does happen, it's bad news for your grass and every other plant that's growing in your yard. Just as we saw with thatch, before you set out to repair compacted soil, it helps to know what caused the problem in the first place. Some of the prime compaction culprits are:

- Constant foot traffic, like the mailman beating the same path to your box every day, or the kids cutting across the same corner on their way to the school bus in the morning—and then back again in the afternoon!

- Work in progress, like the construction crew that spent the summer building your swimming pool—aided by a lot of heavy equipment—or the salt-and-cinder guys who roll their truck across your lawn's edges all winter long. After all, when there's so much snow, how can they tell where the road ends and your grass begins?

- Misguided TLC; in particular, running a heavy roller over an established lawn. A lot of folks do this every spring to produce that velvet-carpet look.

- Working with wet soil, or simply walking on it, makes the soil particles clump together. If you do it often enough, they stay that way.

- Repeated tilling, especially in clay soil, compresses the pores so much that it can actually create hardpan, the most severe form of compacted soil.

Give Me a Clue

Of course, if you notice that your grass is wearing thin in places where people frequently walk, it's a sure bet that the ground below is on its way to rock-hardness. Here are some other clues that you've got a yard full of compacted soil:

1. After a rain, water puddles up on the surface and stays there for hours—maybe even days.

2. After you've had the sprinkler on for only a few minutes, water runs off the lawn and down the street.

3. The grass is turning brown and losing its get-up-and-grow power (because, of course, water isn't getting to the roots). And in some areas, it just plumb disappears.

Fork It Over!

Your first response to compacted soil should be a technique called aeration. It simply involves poking holes in the soil so that air can reach the grass roots—followed quickly by food and water. On a small lawn, or in isolated spots of a large one, you can easily do the job with a garden fork or, better yet, a hand aerator. This useful gadget has a long, tined, horizontal bar at the bottom with a handle at each end. To use it, take hold of both handles, shove the tines 6 or 8 inches into the ground, and stand on the horizontal bar. Then rock back and forth a few times to make nice, wide holes in the soil. Pull up the fork, move it along 3 inches or so, and repeat the performance.

Jerry Baker's Hole Improvement Plan

You might think that in order to soften up a yard full of compacted soil, you'd have to remove your existing turf and dig in mountains of organic matter. Well, you *could* do that, but there's a much easier way: Just implement my hole improvement plan! This technique is so potent, it'll even soften up hardpan. Here's all there is to it: Every time you have some organic matter on hand, dig a hole, toss in your stash, and refill the hole. Then scatter some grass seed on top. Or you can simply wait for the surrounding grass to mosey on over and cover the bare spot.

Holey Moley!

My hole improvement plan (above) isn't just for soil with clay or hardpan headaches. It's a simple way to add get-up-and-grow power to any kind of soil. So what do you toss into your holes? Well, grass clippings, fallen leaves, and vegetable scraps are obvious choices, but here are some hole fillers that you might not normally think of:

- Brown paper bags
- Coffee grounds (filters and all)
- Dead flowers
- Dirty paper liners from the floor of a birdcage
- Eggshells
- Feathers
- Hair from your (or your pet's) brushes
- Matches (new or used, wooden or cardboard)
- Wine corks
- Wood chips

If you have hardpan, it's best if the hole reaches down to that layer, but if you don't have time to dig that far, don't bother; just go deep enough to cover whatever material you're planning to bury. The depth could range from an inch or so for a couple of tea bags to a foot or more for tree and shrub prunings. As the material decomposes, it will eventually make the soil fluffy, fertile, and rarin' to grow gorgeous green grass.

Telltale Trees

If you have trees in your yard and you can see their surface roots on your lawn, that's a certain sign that your soil is compacted. How so? Well, normally, a tree's feeder roots roam through the top 4 to 8 inches of soil in search or air, water, and food—the same territory that grass roots call home. When that ground is compacted, the trees send their roots to the surface in their quest for oxygen—and who can blame them?

Spike It

One ultra-simple way to help keep your soil aerated—and fend off thatch in the process—is to wear spiked golf shoes whenever you mow your lawn. That way, you'll break up the surface tension barrier that develops between the soil and the blades of grass.

Dippity Don't!

Even when your soil is just fine, thank you, there may be times when you need to fill low-lying areas in your lawn. To correct tiny irregularities in your terrain, just fill those micro-mini valleys with a half-and-half mixture of topsoil and compost. If the grass in residence is healthy, it'll grow right up through that topping faster than you can say "Jack and the Beanstalk." When

---

FAST FORMULA

Kick-in-the-Grass Tonic

After you've given your lawn a sod "bandage" (see Step 6 in "Dippity Don't!" at right), apply this timely tonic to get it off to a rip-roarin' start.

1 can of beer
1 cup of antiseptic mouthwash
1 cup of dishwashing liquid*
1 cup of ammonia
1/2 cup of Epsom salts

Mix these ingredients in a large bucket, and pour the solution into a 20 gallon hose-end sprayer. Apply it to your lawn-repair site to the point of runoff, wait two weeks, then administer another dose.

Do not use detergent or any product that contains antibacterial agents.

---

you're faced with deeper dips though, follow this eight-step procedure:

Step 1. Remove the grass in the low area with a sharp, square-ended shovel. Simply dig down about 2 inches, and lift out whatever size pieces you can manage easily.

Step 2. If the sod is healthy, and you plan to finish the job within a day or so, tuck the pieces away in a shady spot and keep them moist. (But don't cover them with plastic— that's like throwing a party for all the foul fungi in town!) If this is a longer-term project, or the grass has seen better days, toss it on your compost pile and order new sod.

Step 3. To lower a bump, simply shovel off enough soil to level the area; then work about an inch of compost into the soil. To raise a low spot, fill it with a half-and-half mixture of topsoil and compost.

Step 4. Rake the area until it's smooth.

Step 5. Water the site lightly to help the soil settle down.

Step 6. Replace the saved sod, or roll out your new strip that's been cut to fit the bare spot.

Step 7. To get your newly installed turf growing on the right root, give it a good soaking with my Kick-in-the-Grass Tonic (at left).

Step 8. Water the area lightly once a day for a week to 10 days, and tread lightly around the new turf until it's well established and showing signs of new growth.

GET OUTTA HERE!

It can take a lot of money, time, and good old-fashioned elbow grease to keep a lawn looking its best. So the last thing you need is to have it bashed, hashed, and mashed to pieces by bad bugs, roving critters—or even your own best pals. Well, never fear: I've got a wheelbarrow full of ways to keep your turf in tip-top condition.

Banish Bad Bugs

In this wide world of ours, there are a whole lot more beneficial bugs than there are destructive ones. But a few multilegged menaces can cause big-time damage. Armyworms, chinch bugs, and sod webworms rank right at the top of a lawn keeper's "Most Unwanted List." Read on for tips on how to give them the boot.

Discharge Armyworms

These nasty Nellies gobble up every grass blade in their path. They dine after dark, and a large horde can destroy a small lawn in a single night. Armyworms generally strike in late summer or fall, leaving round, bald spots in the turf. They conduct maneuvers from coast to coast, sparing only very cold regions of the country. But they do the most damage on warm-season grasses in southern Florida and along the Gulf Coast. (They're especially partial to Bermuda grass.)

There's no mistaking the vile villains when you see them. They're slightly hairy caterpillars, about $1^1/_2$ inches long, with a black head marked with a white Y. Three thin, yellowish white stripes stretch along the back from stem to stern. On each side is a dark stripe and, below that, a wavy yellow line splotched with red. The main body color can be green, brown, or nearly black. Follow my control measures to get rid of these pests:

- If you can be on the scene just after dusk when the worms slither out to feed, blast 'em with my All-Season Clean-Up Tonic (see page 265). Remember, though, that for this treatment to be effective, it has to make direct contact with the target.

- If you prefer a hands-off approach, treat your lawn with either Btk *(Bacillus thuringiensis* var. *kurstaki)* or parasitic nematodes of the species *Neoaplectana carpocapsae*—they've been specially bred to polish off armyworms. You can order both through catalogs and at the click of a mouse on the Internet.

- For long-term protection, dig up the dead turf, and reseed the bare spots with a grass that's resistant to armyworms. New varieties come on the market almost every year, so check with your Cooperative Extension Service to find the best type for your area.

Say Good-Bye to Chinch Bugs

These dark brown and black bugs suck the sap from grass blades and, at the same time, inject a poison that kills the plants, leaving your lawn full of round, yellow patches that quickly turn brown and die. Any turf grass in any climate is a likely target, but certain varieties of St. Augustine and Kentucky bluegrasses are especially vulnerable. Chinch bug nymphs are bright red with a white band across their backs. Adults have dark brown bodies with a black triangle between white, folded wings. Here's how to bid them a fond farewell:

- Make a solution of 2 tablespoons of dishwashing liquid to 1 gallon of water, and pour it on the area, using a sprinkling can to ensure even coverage. (*Note:* When adding dishwashing liquid, do not use detergent or any product that contains antibacterial agents.) Put a white flannel sheet or other soft, white cloth on top of the grass. Wait 15 to 20 minutes, then peek under the fabric. It should be teeming with chinch bugs that've crawled toward the surface to escape the soap. Gather up the cloth, and dunk it into a bucket filled with soapy water. Then, get out the hose, and spray your lawn thoroughly to remove the soap residue.

- If chinch bugs are attacking an area that's too big for the flannel-sheet treatment described above, mix 1 cup of Murphy® Oil Soap with 3 cups of warm water in a bucket, pour it into a 20 gallon hose-end sprayer, and saturate your lawn. Wait for it to dry, then apply gypsum to the infested territory at the rate of 50 pounds per 2,500 square feet of lawn area.

- To avoid future problems, control thatch, keep your lawn well watered, and avoid overfeeding (especially beware of feeding your grass too much nitrogen).

So Long, Sod Webworms!

These culprits are famous (infamous, rather) for chewing off grass blades at the crown and pulling them into silk-lined tunnels in the ground to eat them. The damage first appears as small dead patches (1 to 2 inches in diameter) in early spring. By July or August, they've usually developed into *big* dead patches. Sod webworms wander here and there and yonder, and gleefully chow down on any kind of grass. But their favorite stomping, er, crawling ground is out there in America's heartland. And their idea of a genuine fine dining experience is a lawn full of bent grass or Kentucky bluegrass, covered with a thick, cozy layer of thatch.

The worms are sleek, tan caterpillars with black spots on their backs and a beaklike projection on their heads. Their parents are small, white moths. (You'll know for a fact that webworms have come to call when these little fliers rise up in clouds in front of your lawn mower.) Show them the door with these control measures:

Step 1. When you mow your lawn, wear your golf spikes or lawn sandals. That way, your weapon (or tonic) of choice can better penetrate the layer of thatch down below.

Step 2. Apply either Btk (*Bacillus thuringiensis* var. *kurstaki*) or my All-Season Clean-Up Tonic (at right). Whichever weapon you choose, be quick about it, because with sod webworms, a small problem can turn into a big one in the blink of an eye. And be aware that you may need to repeat the process several times before you see results—but see results you will!

Step 3. Do everything in your power to control thatch, and encourage the slimy squirts' natural enemies. Many good-guy bugs and other critters consider sod webworms a tasty treat, but birds and spined soldier beetles gobble 'em up like there's no tomorrow.

Wave Away White Grubs

These familiar pests eat the roots of your grass and leave you with a lawn full of irregular, brown patches that look burned. If you tug on one of the dead clumps, it'll come right up like a piece of loose carpet—often exposing the culprits in action. Grubs start feeding in early spring, and the damage becomes apparent any time from late spring through early fall, usually during dry spells. Any kind of grass in any part of this great land of ours is fair game for these greedy gluttons.

White grubs are the larvae of many different beetles, including chafer, Japanese, June (a.k.a. May), and Asiatic garden beetles. It's near impossible to tell them apart: They all have fat, whitish bodies that tend to curl up into a C shape. Escort them off of your property by following these tips:

- A few grubs are no cause for panic. The trouble comes when too many of them start munching on the same piece of turf. Here's a simple way to take a census: Cut both ends off of several soup cans and sink each one up to its rim in the soil, spaced about 10 feet apart. Then fill the cans close to the top with water. After 5 or 10 minutes, count the grubs that you find in each can. That number will equal the number of grubs per square foot of lawn. If there are 8 to 10 per can, don't sweat it. Birds can keep that crowd under control without harming your lawn in the process. More than 10 grubs means you've got a major invasion on your hands and you need to strike back—hard!

- To ease your grub woes and aerate your turf at the same time, strap on a pair of aerating lawn sandals (available at **www.jerrybaker.com**) and stroll back and forth across your lawn. You won't get every single one, but you'll polish off enough of them to turn a big problem into a no-worry situation in no time at all.

- Drench your turf with beneficial nematodes (available on the Internet and in some garden-supply catalogs). They'll burrow into the villains, reproduce, and at the same time deliver a bacteria that'll kill the grubs, but harm no other critters. Unfortunately, the

---

FAST FORMULA

All-Season Clean-Up Tonic

This excellent elixir will kill sod webworms and just about any other bad-guy bugs that mistake your yard for the local salad bar.

1 cup of dishwashing liquid*
1 cup of antiseptic mouthwash
1 cup of tobacco tea**

Mix these ingredients in a 20 gallon hose-end sprayer, and give the worms and the turf a good thorough soaking when the worms come out to feed at night.

* Do not use detergent or any product that contains antibacterial agents.

**To make tobacco tea, place half a handful of chewing tobacco in an old pantyhose leg and soak it in a gallon of hot water until the mixture is dark brown. Store the liquid in a glass container with a tight lid.

results are temporary, so you may have to repeat the maneuver the following spring.

- If you know for sure that the grubs in your lawn are baby Japanese beetles (because the grownups are chewin' the daylights out of your shrubs, flowers, and veggies), get some milky spore disease *(Bacillus popilliae)*, available at **www.jerrybaker.com**. All you do is apply it to your freshly mowed lawn according to the package directions, and it stays in the soil for years, killing baby grubs as soon as they hatch, but harming nothing else. Unfortunately, milky spore takes a few years to achieve its full effect, but once it gets up to speed, your grub woes will be gone for good.

The Bigger Bunch

Believe it or not, your neighbor's cat or dog really isn't out gunnin' for your grass. The same goes for wilder creatures like gophers and moles. But in the process of carrying on life as they know it, they sure can make a mess of your lawn! Read on for some super secrets for saying "Not here, please!" to domestic pals and wild pests alike.

Scat, Cat!

As much as I love cats (especially my own), I have to admit that they do have a few unfortunate habits—namely, using freshly seeded lawns as their personal privy, eating or trampling your groundcover plants, and, worst of all, gunning for birds. It's easy to keep your own kitties from making mischief in your yard: Just keep them indoors. To protect your turf from roving felines, try one of these tricks:

- In newly seeded areas, cover the soil with thorny canes cut from rosebushes or bramble fruits, and keep them in place until the baby grass plants have grown big enough to cover the loose ground. Or, if you don't have any prickly branches on hand, use my flashy feline-foiling fence (see the Home Remedy box below).

- Build a flat fence. Just plant seeds of a low-growing groundcover, like creeping thyme or sweet alyssum, around the area you want to declare off-limits. Then, on top of the newly seeded soil, lay 2- to 3-foot-wide strips of chicken wire. When the plants grow up, they'll cover the flat fencing, so you'll hardly notice it. But when Fluffy's paws touch that sharp wire, she'll be outta there! *Note:* If you use this trick to safeguard bird feeders or nesting boxes, just make sure that those shelters are well out of leaping range of tree limbs, porch overhangs, or other handy platforms. Otherwise, the agile assassins won't even notice your fence!

HOME REMEDY

Cavorting cats can destroy a freshly seeded lawn in no time flat. But this flashy foil "fence" will make the felines flee fast! And it's as easy as 1, 2, 3. Here's all you need to do.

1. Half-fill empty 2-liter pop bottles with water, and add a few drops of bleach, just to keep smelly algae from growing.

2. Put two or three long, thin strips of aluminum foil into each bottle.

3. Set the bottles every few feet around the area you want to protect.

The constantly changing reflections from the foil will scare the daylights out of any cat that dares to come prancing onto your turf.

Those Doggone Dogs

The damage you're most likely to see from man's best friend is the brown, burned-looking patches that we call "dog spots." These are simply the result of too much of a good thing—namely, nitrogen and salts. The same damage would occur if you spilled fertilizer on the grass. (By the way, it is not true that female-dog urine is more potent than that of males. It causes more damage only because females tend to urinate all at once, in one spot, while males generally spray a little here and a little there.) Here's how to initiate doggy damage control:

- If you reach the scene while the deed is being done, or shortly thereafter, just grab the hose and flush the site thoroughly; that should stop any damage in its tracks. After a day or so, time is still on your side: Lightly sprinkle gypsum over and around each spot to dissolve accumulated salts, then pour 1 cup of baby shampoo or dishwashing liquid into a 20 gallon hose-end sprayer and overspray the lawn. (*Note:* When adding dishwashing liquid, do not use detergent or any product that contains antibacterial agents.) One week later, overspray the turf with my Lawn-Saver Tonic: Combine $1/2$ can of beer, $1/2$ can of regular cola (not diet), and $1/2$ cup of ammonia in a 20 gallon hose-end sprayer, then saturate your grass to the point of runoff.

- When the grass is dead and brown, your only option is to dig up the affected areas and reseed or resod. And use fescue or perennial ryegrass if it's suitable for your climate; they're the most urine-resistant types.

- Teach your dog to go where her offerings won't hurt anything! While she's learning to use her privy, add a tablespoon or so of brewer's yeast to her food. It seems to alter the chemistry of dog urine, making it less damaging to turf grass. What's more, it helps repel fleas.

- The only sure way to keep neighborhood roamers out of your yard is to erect a good, solid fence. For a temporary solution, though, pour two 8-ounce bottles of hot sauce (the hotter, the better) into a 20 gallon hose-end sprayer, and lightly spray around the areas where canines aren't welcome. Dogs hate the scent of anything hot! (Just be sure to spray again after rain or your sprinklers have washed away the scent.)

Go, Go, Gophers!

These toothy fur balls tunnel through your lawn, killing your grass in the process, and eating just about any plant they encounter. Because gophers operate underground, it's unlikely that you'll see them at work. And at first glance, it's easy to mistake their dirty work for that of moles. To make a positive ID, just eyeball the tunnel entrance. You'll know you've got a gopher on your hands if you see a U- or crescent-shaped mound of moist soil that looks as though it's been sifted. Moles make round mounds at their entrance holes. The damage in your yard will give you another clue: Moles eat no plants at all, so if all kinds of greenery are being munched on, you can pin the blame on the G-men. To stop the feasting:

- Stuff a potent-smelling substance into each gopher hole. (Gophers hate strong scents.) Be sure to wear gloves so you don't transfer your scent to the repellent, and seal all the entrance holes you can find, so the tunnel gets good and smelly. See the Quick Fix box on page 268 for a list of my favorite fragrant offerings.

- Sprinkle my Gopher-Go Tonic around the varmints' *real* targets: all the plants in your yard. When they find that dinner has developed a repulsive aroma, they'll clear out in a hurry. To whip up a batch, combine 4 tablespoons of castor oil, 4 tablespoons of dishwashing liquid, and 4 tablespoons of urine in $^1/_2$ cup of warm water. (*Note:* When adding dishwashing liquid, do not use detergent or any product that contains antibacterial agents.) Then stir the solution into 2 gallons of warm water, and pour the mixture over any problem areas.

- Plant a protective barrier. Just run down to the garden center, and buy as much gopher spurge *(Euphorbia latyrus)* as you can afford. Then plant it all around the perimeter of your garden—or even your whole lawn. The roots produce an acrid, milky juice that gophers can't stand. One whiff, and they'll find another dining establishment!

Move On, Moles

Unlike gophers, moles don't eat plants at all. Instead, they eat insects—and plenty of them, including their favorite of favorites: grubs. The problem is that as they tunnel through the ground in search of dinner, they damage the grass roots, leaving the plants vulnerable to drought, diseases, and other pests. Put a stop to their travels with these techniques:

- Stuff each tunnel entrance with one of the smelly substances listed in the Quick Fix box below. Whichever one you choose, you might have to repeat it a few times, but eventually, the moles will give up and move on.

- Get a bunch of plastic toy pinwheels, and shove them into the ground at regular intervals. Moles are supersensitive to sounds and ground vibrations, and the whooshing of the wheels will send 'em packing.

- Get rid of their food supply—namely grubs. Over the long haul, milky spore disease *(Bacillus popilliae)* is your best bet, but you won't see the full results for several years. For more immediate measures, see my antigrub tactics on page 265. Just beware that once you've sent the grubs packin', your mole problems could get worse before they get better. That's because the little guys, finding themselves without their favorite food, will frantically search for dinner before they head for grubbier pastures.

> ## ⏳ *Quick Fix*
>
> *Both gophers and moles flee from strong-smelling substances. You can buy commercial repellents, but stuffing any of these aromatic goodies into the tunnel entrances should make the terrors take off: rags soaked in ammonia, sticks of Juicy Fruit® gum, rotting garbage, paper towels soaked in rancid oil, dog or cat hair, a few squirts of pine-based cleanser, or a scoop of used cat litter. (**Note:** Don't use this last one anywhere near vegetables, herbs, or any other edibles!)*

WINNING THE WAR ON WEEDS

Botanically speaking, there is no such thing as a weed. But there *is* such a thing as a plant that's growing where it's not welcome. And a whole lot of unwelcome greenery can—and does—show up in even the best-kept lawns. Here's a roundup of my super secrets for keeping the upper hand over these trespassers.

First Things First

One sure way to cut down on the time you spend pulling, digging, or spraying weeds is to keep your lawn mowed at the maximum recommended height for your type of grass. This way, you can wipe out a whole lot of those worrisome plants—thereby leaving yourself more time to spend on the golf course or down at the old fishin' hole. This easy trick works for a couple of reasons. First, tall grass shades and cools the soil, making it harder for weed seeds to get a toehold. Second, mowing high makes for deep-rooted, healthier grass that's better able to crowd out any weeds that do develop.

High mowing is especially effective at controlling low-growing troublemakers, such as annual bluegrass, crabgrass, witchgrass, and yellow nut sedge.

Coming to Terms with Weeds

Before you set out to do battle with wily weeds, it helps to know a little terminology. That's because your best strategy depends in large part on which category—or rather, combination of categories—your resident troublemakers fall into: their appearance, reproductive styles, and germinating schedule.

Starting with appearance, there are two categories:

- Narrowleaf, a.k.a. grassy weeds, look like, well, grasses, and most of them are exactly that. In fact, the grassy "weeds" in your lawn may be somebody else's idea of first-rate turf grass. (Bermuda grass and annual bluegrass are just two examples.) But some of these intrepid intruders are grass look-alikes called sedges.

- Broadleaf weeds include all of our uninvited green guests that are *not* grasses or sedges— even though some of them have leaves that are downright skinny.

When it comes to reproductive styles, here's the scoop:

- Annual weeds germinate, mature, flower, set seed, and die in a single year. In fact, some especially prolific procreators complete that cycle several times each year.

- Perennial weeds live for two or more years. (Unlike flower gardeners, who have a separate category for biennials—plants that complete their life cycles in two years—lawn-weed warriors generally lump these two-year wonders in with their longer-lived cousins.)

It pays to know when your weeds will be in their prime troublemaking period. Here's how you can tell:

- Cool-season weeds germinate in spring or fall. Up North, that's also when they raise the biggest ruckus. In the South, they go on the rampage in the winter, when temperatures are mild and warm-season lawns are dormant.

- Warm-season weeds germinate in late spring or summer, and grow like blazes as long as the hot weather lasts. Come winter, the annuals die (leaving their seed behind to launch the next generation), and the perennials go dormant (to rise again, bigger and stronger, in the spring).

Naming Names

Of course, every kind of weed has a combination of three of the above attributes. What follows is a roster of some of the more common turf-trashing trespassers and where they fall in this three-part classification system:

Cool-season broadleaf annuals: Burclover, a.k.a. black medic; henbit, a.k.a. deadnettle; mallow, a.k.a. cheeseweed.

Cool-season broadleaf perennials: Broadleaf plantain, Canada thistle, clover.

Cool-season narrowleaf annuals: Annual bluegrass, crabgrass.

Cool-season narrowleaf perennials: Quackgrass, wild garlic.

Warm-season broadleaf annuals: Carpetweed, purslane, spurge.

Warm-season broadleaf perennials: Bindweed, a.k.a. wild morning glory; dandelion; Queen Anne's lace, a.k.a. wild carrot.

Warm-season narrowleaf annuals: Foxtail, goosegrass.

Warm-season narrowleaf perennials: Dallis grass, smutgrass, yellow nut sedge.

FAST FORMULA	**Wild Weed Wipeout Tonic**

When you've got weeds that won't take "no" for an answer, knock 'em out with this potent potion.

1 tbsp. of gin
1 tbsp. of vinegar
1 tsp. of dishwashing liquid*
1 qt. of very warm water

Mix these ingredients together, and pour the solution into a handheld sprayer bottle. Then, drench the weeds to the point of runoff, taking care not to spray any nearby plants that you want to keep.

* Do not use detergent or any product that contains antibacterial agents.

But no matter what categories your unwelcome guests fall into, you can bid them all a fond farewell with the following tips.

A Weed Warrior's Bag of Tricks

Some of my favorite ways and means for battling bad plants, both big and small, include:

Boil 'em alive. One of the oldest tricks in the book is still one of the best: Just boil a kettle of water and pour it over the weeds. This works best on shallow-rooted weeds, like spurge and crabgrass, because the danged things will keep coming back unless the boiling water reaches the roots.

Pickle 'em. Plain old vinegar—either cider or white—kills weeds fast, especially if you use it on a sunny day. Just pour the stuff into a handheld sprayer bottle, and fire away. But be sure to aim carefully, because vinegar will kill any plant it touches, not just those weedy ones you find annoying.

Give 'em a drink. Fresh out of vinegar? No problem. Just load up your sprayer bottle with rubbing alcohol. It'll accomplish the same deadly task.

Smother 'em. Got a high-traffic area where the soil is so compacted that nothing but weeds will grow there? Then go with the flow, and install a walkway. But first, smother the weeds by laying cardboard, brown paper bags, or newspaper over the soil. Then spread on pea gravel, shredded bark, pine needles, or any other topping that suits your fancy.

Sweep 'em up. A vacuum cleaner makes a dandy antidandelion weapon. Just put the nozzle over each seedhead, and presto—those menaces-in-the-making will be goners. (Either a wet/dry vacuum or a handheld model will work just fine for this maneuver.)

Let 'em eat veggies. Members of the *Brassica* family—which includes Brussels sprouts, cabbage, broccoli, and kale—all contain thiocyanate, a chemical that's toxic to newly germinated seeds, especially small ones. Brussels sprouts pack the biggest dose, which is why I made 'em the star ingredient in my Brussels Sprouts Weed Brush-Off. All you need to do is this: In early spring, puree 1 cup of Brussels sprouts in a blender or food processor, add enough water to make a thick mush, and whirl 'em for another few seconds. Add 1/2 teaspoon of dishwashing liquid, then pour it on the soil in early spring, and your weed woes will soon be history. (*Note:* When adding dishwashing liquid, do not use detergent or any product that contains antibacterial agents.) This mixture is especially useful for weeds that spring up in hard-to-get-at places, like cracks in your driveway and the gaps between stones in your terrace. Remember, though—don't use this stuff on a newly seeded lawn, or your baby grass plants will never see the light of day!

Get 'em while they're down. Perennial weeds are at their weakest just before they flower. That's the time to give 'em a lethal dose of my Wild Weed Wipeout Tonic. You'll find the recipe at left.

Carry No Passengers

Weed seeds can travel for miles in search of a good home. Some types, like dandelions and prickly lettuce, can just catch a good breeze and fly off like tiny hot-air balloons. Dozens of other kinds are more devious: They get help from unintentional co-conspirators—like you. Here are a couple of simple ways to foil the felons:

- Anytime you borrow a mower or other lawn equipment—especially from someone whom you know has a weedy lawn—clean the machine with a good, stiff broom before you start to work. And if you hire folks to tend your lawn, make sure they follow the same routine. This is especially good insurance against the seeds of crabgrass, plantain, and other low-growing free-seeders.

- At the end of an outdoor excursion, inspect your clothes, the soles of your shoes, and the grille of your car before you head for home. These are all favorite clinging spots for Queen Anne's lace, pigweed, and other prickly seeds.

Go for the Gold

One of the most effective ways to keep weeds out of your lawn is to spread a layer of compost, a.k.a. black gold, over the turf twice a year, in the spring and again in the fall. This simple measure works for a very good reason: A whole lot of weeds perform their best dirty work in soil that's deficient in trace elements—of which compost supplies heaping helpings. By keeping your lawn well supplied with these nutritional nuggets, you deprive the weeds of the poor surroundings they prefer, and give your grass the oomph it needs to crowd out the weaklings.

Besides keeping weeds at bay, compost will provide your grass with essential nutrients and help prevent lawn diseases. If you want to try this approach, you'll need a minimum of 50 pounds of compost for each 1,000 square of lawn area. As for the maximum, well, the sky's the limit—there's no such thing as an overdose of black gold!

CHAPTER 14

Terrific Trees and Shrubs

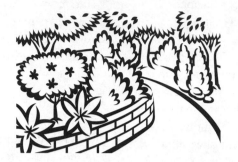

Trees and shrubs are a lot more than just pretty "faces." They
can also help you overcome challenges galore in your yard.
But of course, like every other living thing, they can have
their own share of woes every now and then. In this chapter,
I'll share some of my best secrets for solving your woody
plants' problems—and using them to solve yours.

WOODIES TO THE RESCUE!

Before I give you some hints on
helping your woody plants through
tough times, let's look at how trees
and shrubs can come to the aid of your
green scene. Read on for a roundup of my
favorite ways for using these hard workers
around the old homestead.

Off to Work They Go

Trees and large shrubs give your yard what
garden designers call "structure." In plain English,
that means you can use them to make your yard
into just about anything you want it to be. Some of
the best examples of how you can put "woodies"
to work around your place include:

Create an oasis. A big yard filled with nothing
but grass is about as inviting as the Sahara
desert. But add a few trees and big shrubs,
and bingo—you've got yourself a place that
says, "Come on out and sit a spell."

Divide and conquer. Trees and shrubs make
some of the niftiest "walls" you'll ever hope to
find. Use them to create outdoor "rooms" in
your yard—to divide your flower garden from
the kids' play area, for example.

Block that view. Tired of looking at your
neighbors' camper, or the busy street in front of
your house? Then just plant a few fast-growing
trees and/or shrubs, and presto—you've
turned that old eyesore into a sight
for sore eyes!

Show off that view. In the same way that a picture frame draws your eye into a painting, trees and shrubs can direct your gaze toward a beautiful part of your yard—or the broader landscape around you. For instance, you can use them to highlight your prized flower beds, or a mountain peak over yonder.

Put the Breaks On

If your yard (and your tender plants) get too much wind to suit you, provide some shelter with a row or two of evergreen trees. To make this windbreak as attractive as it is useful, plant a row of flowering shrubs or small, flowering trees along the inside edge of the evergreens. This easy-care pairing is guaranteed to fill your yard with color, season after season. Plus, any plant with white or light-colored blooms will look like a million bucks when it's backed up by a dark green screen!

Bug Off!

Did you know that trees and shrubs can help you solve a whole lot of garden-variety pest problems? It's true! They do it simply by providing food and shelter for birds, which in turn polish off bucket loads of destructive (and disease-spreading) insects. The best plants for welcoming winged warriors are trees and shrubs that are native to your area. The experts at your local native plant society or Audubon Society chapter can steer you toward some real winners. As a general guideline, though, remember that birds will throng to plants that produce bitter-tasting berries, such as barberry, chokecherry, juniper, and Russian olive. And for setting up housekeeping, most feathered fliers prefer the dense, sheltering boughs of evergreens. (For more on welcoming birds into your yard, see Chapter 18.)

The Shrubby Advantage

Make that advantages, plural. Just like trees, shrubs come in both deciduous and evergreen versions. And—also like trees—many kinds boast beautiful, fragrant flowers, colorful, bird-pleasing berries, and showstopping fall foliage. But shrubs have a couple of traits that make them even more versatile problem solvers than their woody cousins:

1. By definition, a shrub is a woody plant that has multiple, often spreading—or even sprawling—stems, rather than a single trunk. This means, for instance, that it generally takes far fewer shrubs than trees to make a living fence.

2. Shrubs range in height from just 10 inches or so to more than 15 feet tall. So they can do the work of small trees, fit right into a perennial flower garden, or even nestle into a window box.

Quick Fix

*Are you ready for some new window treatments? If so—and you like your home decor on the rustic side—just cut straight, slender branches from a tree or shrub, and use them in place of traditional curtain rods. Depending on your taste and the type of plant, you can either strip off the bark or leave it on, but be sure to cut off any protrusions that could snag the fabric. Then slide your curtains onto the branch, and rest your curtain rod on store-bought, wood or metal rod mounts. (**Note:** This trick works best with curtains that hang by tabs or rings, rather than rod pockets.)*

Take Comfort

If you suffer from allergies, as a whopping 38 percent of the population does, you can boost your comfort level a whole lot simply by planting female trees and shrubs. Here's the deal: Many of our country's favorite trees and shrubs are *dioecious*, which means that each individual plant is either male or female. In order to reproduce their kind, the males release huge amounts of pollen into the air. When a female of the same species is close by, her flowers snag most of those particles. But when your yard (or, as is often the case these days, your whole neighborhood) is an old boys' network, the pollen just floats around—until it reaches your sinuses. So do yourself a favor: When you're shopping for woody plants, tell the folks at the garden center that you want a female. (Don't let anyone sell you a so-called "seedless" variety. These are actually male clones, and although they don't produce seeds, fruits, or flowers, they still produce pollen—and plenty of it.) Some of the most popular dioecious landscape plants include:

Ashes (*Fraxinus*)

Bittersweets (*Celastrus*)

Cottonwoods (*Populus*)

Hollies (*Ilex*)

Honeylocust (*Gleditsia triacanthos*)

Junipers (*Juniperus*)

Kentucky coffee tree (*Gymnocladus dioica*)

Maples (*Acer*)

Mulberries (*Morus*)

Poplars (*Populus*)

Smoke tree (*Cotinus coggygria*)

Spice bush (*Lindera benzoin*)

Sumacs (*Rhus*)

Willows (*Salix*)

Yews (*Taxus*)

Hold That Hill!

Does your yard have a slope that's a real pain in the grass to mow? Or, even worse, does the ground tend to slide away in heavy rains? Then here's an idea whose time has come: Cover that hillside with spreading shrubs. Not only will they put a happy end to your mowing chores, but their dense, far-reaching root systems will hold the soil in place. Plenty of shrubs excel at this task. My four-star favorites are:

Abelia

Cotoneaster

Forsythia

Low-growing junipers

Shrub roses

Spirea

Speaking of Roses

You will note that in the list of problem-solving shrubs above (see "Hold That Hill!") I mentioned roses, America's favorite flowering shrub. And you may very well be thinking, "Roses don't *solve* problems—they *have* problems!" Well, think again, my friend. Granted, it *is* true that some types of roses (most notably hybrid teas—the spoiled brats of the plant world) can hand you more woes than a blues singer ever dreamed of. On the other hand, old-time species roses can not only hold your soil in place, but they can also cloak chain-link fences or plain-Jane walls, keep bird nests safe from tree-climbing cats, and a whole lot more. Furthermore, if you plant a species rose that's hardy in your climate and happy in your soil, it'll fend off pests and diseases that would knock its modern cousins flat. What's more, species roses don't even need to be pruned, except to keep them within boundaries that you've set. (Their one character flaw is unbridled enthusiasm.) Here are some of my all-time favorite rosy heroes. You'll find all of these, and plenty more besides, in catalogs that specialize in roses:

Lady Banks Rose (Rosa banksiae). A rugged rambler (a.k.a. sprawling climber) with thornless canes that grow 20 to 30 feet (yes, you read that right). This lady shrugs off salty ocean breezes, says "boo" to diseases that knock other roses flat, and thrives in any light from full sun to partial shade. There are two versions: one with lightly fragrant yellow flowers (*R. banksiae lutea*); the other with stronger, violet-scented white blooms. You'll see this one listed in catalogs as either *R. banksiae banksiae* or *R. banksiae alba-plena*. Lady Banks is hardy only in Zones 8 to 10, but in colder territory, she makes a great container plant if you keep her pruned and move her to a sheltered spot for the winter.

Red-leafed Rose (R. glauca). A real winner for cold climates. This upright shrub is hardy in Zones 2 through 8, but performs best where winter is serious business. And talk about colorful plants! Young canes are an eye-catching purple (and nearly thornless); foliage is copper to purplish in sunny sites, silvery green in partial shade. Flowers—clear pink with white centers—bloom in late spring, followed by bright red hips.

Shining Rose (R. nitida). A groundcover with real pizzazz! If you need to anchor a hillside that wants to slide, this is the rose for you. It grows about 2 feet high, spreads like nobody's business, and performs like a trouper, even in poor soil and partial shade. What's more, it'll give you year-round color with fragrant, pink flowers in spring; glossy green foliage through the summer; scarlet leaves in fall; and bright red hips and reddish brown prickles through the winter. It's hardy in Zones 4 to 6.

Swamp Rose (R. palustris scandens). One of the few roses that not only tolerates poorly drained soil, but actually thrives in it. This winner doesn't demand wet feet, though: It also grows sleek and sassy in ordinary, well-drained garden soil. Hardy in Zones 4 to 8, it has nearly thornless canes that bear fragrant, bright pink flowers and willowlike leaves.

Think Beyond Green

To do their very best problem-solving work in your yard, woody plants need to look good in all four seasons of the year. Of course, evergreens are natural standouts in this department. But so are a whole lot of deciduous trees and shrubs. To get the biggest bang for

HOME REMEDY

Before antibiotic ointments came along, juniper berry tea was often just what the doctor ordered to treat burns, scrapes, and even infected wounds. It still works (of course), and costs just pennies compared to those high-priced ointments. Plus, it's a snap to make. Just put 4 cups of water in a pan and bring it to a boil. Stir in 1/2 cup of juniper berries, remove the pan from the heat, and let the mix steep for one hour. Strain out the berries, and wash the affected area with the brew several times a day.

your landscaping buck, look for some, or all, of these attributes:

- Fabulous flowers

- Bright berries

- Brilliant fall foliage

- Dramatic branching patterns

- Bark with interesting texture or colors

START 'EM OUT RIGHT

As we've all learned (often the hard way), it's nearly always easier to avoid problems than it is to solve them after they've landed on your doorstep. And when it comes to trees and shrubs, the time to start your avoidance measures is before you even bring your plants home from the garden center. Here's everything you need to know about getting your woody plants started off on the right root.

Do Your Homework

All too often, I hear from folks who've fallen in love with a particular kind of tree or shrub, planted it—and then discovered that it was a regular magnet for pests, diseases, and all sorts of other problems. And do you know what? In almost every single case, it turns out that the plant was simply not suited for the growing conditions the site had to offer. The moral of this story is simple: Always select woody plants that will thrive (not simply *survive*) in the growing conditions you can offer them. Before you head off to the garden center, or even start looking at pictures in catalogs, have your soil analyzed by a professional testing laboratory, and study your

site carefully. Consider the amount of sunlight your plant(s) will get, as well as temperature ranges, prevailing winds, and humidity levels. A tree or shrub that's out of its comfort range in any of these conditions is all but guaranteed to give you trouble.

Ask for Help

Trees and shrubs are big investments, in terms of both time and money. To head off problems and simplify your shopping process, consult a professional arborist. (You'll find them listed in the Yellow Pages.) Or, better yet, get in touch with your local native plant society and ask its experts to recommend trees and shrubs that are native to your area and your site's growing conditions.

Time It Right

The time for planting a tree or shrub depends on how the plant has been grown. There are three possibilities:

1. Bare-root plants must go into the ground when they're dormant, in either early spring or late fall.

2. Balled-and-burlapped (a.k.a. B-and-B) woodies can be planted at any time the ground isn't frozen, except the hottest days of summer.

3. Container-grown plants can also be planted at any time the ground isn't frozen. Still, after a lot of practice, I've found that they perform best if you plant them in spring or fall, when the weather won't make heavy demands on them.

Keep Cool

When you plant early-blooming shrubs or small trees in a cold-winter climate, common sense would tell you to site them in a warm, sheltered spot (against a south-facing wall, for example). There's just one problem with this approach: While you will get the earliest possible blooms, chances are they'll be zapped by the cold spells that come from out of nowhere in late winter and early spring. So instead, plant early bloomers in a cooler spot—say, against a north wall or on a north-facing slope. The blossoms will arrive a tad later, but by that time, there'll be much less chance of their getting nipped by Jack Frost.

Trees vs. Turf

Shallow-rooted trees can give grass a real run for its root space, and can cause you a whole lot of headaches if you're trying to grow a lawn around them. Save yourself a lot of frustration by skirting these trees with mulch instead of grass — or, install them outside of your lawn area:

Beeches (*Fagus*)

Birches (*Betula*)

Elms (*Ulmus*)

Norway maple (*Acer platanoides*)

Silver maple (*Acer saccharinum*)

The Hole Truth

When I was a boy, the procedure for planting a tree or shrub started with digging a deep, wide hole and amending the soil with plenty of organic matter and other nutrients. Well, that thinking has gone the way of the dinosaurs. Now, the experts tell us to follow this procedure:

Step 1. Dig a hole that will keep the plant at the same depth it was growing at in the nursery. Make the hole at least three times the width of the plant's root-ball or the container it was growing in.

Step 2. Rough up the sides and bottom of the hole with a digging fork to keep water from pooling up and drowning the roots. Then work a handful or two of my Woody Plant Booster Mix (at left) into the soil in the bottom. But do *not* add any compost, peat moss, or other soil amendments.

Step 3. Take the wrapping and all the strings and wires off the tree or shrub. Then prune off any damaged branches and roots.

Step 4. Make a small mound of raised soil in the bottom of the hole to let water run away from the crown of the plant.

> ### FAST FORMULA
>
> ## Woody Plant Booster Mix
>
> This healthy breakfast supplies just enough nutrients to get your young trees and shrubs off to a good start without encouraging their roots to hang around the planting hole too long.
>
> 4 lb. of compost
> 2 lb. of gypsum
> 1 lb. of Epsom salts
> 1 lb. of dry dog food*
> 1 lb. of dry oatmeal
>
> Mix these ingredients together in a tub or wheelbarrow. Then work a handful or two of the mixture into the planting hole of each tree or shrub. After planting, sprinkle another handful over the soil before you water.
>
> *Use a low-priced supermarket dog food that contains corn gluten (a filler that's lacking in premium brands).

Step 5. Set the tree in the hole so that the base rests on top of the mound and the roots trail down over the sides. If you're planting a dwarf fruit tree that has a graft union (the spot where the trunk has been grafted to the rootstock), you want the graft union to be about 2 inches above ground level.

Step 6. Remove or add soil until the mound is exactly the right height, then set the tree back in place and give the roots a nice drink of my Tree and Shrub Transplanting Tonic (at right). It'll help ease the stress of moving into a new home.

Step 7. Fill up the hole with the remaining soil, and firm it gently with your foot. Water thoroughly after planting and as needed in the following weeks.

What—No Compost?!

My spartan soil-amendment routine for planting trees and shrubs, above, might seem odd if you're used to planting vegetables or perennial flowers, which generally benefit from all the compost and other organic matter you can work into their beds. So consider this fact of plant life: In order to grow big, strong, and sturdy, a tree or shrub needs to send its roots out a long, long way into whatever soil it's growing in. But if you start it out in lush, cozy surroundings, those roots will do their best to stay right there in the hole, where the livin' is easy. The result: a weak, trouble-prone—and possibly even doomed—plant.

The Fruitful Difference

Although the procedure described in "The Hole Truth" on page 277 is just the ticket for giving trees and shrubs a healthy start in life, fruit trees demand slightly different treatment. They can be mighty finicky about their home ground. If you have young fruiters that are refusing to get

---

FAST FORMULA

Tree and Shrub Transplanting Tonic

For any woody plant, being transplanted is a shocking experience. This soothing drink will ease the stress of going from a nursery pot, or bare-root wrappings, to the wide open spaces of your yard. (It works like a charm for fruit-bearing bushes, too.)

$^1/_3$ cup of hydrogen peroxide
$^1/_4$ cup of instant tea granules
$^1/_4$ cup of whiskey
$^1/_4$ cup of baby shampoo
2 tbsp. of fish fertilizer
1 gal. of water

Mix all of these ingredients in a bucket, and pour the solution into the hole when you plant a tree or shrub.

---

up and grow, chances are the blame lies with one—or all—of these factors:

It's the wrong time. Fruit trees prefer to be planted in early spring, when they're completely dormant. If you can't do the job then, or if the nursery can't guarantee delivery before the buds begin to open, wait until next year before you buy.

It's the wrong place. Most fruit trees like full sun, and they demand plenty of elbow room. Catalogs list the spacing requirements for full-size, semidwarf, and dwarf trees. Choose whichever size you've got room for, and if there's any doubt, go with a smaller version. And, whatever you do, keep new, young trees away from mature ones, which will compete with them for water and nutrients.

It's the wrong soil. All but a few kinds of fruit trees insist on near-perfect drainage. If the ground is the least bit soggy, they'll just sit in their holes and pout. Or rot. When you plant your new arrivals, mix plenty of compost and manure into the soil, and add a handful or two of my Woody Plant Booster Mix (see page 277).

Some Like It Damp

Not all fruit trees need well-drained, loamy soil. In fact, elders (*Sambucus*) thrive with damp roots, and quince (*Cydonia oblonga*) trees, as well as pear trees grafted to quince rootstocks, are happy as clams to grow in clay soil with so-so drainage.

Say "No" to Stakes...

if you possibly can. Young trees grow stronger, sturdier—and less prone to problems—if they're left to their own devices. Of course, if your woody youngster can't stand on its own, you will have to stake it, using this procedure:

Step 1. After you set the root-ball into the planting hole, drive in two posts (either wooden or metal is fine), one on each side of the hole.

Step 2. Attach the tree to the posts with soft fabric or broad strips of rubber. *Never* use cord or wire, even if it's covered by pieces of rubber hose—it can girdle the bark. And make sure the straps are loose enough so the trunk can move 2 inches in every direction.

Step 3. Remove the support system about a year or so after planting.

Great Starts Made Simple

While it doesn't pay to pamper trees and shrubs when you're making their beds, it's good green-thumb sense to give them some extra TLC *after* you've got them in the ground. Follow this simple, three-part routine:

1. Use the leftover soil to form a raised ring around the edge of the planting hole. This will direct water down to the roots, instead of letting it run off to who knows where.

2. Using a gentle flow from a hose or watering can, fill the basin with water, and let it soak into the soil. Then repeat the process one or two more times.

3. Finish up by covering the soil with a 2-inch layer of mulch, such as shredded bark or chopped leaves, to hold moisture in the soil and keep wicked weeds at bay. Just be sure to keep the material at least 4 inches away from the trunk (or shrub stems). Otherwise, moisture will be held against the base of the plant, possibly causing the bark to rot and providing a dandy breeding ground for pests and diseases.

Movin' On

A problem I hear about from a lot of folks is that they've just bought an old house with a garden that's been neglected since Heaven knows when. Among all the overgrown mess, they've found a beautiful, very old climbing rose. The only problem is, it's growing in an out-of-the-way place where no one can enjoy it. Well, if that's a situation you've found yourself in, take heart: Old climbers are rugged, and they can take some pretty rough treatment. I've moved plenty of 'em, and I've never lost a one. In mild climates, the best time for transplanting is midwinter, when roses are dormant. In colder territory, you can do the job in early spring, but I like to wait until late spring, just after the flowers fade. That way, I get to enjoy the big, bloomin' show, and the plant still has several months to get growin' strong again before winter sets in. Here's the game plan:

Step 1. First, get the new planting hole ready. That way, you'll minimize the time the roots are exposed to the air.

Step 2. Cut all the stems back to within a foot of the ground. This will make the plant less prone to dehydration.

Step 3. Dig a circle around the plant, 18 inches out from the stems, and at least 1 foot deep. Then reach under with your shovel, and lift out the plant. A lot of the soil will fall away from the roots, but don't worry about that; just do the best you can.

Step 4. Rush the old-timer to its new home, and get it in the ground, pronto! Then give it a good, deep drink of my Rose Start-Up

Tonic (below). Before you know it, new leaves will be sprouting all over those old canes!

Step 5. Water the plant every other day for the first few weeks, then once a week for the rest of the growing season.

TENDER LOVIN' TREE AND SHRUB CARE

Just like any other plants, trees and shrubs need certain basic care if they're going to stay happy, healthy, and handsome. I've rounded up a bunch of my favorite tricks for delivering that essential TLC.

Feed Me, Please!

To perform their best, early-blooming trees and shrubs need a hearty spring breakfast. And serving it up is as easy as 1, 2, 3! Here's all you need to do:

1. Scatter a bit of organic fertilizer around the base of each plant.

2. If your soil tends to be acidic, add a dusting of lime to help keep the pH near neutral.

3. Finish up with $1/4$ cup of Epsom salts for every 3 feet of plant height. Sprinkle it on the ground in a ring around the plant, out at the tips of the farthest branches.

This trio of fertilizer, lime, and Epsom salts will deepen flower and leaf colors, thicken flower petals, improve your plants' root systems—and help give you the best-lookin' landscape in the neighborhood!

FAST FORMULA	**Rose Start-Up Tonic**

Here's the perfect meal to get your roses off to a fantastic start.

1 tbsp. of dishwashing liquid*
1 tbsp. of hydrogen peroxide
1 tsp. of whiskey
1 tsp. of vitamin B_1 plant starter
$1/2$ gal. of warm tea

Mix all of these ingredients together in a watering can. Then pour the solution all around the root zone of each newly planted (or replanted) rosebush.

Do not use detergent or any product that contains antibacterial agents.

We'll Eat Later, Thanks!

There are a couple of exceptions to that spring breakfast rule in "Feed Me, Please!" at left—azaleas and rhododendrons. You want to feed these floriferous beauties after they bloom. Then give them a fertilizer that's especially formulated for plants that prefer acidic soil. And don't forget to toss your used coffee grounds around these shrubs, too—they'll love you for it!

Don't Forget About Us!

Big, established shade trees need to eat, too. Start their spring breakfast by mixing 25 pounds of organic fertilizer (5–10–5) with 1 pound of sugar and $1/2$ pound of Epsom salts. Then drill holes in the ground out at the weep line (at the tip of the farthest branch). Make the holes 8 to 10 inches deep and 18 to 24 inches apart. Then pour 2 tablespoons of the breakfast mix into each hole, and sprinkle the remainder over the soil. That's all there is to it!

Liquid Refreshment

Like any other plants, trees and shrubs need to drink as well as eat. How much water they need varies, depending on the age of the plant and the variety. But here's my general rule of thumb for supplying this life-giving elixir:

Trees. For the first three years or so after planting, water deeply and thoroughly once a week (that is, unless steady rains are supplying plenty of moisture). The most efficient way to serve drinks to newly planted trees is to lay a soaker hose in a circle around each tree at the far edge of the branches. Then turn on the water and let it slowly drip for an hour or two. After the first few years, you should have to water only during prolonged dry spells to keep your trees happy and healthy.

Shrubs. Water daily for the first three or four days after planting (again, a soaker hose is your best option for delivering deep-down moisture). Following that, shrubs differ greatly in their need for liquid replenishment, so ask for guidance at the nursery where you bought them, or check a comprehensive book on the care of woody plants.

It's in the Pipeline

A climbing rose—especially one of the old-timers—looks great growing up the trunk of a tree and into the branches. There's only one problem: The tree's roots tend to drain off most of the moisture, and the rose's roots dry up. Here's a simple way to make sure the rose gets its thirst quenched: Just sink a 2-foot length of 2-inch-diameter pipe into the ground near where you've planted the rose. Rain will fall into the pipe and travel straight to the rose's roots. Then during dry spells, shove your hose nozzle into the pipe and let it trickle slowly for 15 minutes or so.

Don't Touch That Hose!

Rather, don't put it away at the end of the summer. It's important to keep watering right through the dry spells of fall, because autumn is prime time for good root growth. But keeping the soil moist at this time of year serves another purpose, too: It ensures that evergreen trees and shrubs have enough water in their leaves to survive the drying winter winds.

A Little Mulch Magic

Here's a question for all you crossword-puzzle fans: What's a five-letter word for landscape problem solver? The answer: m-u-l-c-h! What's so special about this stuff? I'll tell you:

- Mulch helps keep the soil moist and at an even temperature—in other words, exactly the right conditions for healthy root growth.

- Organic mulches, such as shredded bark and chopped leaves, release plant-pleasing nutrients as they break down.

- A thick layer of mulch stops most weed seeds from sprouting, and the ones that do pop up are easy to pull out.

- Take it from me, nothing looks better than a neatly mulched yard!

Make the Most of Mulch

Now that I've sold you on the whys of mulching trees and shrubs, follow this trio of tips to help you maximize your mulch magic:

1. You want to keep a 2- to 3-inch layer of mulch on the soil at all times. If you're using an organic material, you'll need to renew it at least once a year, and maybe twice. Apply the first layer in spring and again in mid- to late summer, if needed.

2. Before you lay down a winter mulch, wait until the ground has frozen solid. That way, you'll prevent the root damage that can happen when midwinter thaws cause the soil to shift.

3. Don't think that if a little mulch is good, a lot is better. In particular, piling mounds of the stuff around the base of any tree or shrub is like throwing an open house for fungal spores and plant-munching pests.

Try Bug-Busting Bark

If you can lay your hands on shredded cedar or eucalyptus bark, go for it! These mulches are terrific for keeping bad bugs at bay. To make it go farther (in case you're not able to find much), just spread an inch or so over the soil, then top it with another mulch material.

Don't Prune Too Soon

Instead, go to work on your early-flowering trees and shrubs *after* they're done blooming. Many of these plants need a whole year to develop new flower buds, so if you snip off the shoots *before* they bloom, you'll be cutting yourself out of a spectacular display this year! These are some prime candidates for after-flowering "haircuts":

Early spireas *(Spiraea)*

Flowering quinces *(Chaenomeles)*

Japanese rose *(Kerria japonica)*

Lilacs *(Syringa)*

Weigelas *(Weigela)*

Spring Into Action for Summer Bloom

The exceptions to the "no spring pruning" rule are shrubs that bloom on "new" wood (stems that are produced in the current growing season), such as butterfly bush *(Buddleia davidii)* and chastetrees *(Vitex)*. Go ahead and gives these plants a good hard trim—back to a foot or so above the ground—and they'll reward you with fountains of flowers to brighten up the dog days of summer.

Two, Four, Six, Eight...

when do we procrastinate? When we need to prune certain shade trees, including beeches, elms, and maples. How come? Because if you cut into these woody guys in the spring, they tend to "bleed" a whole lot of sap, and the wounds can take a long time to heal. And in the meantime, the poor trees become sitting ducks for pests and diseases. The simple solution: Wait until early or midsummer to do any needed trimming on these heavy bleeders.

FAST FORMULA

Spring Shrub Restorer

This elixir is just the ticket for perking up tired old shrubs and getting them started on their way to a robust new life.

1 can of beer
1 cup of ammonia
½ cup of dishwashing liquid*
½ cup of molasses or clear corn syrup

Mix all of the ingredients in a 20 gallon hose-end sprayer. Drench your shrubs thoroughly, including the undersides of the leaves. And if you have any left over, spray it on your trees, too!

Do not use detergent or any product that contains antibacterial agents.

Warm Thoughts

If you're tired of freezing your fingers pruning your fruit trees in winter, I have good news for you: Contrary to conventional wisdom, fruit trees will not "bleed" to death if you cut into them during the growing season. Wait until late summer, though, when the peak growth period has passed. And make sure you do the job at least two to five weeks before you expect the first frost. That way, the pruning cuts can heal, and any new growth will have time to harden off before Old Man Winter arrives.

New Life for Old Shrubs

At one time or another, most of us have to deal with an old, overgrown shrub that's simply gotten too big for its (and our) own good. But instead of hiring someone to remove it, or using your own time and energy to dig it out, I've got a better plan: It's called renewal pruning, and it's a piece of cake!

Here's all you need to do: Every year for three years running, cut out one-third of the branches close to the ground. By the second spring, you'll already see lots of new growth eager for the room you're about to create with your pruning saw. By the third (and final) rejuvenation pruning, you'll be taking out the last of the old wood—and your vigorous new shrub will have a whole new lease on life.

It's So Complicated!

Lots of folks tell me they'd love to grow raspberries, but they're confused as all get out by the training and pruning process. Well, if that's the reason you're denying yourself these sweet treats, I have good news for you: There's nothing complicated about it! Here are two simple secrets for keeping your raspberries in line and your harvest basket full—without turning berry tending into a second career:

You don't need a trellis. Unless you want an ornamental effect, you can just let the canes grow naturally in place.

Pruning's a piece of cake. There's nothing to it with these three easy steps:

Step 1. In the spring, remove all of the dead or weak-looking canes.

Step 2. As soon as any cane finishes bearing fruit, cut it off at ground level. That way, the plant will put all its energy into canes that will produce the next batch of fruit.

Step 3. If the bed gets too deep to harvest easily, or you get busy and don't prune at all for a year, don't fret. Just chop the whole thing to the ground and let it grow back.

KEEP MUNCHING MARAUDERS AT BAY

No matter how well you tend your trees and shrubs, they can still fall victim to a multitude of multilegged munchers. Here's a roster of some of the most troublesome diners—and some foolproof ways to say, "This restaurant's closed!"

Public Enemy No. 1

It happens every year: In early summer, hordes of Japanese beetles appear from out of nowhere (or so it seems) and start munching on every shrub in sight—and your other plants, too. Unchecked, they can turn leaves, buds, and flowers to shreds in the blink of an eye.

There's no mistaking these voracious villains: Japanese beetles are about $1/2$ inch long and $1/4$ inch wide, and they're a dramatic, metallic copper color with green and white markings. In fact, they're good-lookin' bugs; it's a shame they've got such big, ugly appetites! Try some of these super secrets to end their dining pleasure once and for all:

The shakedown. Japanese beetles hate to eat alone. Generally, hundreds of them will zero in on one plant and ignore the bush right next to it. That makes them prime candidates for mass drowning. All you need to do is fill a wide bowl with water, and add a few drops of dishwashing liquid (to break the surface tension). Then hold the bowl under a beetle-infested branch and shake it gently; the pests will tumble into the soapy water, and that'll be all she wrote. Just one note: Perform this maneuver in the morning or evening, when the beetles are sluggish and likely to drop straight down; if they're disturbed at midday, they generally fly off.

The cocktail party. If you'd rather not stand around shaking buggy branches, this is the method for you. Just set a pan of soapy water on the ground about 25 feet from a plant you want to protect. In the center of the pan, stand a can or jar with an inch or so of grape juice in it (Japanese beetles go gaga for grape juice!). Then cover the top of the can with a piece of window screen. The beetles will make a beeline for the juice, fall into the water, and die happy.

The hit squad. You don't have to fight the beetle wars alone. In fact, you have some powerful allies in both the plant and animal kingdoms. For instance, garlic, rue, tansy, catnip, and larkspur are all plants that release chemicals that'll send Japanese beetles packin'. On the animal side, a whole lot of birds eat the pests by the bushel, and even bugs get into the act—two kinds of tachinid flies (available over the Internet) kill 'em off for good.

Quick Fix

If you want a really simple (and very attractive) way to get rid of Japanese beetles, just plant plenty of Geranium maculatum in your yard. It's a delicate-looking perennial with pretty little pale pink flowers, and it's hardy in Zones 4 through 8. And here comes the best part: Japanese beetles are drawn to it as if by magic, and when they chow down on the leaves, they die!

Aphids in Action

Aphids go gunnin' for just about every kind of plant under the sun, but they can be especially troublesome in trees. If the leaves on your trees pucker, curl up, and turn yellow, chances are these little suckers are hard at work. To confirm the diagnosis, look around for ants scurrying up and down the tree trunk. They're so crazy about aphid honeydew—and so smart—that they tend to herds of aphids, to ensure a steady supply of the sticky stuff.

To move out the aphids *and* the ants, give your trees (or shrubs) a good blast of water from the garden hose. Then spray twice more, every other day. That'll send most of the little critters tumbling to the ground.

Close the Farm!

The secret to closing the aphid farm in your tree is to fire the farmers. If you can keep the ants out of your tree for just a couple of months, good-guy bugs will take over, and your aphid woes will be history. Just follow my favorite ant-removal plan:

• First (if necessary), prune your tree so that only the trunk is touching the ground.

• Wrap a band of carpet tape or double-sided masking tape around the trunk. The tape won't harm the tree, but it will trap the ants as they try to scamper up.

• For added protection, sprinkle bonemeal or diatomaceous earth around the trunk. The ants won't cross the scratchy stuff.

• If a colony of ants has set up housekeeping near your tree, spray the nest with water. Then spray again. After being doused a few times, the ants will pack up and move elsewhere.

• Repeat any or all of these measures until the ants ride off into the sunset.

Don't Coddle 'Em!

You know the old joke that goes "What's worse than biting into an apple and finding a worm?" Well, the culprit that's responsible for that worm—or half-worm—is the codling moth. And if you've ever grown apples, you know that moth is no joke! Although apples get most of the attention from would-be comedians, codling moths also lay their eggs on the branches of pear, quince, and walnut trees. When the eggs hatch, the larvae burrow into the fruit and feast on the core. The good news is that stopping codling moths in their tracks is easier than most folks think. This three-part battle plan is foolproof:

Early spring. Scrape off any rough bark from the lower 3 feet of the trunk. Underneath, you'll find cocoons—the winter home of codling moths. Pull the cocoons off and drop them into a bucket of soapy water.

Late spring. When the first infected fruit drops, pick up every single piece and destroy it. That way, you'll make a sizeable dent in the next generation of would-be moths.

Early summer. Wrap a band of corrugated cardboard around the tree trunk, about 3 feet off the ground and fasten it with duct tape. As the caterpillars crawl down the trunk to spin their cocoons, they'll be trapped in the cardboard. Then, you can peel it off and drop it into a bucket of soapy water. Or, if the thought of all those scampering caterpillars makes you squeamish, spray the creepy things with rubbing alcohol. Either way, when the larvae are good and dead, toss 'em in the trash can.

HOME REMEDY

Codling moths have a sweet tooth the size of Toledo. And that's the good news. Take advantage of their sugar cravings by whipping up a batch of my Drink of Death Traps. I make a bunch of them each spring, when the apple blossoms are just beginning to open. You'll need some 1-gallon plastic jugs, and a half-and-half solution of molasses and vinegar. Pour an inch or two of the solution into each jug, tie a cord around the handle, and hang the trap from a branch. The moths will fly in for a drink, and that'll be all she wrote! *Caution:* To keep bees from joining the fatal party, cover the jug opening with 1/8- to 1/4-inch mesh screen.

Hang It All!

To get codling moths both coming and going, hang these two pieces of ammunition in your fruit trees:

Suet. It'll attract woodpeckers, which will then have a field day feasting on the larvae as they hatch from their eggs.

My Drink of Death Traps. The moths will flit in for a little nip, and they won't flit back out! (See the Home Remedy box above.)

Vamoose, Varmints!

All kinds of toothsome critters love to chew on the bark of young trees, especially in winter, when they have few other dining options. To protect your treasures, just circle the trunks with fine-mesh screen or hardware cloth up to about 2 feet above the ground. It'll keep the critters' teeth at bay, without giving safe haven to bad-guy bugs.

Broader-Reaching Measures

If you have shrubs as well as young trees to protect, or you want to keep unwelcome visitors out of your whole yard, try any or all of the following tricks. They work like a charm to bid bye-bye to all kinds of small, four-legged pests, including gophers, rabbits, groundhogs, squirrels, rats, mice, and voles:

Call out the archenemy. Or at least make the pests think you've done that. Get some ferret droppings from a zoo, pet shop, or ferret-owning friend, and sprinkle the stuff around your yard. It'll make 'em scurry in a hurry!

Sound 'em out. Gather up six or eight empty glass bottles and half-bury them, top ends up, in a line near the critters' hangouts. When the wind passes over, it'll make a scary sound that will send them packing.

Shine light in their eyes. Fill 1-gallon glass bottles with water and set them around your yard. Sunlight (or at night, artificial light) bouncing off the glass startles the animals and makes them flee.

Make 'em smell danger. Round up all of the old shoes you can find, and scatter them among the critters' targets. Set out a new supply every few days, so the human odor is, shall we say, always fresh.

Give 'em the hair of the dog. And the cat. And the human. Lay circles of it around your plants, and hang bags of it from fences, trellises, and branches. I've found that hairdressers and dog groomers are always happy to supply as much hair as you care to carry off.

Two-time it. When you give your lawn its fall feeding, mix diatomaceous earth and Bon Ami® cleansing powder in with the lawn food. You'll clear a lot of varmints (and especially voles) out of your yard and pep up the grass at the same time!

Pour it on. Drench the area around your trees and shrubs (or even the perimeter of your whole yard) with my All-Purpose Pest-Prevention Potion (see page 289). It'll make just about any critter turn tail and run!

Bye-Bye, Birdies

As I said earlier in this chapter, birds are some of the best pest-control workers you'll ever find—not to mention the fact that they provide some mighty fine outdoor entertainment. Unfortunately, many of these winged wonders have one regrettable trait: a big appetite for cherries and other fruits. These super-simple solutions will send them elsewhere for dinner:

- Wind black cotton thread among the branches of your fruit trees. When the birds see the thread against the sky, they can't judge the distance between strands, so they won't land. Just make sure that you string the thread before a bird family builds a nest and fills it with eggs!

- Put up a wren house near your vulnerable trees or fruit-bearing bushes. Wrens eat no fruit or berries, only insects. And when they've got young 'uns in their nests—which is the same time you'll have fruit on many of your plants—they won't let any other birds within 50 feet of the place. (Don't try this trick in your vegetable garden because the wrens will chase off all the other insect-eating birds that you need for crop protection.)

- Instead of full-size fruit trees, grow dwarfs or miniatures. They deliver a full-size, full-flavored crop on plants that are small enough to cover with a sheer curtain or two. The birds won't get so much as a nibble!

Use Some Culinary Psychology

When dinnertime comes, birds target red fruit more than any other color. And, given their druthers, they'll go for wild, bitter fruit and leave the cultivated, sweet stuff to us humans. So put this knowledge to good use in one of two ways:

1. Instead of red cherries or raspberries, plant yellow ones. (You'll find some mighty tasty varieties in catalogs.) Unless the birds have no other dining options, they'll fly right on by.

2. Give 'em other options. Plant one or two of their favorite fruits, such as the ones mentioned in "Bug Off!" on page 273. Or contact your local native plant society for some great choices for down-home dining, avian style.

Make a Snake in the Grass

Birds are as scared of snakes as a lot of people are, and for better reason: There's nothing most snakes like better than a plump, juicy bird. If you don't have a lot of real snakes in your yard (and are just as glad that you don't!), a rubber stand-in works as well as the real thing—and, for my money, at least, it's a lot more pleasant to have around!

You can buy realistic, fake snakes in garden centers, but I make my menacing pretenders by cutting old black or green garden hoses into 4- or 5-foot lengths. Then I wrap strips of red and yellow tape around the hose every few inches to look like stripes. If you really want to be authentic, check out a book on snakes that are native to your area and use paint or tape to make that piece of rubber look *just* like your local serpents. Get the kids to help you, and you can turn it into a biology lesson!

Just remember to move your slinky reptiles around every day or so; otherwise, the birds will catch on to your game, and you'll be right back where you started from!

Be a Quick-Change Artist

Whatever kind of tactics you use to scare away birds or other uninvited diners, remember to change your methods frequently. Our fellow members of the animal kingdom are a whole lot smarter than you may think, and they quickly get accustomed to anything in their day-to-day environment that doesn't gobble them up— including predators that leave their scent on the ground, but never appear.

Trouble on the Hoof

There's nothing more frustrating than looking out your window and seeing a couple of deer helping themselves to your trees and shrubs. A fence would guarantee protection, but if you can't—or don't want to—fence in your whole yard, take heart. Big woody plants are tailor-made for deterrents that can hang from their branches. My all-time favorite deer chasers include these odiferous items:

- Athlete's foot powder or baby powder, sprinkled on a cotton cloth

- Dog or human hair

- Smelly socks

- Strong deodorant soap

It's a Washout

Unless deer are on the brink of starvation, any of the aromatic wonders listed in "Trouble on the Hoof" (at left) will send them scurrying. There's just one drawback: Rain or snow will wash away the scent (and in the case of soap, the whole shebang). That means you can spend a lot of time replacing your deer deterrents. The simple solution: Before you hang them in the tree, put each one in a mini garage. Here's the simple, three-step process:

Step 1. Tuck your deterrent of choice into an old pantyhose toe, or a mesh onion bag, and tie the pouch closed with a string.

Step 2. Poke a hole in the bottom of a 12-ounce foam or waxed-paper drinking cup. (Or use an old plastic flowerpot that has a drainage hole.)

Step 3. Tuck the pouch into the cup, pull the string through the hole, and tie it into a loop. Then fasten the loop to a tree or shrub branch, and you're good to go. Your odiferous deterrents should keep their deer-chasing power for about a year, through rain, sleet, snow, or dark of night!

Deer-Buster 'Nog

If deer are sniffing around your trees and shrubs, and maybe taking a nibble here and there, it's time to lay out the unwelcome mat. Here's an un-tasty eggnog that will send them scurrying: Simply puree 2 eggs, 2 cloves of garlic, 2 tablespoons each of hot sauce and cayenne pepper, and 2 cups of water in a blender. Let the mixture sit for two days, then spray or pour it around any particularly tasty trees and shrubs.

Aw, Nuts!

It's no secret that squirrels love nuts—any

FAST FORMULA

All-Purpose Pest-Prevention Potion

Voles, rabbits, and just about any other critter I can think of will run away when they get a whiff of this powerful potion.

1 cup of ammonia
$^1/_2$ cup of urine
$^1/_2$ cup of dishwashing liquid*
$^1/_4$ cup of castor oil

Mix all of these ingredients in a 20 gallon hose-end sprayer. Then, just before the first snow flies, thoroughly saturate the area around each of the young trees and shrubs you want to protect.

Do not use detergent or any product that contains antibacterial agents.

kind of nuts—and fruits, too. I'll be the first to admit that it's not easy to foil these clever acrobats, but here's how I defend my fruit and nut trees:

- Prune your trees so that the lowest branches are at least 6 feet above the ground. Then about a foot below the lowest branch, circle the trunk with a 2-inch-wide piece of aluminum roof flashing. As the tree grows and the trunk increases in diameter, replace the flashing with a longer piece.

- Make sure the squirrels' target is at least 10 to 12 feet away from other trees, fences, or deck railings. That may mean pruning branches, or even removing trees, shrubs, or anything else that serves as a launching pad.

Mice Aren't Nice

For as tiny as they are, mice can cause mighty big damage to woody plants. Fortunately, you don't have to just sit back and hope for the best. Any one of these simple maneuvers will go a long way in protecting your trees and shrubs from these minute marauders:

- Whenever you mulch your trees or shrubs, keep the material at least 6 inches away from the trunks. That way, you'll deprive the munchkins of one of their favorite hiding places.

- Don't rush to apply winter mulch. Instead, wait patiently until the ground has frozen solid. That way, even if the mice snuggle down in the cozy blanket, they won't be able to tunnel into the soil.

- Before winter sets in, wrap the trunks of your shrubs and young trees loosely in aluminum foil to a height of 18 inches to 2 feet. The glittering, rattling surface will send the gnawers looking elsewhere for food!

- If aluminum foil isn't your idea of pleasing garden decor, guard your woody plants with a mini fence. Just circle your shrub bed, or the root zone of each plant or young tree with fine mesh wire that extends 3 to 4 inches above the ground and 6 to 8 inches below it.

Make Mine Mint

There's nothing mice hate more than the cool, clean scent of mint. They'll flee if you plant it among your shrubs, but there's an easier way to put mint power to work in your yard. Just mix 2 tablespoons of peppermint extract or oil of peppermint in a gallon of warm water. Pour the solution into a handheld sprayer, and thoroughly spritz the crown and lower stems of your shrubs and young trees. To protect woody plants growing in containers, simply saturate a cotton ball in the oil or extract, and tuck it into the pot at the base of the plant. (For large specimens, use two or three cotton balls.)

How Dry They Are

To us, a dryer sheet might smell like the freshest thing this side of a violet patch. But luckily that strong, flowery aroma sends mice scurrying. The sheet's go-away power lasts longer indoors (I use them to safeguard the contents of my garden shed), but as a temporary measure, tie a few sheets to the lower trunks of your shrubs. They'll keep mice and other small critters at bay at least until the next rain washes the scent away.

Bribery Might Get You Somewhere

If your yard is large enough, you should consider sowing a big patch of alfalfa, soybeans, clover, or lettuce well away from the trees or shrubs the rabbits are gunnin' for. It's not guaranteed protection, but chances are reasonably good that the bunnies will be so busy romping and nibbling in their very own field that they'll give your favorite plants the cold shoulder.

Banish Bunnies

Mother Nature blessed rabbits with the cutest looks this side of a teddy-bear store. Unfortunately, she also equipped them with razor-sharp choppers and a hearty appetite for any plant material under the sun—including the bark of trees and shrubs. Your anti-bunny arsenal begins with the maneuvers described earlier (see "Broader-Reaching Measures" on page 286). But when more decorative measures are called for, consider planting one of these beautiful, natural repellents close to any of your vulnerable woody plants:

Ornamental alliums. One of my favorites is *Allium giganteum*, a real stunner with soft-ball-size globes of lilac flowers, and stems that reach to 5 feet high. If your space can't handle a plant quite that tall, try a shorter variety like *A.* 'Globemaster', which only grows to about $2^1/_2$ feet.

***Coleus canina* 'Bunnies Gone'.** It gives off an aroma that sends rabbits running, but one that humans can barely detect. Plus, this annual makes a fine addition to any yard. It grows to about 2 feet tall, with dark green foliage and spikes of blue flowers in summer. It's drought-tolerant and thrives in any kind of light from full sun to partial shade—unlike most coleus, which demand shade. *Note:* Catalogs and garden centers also sell this plant under the name of either *C. canina* 'Scardy Cat' or 'Dog Gone' (because it also repels cats and dogs). But they're all the same plant.

CHAPTER 15

Fabulous Flowers

It's no secret that annuals, perennials, and bulbs can fill your yard with vibrant color and delightful scents from spring through fall. But if you've ever grown so much as a potted petunia, you know that flowers can also attract their fair share of trouble. In these pages, you'll find tons of terrific tips for solving your posies' problems, both big and small.

KNOWLEDGE IS POWER

As any experienced gardener will tell you, you can avoid an awful lot of trouble simply by putting the right plant in the right place. But before you can do that, you need to know as much as possible about the kind of place you've got. In other words, you need to analyze the growing conditions in your yard, so you know just what kind of hospitality you can offer to your green, rooted friends. Don't worry! That's not nearly as complicated as it may sound. And if your flowers are already giving you cause for concern, these tips, tricks, and tonics will help you correct whatever is wrong.

Two for the Show

Whether you're setting out to plant a new flower garden or you're struggling day and night just to keep your current one alive, the road to less trouble and lower maintenance begins with two simple actions on your part:

1. Decide on a garden size that you're sure you can handle comfortably and cheerfully, then reduce it by a third. You can always expand it later if you want to. If you already have more garden than you care to care for, dig up your excess plants and give them to friends, or pack them off to a charity plant sale.

2. Choose plants that thrive in the growing conditions you have now. Don't struggle to make a home for whatever strikes your fancy in a catalog or garden center.

The Root(s) of the Matter

Many flowering plants have definite ideas about the kind of soil they like to sink their roots into, and if it doesn't measure up to their standards, they can cause a ton of trouble. Fortunately, getting the lowdown on your home ground couldn't be easier: Just dig up several soil samples from your intended garden site and send them off to your Cooperative Extension Service or a private testing lab. You can also buy do-it-yourself testing kits at any garden center. By turning the job over to pros, however, you'll get a much more thorough analysis, along with instructions for correcting any problems. There's just one catch: If you're new to the gardening game, some of the terms you'll see on the report (and hear other gardeners tossing around) may be a little confusing. So a brief language lesson is in order. After all, it's hard to correct a problem when you're not even sure what to call it!

Texture and structure refer to the relative amounts of sand, silt, and clay particles the soil contains. Sandy, or light, soil drains quickly and doesn't hold nutrients well. Clay, or heavy, soil holds nutrients like a dream, but it also holds water too well. When it gets wet, it sticks together like two sides of a peanut butter sandwich—and that's hostile territory for almost any plant's roots. A gardener's (and your average plant's) dream soil is loam: a nicely balanced mix of sand, silt, clay, and organic matter. Loam holds a good supply of nutrients, doesn't dry out too fast, but doesn't stay soggy, either.

pH (short for potential of hydrogen) measures acidity and alkalinity on a scale that runs from 0 (pure acid) to 14 (pure alkaline), with 7 being neutral. Although there are many exceptions, most garden plants tend to perform best when the pH is close to neutral,

---

FAST FORMULA

Natural Nutrients for Neglected Soil

Unless you're sure that your soil is naturally very fertile, don't take chances: Give it a big nutritional boost with this all-natural, home-blended soil builder. It's just what you need to keep your flowers looking great and growing their best.

6 parts greensand or wood ashes
3 parts bonemeal
3 parts cottonseed meal
Gypsum
Limestone

Mix together the greensand or wood ashes, bonemeal, and cottonseed meal. Add 2 cups of gypsum and 1 cup of limestone per gallon of the resulting mixture. Apply 5 pounds of the mix per 100 sq. ft. of garden area a few weeks before planting, or work it into the soil around established perennials.

---

because that's when the nutrients in the soil are most available to the roots. Beneficial soil bacteria also seem to be most active in the 6.0 to 7.0 range.

Rich and lean have to do with fertility. Rich soil is chock-full of all the nutrients, including trace elements, that plants need for healthy growth. Soil that's lean has a low supply of nutrients.

Secrets to Success

When you contact a lab about soil testing, it will send you detailed instructions for taking your samples. Follow them and these general pointers to ensure the success of your test:

- When you send in your soil sample, include a list of all the kinds of annuals, perennials, and/or bulbs you'd like to grow in the bed. That way, the folks who do the testing can give you specific recommendations for giving each plant the nutrients and pH range it needs. (This is especially important if you're hankering to mix herbs, shrubs, or ornamental vegetables in with your flowers.)

- Make sure your sample contains nothing but soil. A stick, stone, or scrap of mulch can skew the test results. In fact, even using a trowel that has iron in it can throw off the nutrient reading. So work with a non-iron tool, fish out all foreign objects before you pack up your samples, and don't take your sample for at least 30 days after you've added fertilizer or soil amendments of any kind.

- Dig only as deep as the soil your plants' roots will be feeding from. For flowers (and vegetables, too) stay within the top 5 to 6 inches of soil.

- If part of your future flower garden includes an atypical spot, such as the place where your home's former owners had a compost pile, or a low area where puddles form after a rain, don't include any of that soil in your sample. You want your analysis to reflect the condition of the normal soil in your bed-to-be.

- When your plans call for two or more flower beds in different parts of your yard, order a separate test for each one—the soil characteristics could vary considerably from one spot to the next.

The Results Are In

If your soil-test report says that you need to alter your pH, the lab will most likely recommend adding sulfur to make your alkaline soil more acid, or ground limestone to make your acid soil more alkaline. There are only two problems with this method. First, although sulfur and limestone are good quick fixes, they don't last forever. Eventually, you'll have to crank up the old spreader all over again. Second, neither of these minerals does a thing for the soil structure.

I have a better plan: Add the right kind of organic matter at the outset. You'll get longer-lasting results and improve the soil structure at the same time. Some of my favorite sweet and sour condiments are:

To make the soil more acid (lower the pH), add: Aged sawdust, coffee grounds, cottonseed meal, fresh manure, oak leaves, or pine needles. *Note:* Fresh manure is fine if you're making up a new bed (especially for roses—they love manure). But don't use the fresh stuff on established plantings of *any* kind because it'll burn the plants' roots.

To make the soil more alkaline (raise the pH), add: Bonemeal, ground clamshells, ground eggshells, ground oyster shells, or wood ashes.

Doing the Numbers

Of course, the right soil isn't the only thing plants need to help them deliver trouble-free performance. Plenty of other growing conditions come into play, too. Three of the most important ones are as easy as pie to figure out because they're expressed in numbers. And (to paraphrase Yogi Berra), you can look 'em up. Here's the timely trio and where to find them:

How cold it gets. Your USDA Zone number tells you the lowest temperature that strikes your region in an average winter. It's a crucial statistic to remember when you're dealing with perennials and bulbs, which live for more than a single growing season. The newest Plant Hardiness Zone Map shows this information for every single county in the United States. To find out how your climate stacks up, log on to **www.jerrybaker.com** and click on Zone Finder.

How hot it gets, and for how long. That's important knowledge whether you're growing annuals or perennials, because some plants need all the heat they can get for as long as they can get it. Others turn into pest and disease magnets when the temperature climbs much above 80°F—or, in some cases, they simply stop producing flowers (or fruits or vegetables). To find these figures, check out the American Horticultural Society's Heat Zone Map. It's based on the average number of days in a year with temperatures above 86°F. You can find it on the Society's Web site at **www.AHS.org**.

The length of your growing season. It begins with the last frost in the spring and ends with the first frost in the fall. Those dates tell you a lot more than simply when to sow seeds or stand by with warm covers. Your allotment of frost-free days determines whether flowers will have time to bloom in your climate. Often, the answer is a clear-cut yes or no. At other times, it's "maybe." You may or may not decide to gamble with marginal plants, but be forewarned: Chances are you'll have to do a lot of coddling—and still risk failure—at the beginning of the growing season, the end, or both. To find the typical frost dates for your area, contact your Cooperative Extension Service.

Think Colder

Plant hardiness zone numbers are based on the coldest temperature in an *average* winter. So why take chances? Go with plants that are hardy to at least one zone colder than yours. That way, you won't have to panic when your local

HOME REMEDY

This may sound too good to be true, but there is an honest-to-gosh wonder drug that's guaranteed to make soil drain well, retain just the right amount of water, and serve up wholesome, well-balanced meals to your plants. What is it? Organic matter. All you need to do to improve drainage, soil structure, and fertility is dig in plenty of Mother Nature's bounty like leaves, grass clippings, straw, or well-aged manure.

weathercaster says, "We'll have a record low tonight, folks!"

Beyond Numbers

Although it is important to know your region's climatic statistics, garden-variety problem prevention doesn't end there. Plenty of other factors, such as wind, rainfall, altitude, humidity, and even air quality, affect a plant's health and well-being. Those details vary like night and day within both hardiness and heat zones. Even within your own yard, growing conditions are different from one place to the next. So what's the secret to winning the planting game? The same as it was for acing an exam in school: Do your homework! Before you even start perusing catalogs or strolling through a garden center, study your yard and take notes. Here are some of the things to jot down:

Places sheltered by walls or buildings. Most likely, they're warmer than the open space that's only a few feet away.

Strips of ground beside busy streets. They'll receive more pollution than areas that are blocked by the house or a solid fence.

Low spots where frost gathers. They'll get cold earlier in the fall, and stay cold later in the spring. Low spots also tend to stay moist longer, even if the soil is well drained.

Areas that warm up early in the day. They'll also warm up earlier in the spring.

The direction of slopes. A north-facing slope gets less sunshine, and stays cooler than one that faces south.

Blowin' in the Wind

A plant with the wind blowing on it is a plant that's under stress. And a stressed-out plant is a prime target for every kind of trouble under the sun. But before you can put up an effective windbreak, or take advantage of a structure that's already in place, you need to know which way the wind generally blows. Try either of these two simple ways to find out:

- Pound several 3- to 4-foot stakes into the ground in your prospective planting area, and tie a banner, bandanna, or piece of lightweight fabric to each one. Then keep an eye on those flapping flags, and take note of which way the breezes blow them.

- If you live in a cold-winter region, just look out the window during a snowstorm. The blowing and piling flakes will show you exactly which direction the wind is coming from, and what walls, fences, or other obstacles stop it in its tracks.

Who Dimmed the Lights?

Some folks think of a shady site as a major pain in the grass. And, actually, it *can* be just that if what you want to grow in that area *is* grass. But with flowers, shade is another matter altogether, because some of the finest plants around are shade lovers. The key to success is to figure out which kind of shade or light you've got, so you can find plants that like it. Keep this checklist in mind:

- Dense shade is cast by north-facing walls, or the low, dense branches of evergreen trees. This is a good spot for a shade-loving vine, such as trumpet honeysuckle, Dutchman's pipe, climbing hydrangea, or English ivy.

- Dappled shade is what you get from large-leaved trees like oaks, maples, or elms. The foliage blocks the sun, but still lets in light. It's just the ticket for hostas and ferns, as well as early-blooming bulbs and wildflowers like Jack-in-the-pulpit.

- Filtered light falls through the openings in an arbor, the small leaves of trees such as willows or birches, or a translucent structure like a fiberglass overhang. A whole passel of winners, including lamiums, bleeding hearts, hostas, astilbes, and goatsbeards, perform like troupers in these sites. And here's a word to the wise: When catalogs say that a plant likes "shade," what they often mean is filtered light.

- Bright light is common in city gardens, or on the north sides of houses. No direct sun reaches the site, but nothing blocks the sky, either, and light is magnified as it bounces off of walls on its way to the ground. Violas, ferns, pulmonarias, and lilyturfs all thrive in bright light.

- Partial shade, a.k.a. part shade or part sun, means that a site gets direct sun for anywhere from two to five hours a day. (Six or more hours is generally described as full sun.) This is the trickiest kind of shade to work with, but it can also be a lot of fun—at least if you like to experiment. That's because the effect of sunlight on plants depends not only on how long it lasts, but also on how intense it is. And that varies a lot, depending on the time of day, the time of year, and where you live. For instance, in northern regions like Alaska and the Pacific Northwest, you can grow real sun worshippers in shady spots. During those long summer days, the extra hours of light more than make up for the lack of direct sunshine. And in the South and Southwest, or at high altitudes, Ol' Sol is so intense that most sun lovers not only tolerate shade—they need it, at least during the hottest part of the day.

FINDING HAPPY CAMPERS

Once you know all about the growing conditions in various parts of your yard (what we gardeners call "microclimates"), you're well on your way to stress-free gardening. The next step is to find plants that will please you *and* thrive in the niches you want to put them in. Read on for some terrific tips to help launch your search.

A Little Latin Goes a Long Way

How many times have you ordered a plant from a catalog, or taken a young one home from the garden center—then watched it grow up into something you hadn't bargained for at all? Or worse, watched it go straight downhill because it just wasn't suited to your site? If you're like most folks, the answer is "way too often."

That's why it's mighty helpful to know a little botanical Latin—or at least know where to look it up. Among other things, a plant's Latin name can tell you what it looks like, where it came from, or under what conditions it grows in the wild. For instance, a plant with *alpinus* in its name hails from a mountain region. So it might be right at home on your range in the Rockies. *Altus* means tall, and that's probably not what you want for a container on your breezy deck. Plants from the hot, dry Mediterranean region often sport the word *mediterraneus* in their names. They can be your best friends if your weather is hot and dry, or if you need to conserve water. On the other hand, those plants are likely to need some serious TLC if you live in a cold, rainy, or humid climate.

And where should you look up these scientific monikers? There are a number of books on botanical Latin that are specifically aimed at the home gardener. If your local bookstore doesn't have any in stock, the friendly folks there can usually order one for you, or check your favorite online book supplier.

Go Native

The simplest way to head off all kinds of problems in your flower garden (and all through

---

Quick Fix

Some of the best places to discover problem-free perennials (and roses, too!) are old, abandoned graveyards, churchyards, or homesteads in your area. There you'll see plants that have been thriving for decades with no TLC whatsoever! Of course (I hope this goes without saying), you won't be selfish enough to dig them up, but chances are no one will mind if you take a few cuttings and root them. For the simple directions, see "Cutting Remarks" on page 301.

your yard) is to find plants that are native to your region and the kind of microclimates you have in your yard. It's easy, too, because in every part of the country, there are nurseries that specialize in breeding flowers, trees, shrubs, and even fruits and vegetables that grow, or once grew, naturally in that area. To find a native-plant nursery near you, just search the Internet for "native plants."

A Little of This and a Little of That

As the old saying goes, variety is the spice of life. Well, in a flower garden (or any other kind), variety can also help you avoid a whole lot of pest problems. That's because most plant-eating insects have definite food preferences. When they look down on a big patch of their favorite vittles, they'll drop in for a feast. But when they see a whole lot of different plants—some good, some so-so, and some they wouldn't touch even if they were starving—they generally take their appetites elsewhere. So, when the time comes to shop for plants, do yourself a favor and buy as many different kinds as your space (and your taste) allow.

Wave Good-Bye to Water Worries

Lots of folks tell me their major problem concerns water—or, rather, the frequent lack thereof. If conserving H_2O is at the top of your new-garden priority list—or if you and your bank account are simply tired of catering to a crowd of thirsty plants—reach for any of these modest imbibers. But remember: Even drought-tolerant plants need a steady supply of moisture until their root systems are established. After that, though, you can watch your water bills plummet, while your garden stays lush and lovely. (For more on dealing with dry soil, see "Planting Perennials in Parched Patches" on page 305.)

Annuals

California poppy (*Eschscholzia californica*)

Cosmos (*Cosmos bipinnatus, C. sulfureus*)

French marigold (*Tagetes patula*)

Globe amaranth (*Gomphrena globosa; G. haageana*)

Lantana (*Lantana camara*)

Melampodium (*Melampodium paludosum*)

Moss rose (*Portulaca grandiflora*)

Snow-on-the-mountain (*Euphorbia marginata*)

Vinca, a.k.a. Madagascar periwinkle (*Catharanthus roseus*)

Zinnias (*Zinnia*)

Perennials

Black-eyed Susans (*Rudbeckia*)

Blanket flower (*Gaillardia* x *grandiflora*)

Butterfly weed (*Asclepias tuberosa*)

Coreopsis (*Coreopsis*)

Moss phlox (*Phlox subulata*)

Perennial candytuft (*Iberis sempervirens*)

Russian sage (*Perovskia atriplicifolia*)

Sundrops (*Oenothera fruticosa*)

Wormwoods (*Artemisia*)

Yarrows (*Achillea*)

Yuccas (*Yucca*)

Look at the Leaves

Although the plants I've listed above are definitely some of the least thirsty ones you're likely to find, there are also plenty of other drought-tolerant plants out there to choose from.

It's easy to spot them in the garden center, too. Just check their leaves for any of these clues: a covering of fuzz or dense hairs; a rubbery or waxy appearance; a silvery or blue color; or a slender, needlelike shape. If you see any one or more of these signs, there's a good chance that you've found yourself a water-thrifty winner.

At the Opposite Extreme

What do you do about plant selection when your problem isn't too little natural water, but rather, too much? In a word: Experiment. That's because, just as we saw with shady areas, there are different kinds of wet-soil sites. You'll find very few annuals or bulbs that can survive without good to excellent drainage, but plenty of perennials can cope just fine. A list of the best would include:

For Moist Soil

Astilbes (*Astilbe*). Showy flower plumes in white, pink, red, or salmon. Partial shade. Zones 4 to 8.

Bee balm (*Monarda didyma*). Shaggy heads of red, pink, white, or purple blooms. Full sun to partial shade. Zones 4 to 8.

Goatsbeard (*Aruncus dioicus*). Creamy white flower plumes on shrub-size plants. Partial shade. Zones 3 to 7.

Japanese iris (*Iris ensata*). Large, showy blooms in shades of purple, blue, pink, and white. Full sun. Zones 4 to 9.

For Soggy Soil

Ligularias (*Ligularia*). Four- to 5-foot-tall stems topped with clusters of orange-yellow daisies or spikes of bright yellow blooms in late summer. Partial shade. Zones 4 to 8.

Lobelias (*Lobelia*). Cardinal flower (*L. cardinalis*) has rich red blooms; great blue lobelia (*L. siphilitica*) has blue flowers. Both bloom in dense spikes atop leafy, 2- to 4-foot stems from late summer into fall. Partial shade. Zones 3 to 8.

Rodgersias (*Rodgersia*). Looking like astilbes on steroids, these bold beauties produce huge, creamy plumes at the tops of 4- to 6-foot stems in mid- to late summer. Partial shade. Zones 5 to 8.

Slow Drain, Their Gain

Although most bulbs become pest and disease magnets if they don't have near-perfect drainage, there are some exceptions. This trio all thrive in moist soil:

Camassias (*Camassia*). Spikes of star-shaped flowers bloom in late spring, in shades of blue and white. Stems range from 14 to 36 inches tall, depending on the variety. These bulbs thrive even in heavy clay soil, but they do need full sun. Zones 5 to 8.

Checkered lilies (*Fritillaria meleagris*). The flowers look like upside-down tulips on 12- to 15-inch stems, and they really *are* checkered, in either white or green against a base color that ranges from light purple to almost black. (There's also an all-white version called *F. meleagris* 'Alba'.) Checkered lilies bloom in midspring; they like shade and soil that's evenly moist. Zones 4 to 8.

Snowdrops (*Galanthus*). Bell-shaped white flowers bloom in very early spring on 4- to 10-inch stems. They prefer moist, shady sites, but will tolerate sun. Zones 3 to 8.

FAST FORMULA

Bulb Bath

No matter what kind of soil your bulbs will call home, treat them to this nice, warm bath before tucking them into their planting bed.

2 tsp. of baby shampoo
1 tsp. of antiseptic mouthwash
$1/4$ tsp. of instant tea granules
2 gal. of warm water

Mix all of the ingredients in a bucket, then carefully place your bulbs into the mixture. Stir gently, then remove the bulbs one at a time, and plant them. When you're done, don't throw the bath water out with the babies! Instead, pour it onto your perennial bed—those plants would love a little taste, too.

Shop Smart

A healthy garden starts with healthy plants. So, whether you're shopping for annuals or perennials, check them over very carefully before you buy. Follow this inspection procedure to make sure you buy the best:

Step 1. Consider the overall condition of the place where you're shopping. If you see dead, wilted, or obviously neglected plants, walk away! It's not worth taking a chance on a plant that hasn't been well cared for.

Step 2. When you start looking at individual plants, first examine the top growth. Are the leaves an even green shade (or whatever color they're supposed to be), or are they discolored? Pale leaves may indicate a nutrient deficiency, which you can fix easily. But if the leaves are browned or show distinct streaks or spots, then there may be a more serious problem at work.

Step 3. Inspect the stems and the undersides of leaves. Pests like to hide in these sheltered spots. It goes without saying (I hope!) that you won't buy any plant that has obvious pest problems.

Step 4. If possible, gently slide the plant out of its pot to check for pests or dead and/or discolored roots. Roots that are heavily matted or are spiraling around the outside of the soil ball indicate that the plant has been in its pot too long. It may recover with a little extra TLC from you, but during its convalescence, it's a sure bet that plant will be a magnet for pests and diseases.

Step 5. Even if you don't find obvious signs of pests or diseases, check very carefully for any chemical odor or white powder on the leaves or soil. If you find any, it's a sign that either the grower or the seller has problems that you don't want in your garden—so take your business elsewhere!

Annual Allure

Walk into any garden center in the spring, and you'll see table after table covered with annuals, already covered with big, beautiful blooms. So of course, you're going to grab these for your garden. My advice: Don't buy them! Why not? Because those plants are sure candidates for transplant shock—which means they'll probably just sit in their planting holes, not doing much of anything (except being sitting ducks for problems of all kinds). The reason: Producing flowers depletes a young plant's energy, leaving it too tuckered out to put down new roots in your garden. So always look for transplants that have good, healthy roots, and few flowers.

Bulb Buyers, Beware

When your shopping list includes bulbs—either spring- or summer-blooming types—steer clear of any that have mushy gray spots on them. They're not worth carting home at any price, because they're unhealthy and won't recover. But don't worry if the bulb's papery skin is loose; that's normal. Likewise, don't be concerned about a few nicks. That won't affect the development of otherwise healthy bulbs.

But I Already *Have* a Mortgage!

For a lot of folks, one of the biggest flower-garden problems is measured not in numbers on a thermometer or a pH scale, but in dollar signs. If you've perused a plant catalog lately, or shopped for perennials in a garden center, you probably got a first-class case of sticker shock. Even buying annuals can set you back by a pretty penny if you need to fill more than a few pots. Well, rest easy, friends: You can have a flower garden that's the talk of the town—at a cost that'd please old Scrooge himself. Just try some of these budget-pleasing ideas:

Think small. When you're in a hurry to get your garden up and growing, it's tempting to reach for perennials in 1-gallon containers. Don't do it! For what you'll pay for one of those, you can buy three or four in 3-inch pots, and once those babies are in the ground, they'll take off like racehorses out of the starting gate. In no time at all, they'll catch up to the big guys.

Get it wholesale. You don't have to own a garden center to buy plants wholesale. A number of catalogs sell to anyone who places a big enough order. Usually, the minimum is 25 to 50 plants of a particular kind—but the price will be less than half of what you'd pay at retail. If you don't need that many plants at any price, team up with friends or neighbors.

Wholesale nurseries advertise in many gardening magazines. You can also find them via your favorite Internet search engine.

Hold a swap meet. The concept is simple: Folks come bearing plants, cuttings, bulbs, or seeds from their gardens. Then everyone trades what they've got for what they want. If you're starting from bare ground, and you have absolutely no plant material, offer something else in trade—say, homemade grape jelly, your world-famous chocolate chip cookies, your babysitting services, or even that fancy iron bed frame that's been sitting in the attic since the first Eisenhower administration.

Read all about it. In spring and fall, all over the country, local garden clubs, plant societies, and botanical gardens hold fund-raising plant sales. The prices are generally much lower than they are at garden centers. What's more, the plants sold at most of these affairs started life right in the neighborhood, so you know they've got the right stuff to perform on your home ground. Best of all, the folks doing the selling are usually the same ones who did the growing—which gives you a perfect chance to pick up a passel of problem-solving pointers.

Start your own plants. Most annuals and many perennials are a snap to start from seed, sown either directly in the garden, or indoors under lights. (You'll find the simple procedure in Chapter 16.) Other perennials, including tender types such as petunias and impatiens, which are commonly treated as annuals in cold climates, root easily from cuttings. For the easy directions, see "Cutting Remarks" (at right).

Comeback Kids

By definition, an annual is a plant that sprouts, grows, flowers, sets seed, and dies in a single season. But not all annuals are one-year wonders. A whole lot of them come back year after year from their own self-sown seed. And that gives you the advantage of long-lived perennials without the high price tag. Some of the most prolific—and delightful—self-sowing annuals around include:

California poppy *(Eschscholzia californica)*

Corn poppy *(Papaver rhoeas)*

Cosmos *(Cosmos bipinnatus)*

Larkspur *(Consolida ajacis)*

Love-in-a-mist *(Nigella damascena)*

Shoo-fly plant *(Nicandra physalodes)*

Spider flower *(Cleome hasslerana)*

Sweet alyssum *(Lobularia maritima)*

Cutting Remarks

One of the easiest ways to cut the high cost of flower gardening is to start perennials from stem

---

Quick Fix

When you're looking for plants that are a little out of the ordinary, you'll find a lot more choices in catalogs and over the Internet than you're likely to find at even the biggest garden center. But do yourself a favor: When you buy from any mail-order nursery for the first time (no matter how stellar its reputation is), limit yourself to three or four plants at most. If you're pleased with the merchandise and the service, you can always go back for more; if not, at least you won't have gambled (and maybe lost) your whole garden.

---

cuttings. The resulting plants will be identical to the plants you collected them from, and they'll reach flowering size much more quickly than seed-grown perennials will. The process is simple, but it is important to do the job in exactly the right way, or your little shoots could fall victim to a fungal infection called blackleg. (You'll know it's struck your crop if the stems suddenly turn dark at the base.) There is no cure for blackleg, but you can prevent this dastardly disease. Here's how:

1. Before you take your cuttings, go to the garden center and buy two things: a sack of sterilized rooting medium made especially for starting cuttings, and a rooting hormone that contains a fungicide.

2. If your flats or pots have been used before, give them a good cleaning. Soak them for 15 minutes or so in a solution of 1 part household bleach to 8 parts hot water.

3. Take cuttings only from plants that you know are strong and healthy. Otherwise, you're asking for trouble right from the get-go! Cut pieces that are about 4 to 6 inches long from semi-mature stems.

4. Use a clean, sharp knife or clippers; a ragged or torn stem is an open invitation for fungi. After every cut, dip the tool in a solution of 1 part household bleach to 8 parts water. As you cut each group of stem pieces, wrap them loosely in wet paper towels, and tuck them into a plastic bag. And keep that bag in the shade!

5. When you're back inside, cut each stem about 1/4 inch below a node (the place where a leaf or pair of leaves meets the stem). Use a sharp knife, and again, dip it in the bleach and water solution between cuts.

301

6. Pinch off the lower leaves, so the bottom third to half of the cutting stem is bare. Keep the upper leaves in place, but pinch off any buds or flowers. That way, all the shoot's energy will be directed toward forming roots.

7. Dip the bottom of each cutting in rooting hormone, then tuck the bottom third to half of the stem into the rooting medium. With a spoon or the eraser end of a pencil (again, dunked in the bleach solution), press the rooting medium firmly around the cutting. Water lightly, then wrap each pot or flat with a plastic bag to keep the humidity high. (To keep the plastic well above the cuttings' heads, make hoops from old wire coat hangers, and stick them into the rooting medium.) Take off the cover for an hour or so every day to fend off mildew. Keep the rooting medium moist, but not soggy.

8. When you see new shoots forming (usually within three to five weeks), it means the roots are starting to grow, too. Wait a week or so, then start leaving their plastic cover off for several hours a day.

9. Once the cuttings are well rooted, move them to individual pots filled with a good commercial potting mix, and give 'em a drink of my Repotting Booster Tonic (at left). Then set the pots in a cold frame, a sunny, enclosed porch, or another protected spot where they can ride out the end of winter in comfort. Come spring, move 'em to the garden, and they're on their way!

PLANTING FOR PERFECTION

Well, maybe not perfection, *exactly.* (After all, plants are living things, not decorative objects.) But you will find that your flowers will hand you far fewer problems if you get them off and growing in just the right way. So follow my practically perfect posy-planting pointers.

Plant Up or Plant Down?

It seems that every time you turn around, you hear somebody (including yours truly) raving about raised beds as the answer to all kinds of garden-variety soil problems. Well, these elevated planting sites can work wonders, all right, but there actually are times when you want to sink your beds, not raise them. So how do you make the call? It's easy: You just need to understand how each type works. In the simplest terms:

Raised beds improve both drainage and air circulation, and make the soil warm up faster in the spring. This is the way to go if you have heavy, damp soil; you live in a humid climate; or you want to grow plants that need all of the warmth they can get for as long as they can get it.

Sunken beds capture and hold moisture, and provide some protection from the wind. They're your answer if you have very sandy soil, or your climate is hot, dry, and windy.

Timely Transplanting

Time to plant annual or perennial seedlings? Whether you've bought your little gems at the garden center or started them yourself from seed or cuttings, the process is the same—and it's as easy 1, 2, 3. First, harden off your transplants by setting them outside for longer periods each day (see "Toughen 'Em Up" on page 321). Then wait for an overcast day, if you can, and proceed with your planting as follows:

1. Dig a small hole for each transplant. (I suggest digging all the holes first, so you can make sure you have enough plants to fill the space.)

2. Set each plant into its hole so that it's at the same depth it was growing before. Then gently firm the soil around the roots.

3. Water thoroughly, then give each plant a dose of my Transplant Tonic (see "Ready, Set, Go!" on page 304) to get it off and growing on the right root.

The (Bare) Root of the Matter

When you order perennials through the mail, you usually get dormant, bare-root plants delivered to you. And you may get your own version of "transplant shock" when you open the package, because what you see will be a tangled mass of roots topped with a tiny tuft of foliage. Well, don't worry: They may look like death warmed over, but with just a little care, those plants can repay you with loads of beautiful blooms for years to come. The key to success is fast action. If possible, have their bed ready to go *before* they arrive, so you can get them into the ground immediately. If you can't plant within three days of their arrival, put them in pots until you have time to set them into their permanent homes.

Four Steps to Planting Success

Are you ready to plant? If so, then remove the wrappings from your bare-root perennials, and follow these simple steps:

Step 1. Using sharp shears, clip off any broken or discolored roots, and then put the plants into a container filled with a mixture of $1/4$ cup of tea, 1 tablespoon of dishwashing liquid, and 1 tablespoon of Epsom salts per gallon of water. (*Note:* When adding dishwashing liquid, do not use detergent or any product that contains antibacterial agents.) Let the root clumps soak for 24 hours before planting; this will revive the plants and get them up and rarin' to grow.

Step 2. Dig a planting hole that's large enough to hold all the roots without bending them.

Step 3. If the plant has many roots, replace some of the soil to make a mound in the center of the hole. The top of the mound should be close to the level of the surrounding soil, so the plant's crown (where the top growth joins the roots) will be at the right level after planting (see "Perennial Depth Perception" on page 304). Spread the roots as evenly as possible over the mound, then fill in around the roots with the remaining soil.

If the plant has one main root, hold the crown at the right level with one hand, while you fill in around the root with the soil you removed from the hole.

Step 4. Firm the soil around the crown, water generously, and give each plant a drink of my Transplant Tonic (see "Ready, Set, Go!" at right).

Perennial Depth Perception

Perennials tend to be mighty particular about how deep they sit in the ground. If you plant them either too far down or too close to the surface—and you're lucky—they'll repay you by blooming poorly (or maybe not at all). If you're *not* so lucky, the crowns could rot away. Fortunately, you don't have to guess at the correct planting depth. Just follow these simple planting guidelines:

Most common perennials, including coreopsis, hostas, and phlox: Plant with the crown just at, or a smidge above, the soil surface.

Most perennials with taproots, such as baby's breath *(Gypsophila paniculata)*, blue false indigo *(Baptisia australis)*, and hollyhock *(Alcea rosea)*: Plant with the crown just below ground level.

Perennials with eyes, for example, bleeding hearts *(Dicentra)*, Oriental poppy *(Papaver orientale)*, and peonies *(Paeonia)*: Plant deep enough so that the tips of the eyes (new buds emerging from the crown) are about 2 inches below ground level.

Special Handling

When you buy bearded irises by mail, look for them to arrive in late summer as bare-root rhizomes with close-cropped leaves. These thick, fleshy roots call for a slightly different planting strategy than other bare-root perennials because unless the rhizomes are exposed to sunlight, they won't grow well at all.

First, dig a hole that's wide enough and long enough to accommodate one rhizome, then build up a little ridge of soil in the center of the hole. Set the rhizome flat on top of the ridge, so it's about even with the soil surface in the rest of the garden. Let the smaller roots hang downward, spreading them out as best you can. Holding the rhizome in place with one hand, scoop soil back into each side of the ridge to cover the roots (but not the rhizome!), and pack it down firmly. Repeat the process until you've planted all of your irises.

Ready, Set, Go!

To get all your annual *and* perennial transplants off to a superfast start, serve them a planting-day drink of my simple Transplant Tonic: Mix $1/2$ can of beer and 1 tablespoon *each* of ammonia, instant tea granules, and baby shampoo in 1 gallon of water. Use 1 cup of the solution to water each transplant, and then step back and get ready to watch 'em grow!

Quick Fix

No matter what kind of perennials you're planting, make sure you leave enough space between them—crowded plants are easy targets for disease problems. The plant tag or catalog description should specify the ideal distance; if not, check a comprehensive gardening book. (If you find that your flower beds look a tad sparse at first, just fill in the gaps with annuals until your perennials take off.)

Planting Perennials in Parched Patches

If you've got dry soil, your plants will let you know it in a hurry. They'll grow up short and stubby—or they may not grow at all—and they'll wilt dramatically whenever rainfall is scarce. Fortunately, you don't have to spend your summers with a hose grafted to your hand, and you don't have to settle for cacti, either. All you need to do is remember these six secrets to dry-soil success:

1. Choose plants that are naturally adapted to growing in dry soil—and there are plenty of them. For some of my favorites, see "Wave Good-Bye to Water Worries" on page 297.

2. Work lots of organic matter into the planting area. Two inches of compost, dug into the top 6 to 8 inches of ground, will help the soil hold on to whatever moisture it gets from rainfall or irrigation.

3. Plant and move perennials only in the fall, when temperatures are moderate and rainfall is generally more abundant.

4. After planting, snake a soaker hose around the clumps, so it comes within a few inches of each one. If necessary, use wire pins made from old clothes hangers to hold the hose in place.

5. Mulch with 2 to 3 inches of organic matter (such as chopped leaves, pine straw, or whatever's handy) to cover the soaker hose. This will help keep moisture in the soil, rather than evaporating into thin air. Reapply the mulch as needed, each spring and fall, to keep the soil covered.

6. Water regularly for the first year after planting, to give your plants time to get their roots established. After that, you can let Mother Nature take over most of the watering chores. But to play it safe, leave the soaker hose in place; chances are you will need to use it at least once or twice during the growing season—especially if you live where rain clouds seldom darken the sky in summer.

The Homemade Alternative

What's that? You're all set to plant your dry-soil bed, but you don't have a soaker hose on hand? Well, if you *do* have a regular garden hose that's seen better days, you're in luck. Using a hammer and nail, punch holes along the length of it at roughly 1-inch intervals. Block one end with a wine cork or duct tape, and arrange the hose in your planting bed. When it's time to water, attach the open end to an outdoor tap, or—depending on the distance involved—to a regular hose, and turn the faucet on gently.

Bulb-Planting Basics

Inside each bulb is a small-but-perfect plant just waiting to bloom and grow. But it won't do that unless you follow these few simple, but vital, guidelines:

- Handle with care. Bulbs may look tough (well, actually, they look dead). But they're really very much alive—and extremely delicate to boot. So never simply drop them into the bottom of a box or shopping bag. If you do, you'll bruise more than their egos, and chances are, they won't recover.

- Plant spring-blooming bulbs in the fall. Tulips, daffodils, hyacinths, and other spring bloomers need a good, long time to settle in and get their roots established. And if they don't get it, they simply won't perform. (The best time to plant depends on where you live; for the zone-by-zone schedule, see "Early Birds Get the Best Bulbs" on page 306.)

HOME REMEDY

If you live in one of our country's mild-climate regions, take note: In order to grow properly, some bulbs—notably tulips and hyacinths—need a period of chilling, and they don't get it in soil that stays warm in the winter. You can buy "precooled" bulbs (at a premium price), but don't waste your money! Instead, buy regular, garden-variety bulbs in early fall, pop them into your refrigerator's vegetable bin, and leave them there for five to six weeks. Then plant them in December, and they'll appear in spring, right on schedule, to brighten your beds and borders.

- Don't cut the foliage until it's turned brown. Otherwise, you'll rob the bulbs of the food they need to produce next year's flowers.

- Do cut the flowers. If you don't clip this year's blossoms for indoor bouquets, at least make sure you snip them off as soon as they've passed their prime. That way, they won't waste their strength making seeds; instead, they'll use all of their energy to store food for next spring's big show!

Early Birds Get the Best Bulbs

If your spring-flowering bulbs aren't putting on the big extravaganza that you'd hoped for, the problem could be that you put them into the ground at the wrong time. So what's the right time? That depends on where you live. Here's a simple schedule to help you get on track:

Zones 2 to 4: September

Zones 5 to 7: October or November

Zones 8 and 9: December

Make 'Em Touch Bottom

There is one more thing you need to remember about planting bulbs (both spring-and summer-blooming types): Always make sure the bottom of each bulb makes firm contact with the bottom of its hole. If it doesn't, there will be an air pocket between the two. The roots won't develop properly, and the bulb will rot—a mighty sad return for all of your effort!

FABULOUS FLOWER CARE

No matter how carefully you've studied your site, chosen suitable plants, and tucked them into your beds and borders, one fact remains: The better day-to-day care you give them, the fewer problems they're likely to give you. These terrific tips will help you deliver that essential TLC in a way that will keep all of your floral friends fit as a fiddle—and your labor light.

Weather-Wise Watering

Watering wisely means paying attention to your plants, instead of just dumping water on them on a set schedule. As a rule of thumb, flowering plants need 1 to $1\frac{1}{2}$ inches of moisture every 7 to 10 days, from either rain or irrigation. If you get a rainy spell, or a week or two of cloudy weather, you probably won't have to worry about watering at all. But if the weather is hot and sunny, or if a stiff breeze sets up for a few days, you'll have to serve drinks more often.

Soak, Don't Sprinkle

The first rule of smart watering is to make sure you water deeply. Frequent, shallow watering actually does more harm than good, because it encourages plants to keep their roots close to the soil surface—and that can cause *big* trouble during prolonged dry spells! To do the job right, thoroughly soak the top 6 to 8 inches of soil, then wait until the top 2 inches dry out before you reach for the hose again. This will encourage your plants to send their roots down deep, so they'll be better able to handle whatever dry weather Mother Nature sends your way.

The Old One-Two Punch

These are the two surest, simplest ways to keep your plants well watered and conserve precious (and expensive) H_2O at the same time:

1. Keep your soil well-stocked with organic matter—especially compost. Besides adding essential nutrients, it will increase the soil's water-holding capacity by one-third or more.

2. Give each of your flower beds a thick blanket of mulch. A 2- to 3-inch-deep layer of this magical material shields the ground from sun and wind, so any water that's already in the soil stays there, instead of evaporating.

Food, Glorious Food

The way a lot of folks talk, you might think that keeping a flower garden well nourished demands constant effort and all kinds of specialized fertilizers. Well, that's just not so. It's really fast, fun, and easy:

Annuals. These one-year wonders use a lot of energy keeping their flowers on parade. At planting time, sprinkle a few pinches of dry, organic fertilizer (5–10–5 is best) around each one, or give the whole bed a light dusting.

Bulbs. In any garden center, you'll see products specifically labeled "bulb food." This is usually nothing more than ordinary garden fertilizer that has a hefty dose of bonemeal added to it. So who needs it? Instead, just work a handful of compost and a teaspoonful of bonemeal into each hole at planting time. Then, just as the shoots emerge from the ground, mix 2 pounds of bonemeal with 2 pounds of wood ashes and 1 pound of Epsom salts, and sprinkle this mixture on top of beds where bulbs are growing.

Perennials. In early spring, sprinkle a handful of dry, organic fertilizer (5–10–5) on the soil around the base of each plant, or spread a thin layer over the whole perennial bed. (Either pull any mulch aside and replace it after you apply the food, or feed the plants *before* you mulch.)

Vegetable Soup

Fruits and vegetables can do the same things for your flowers that they do for you—that is, they can make the plants healthier, stronger, and therefore better able to fend off any trouble that comes their way. Of course, you need to serve this nourishment to your green friends in a different way than you do to your family! Just take any combination of plant-based kitchen waste like table scraps (no meats, fats, or sauces), potato peelings, and banana peels, and put them into an old blender. Fill it with water, whirl it all up into a soup, and pour it around the base of your plants. Perennials especially benefit from this liquid health food.

I'll Drink to That!

Fruit-and-veggie-scrap soup (see "Vegetable Soup" above) isn't the only nutritious health food you can give to your flowers. When you change the water in your fish tank, or toss an over-the-hill floral arrangement onto the compost pile, don't send the used H_2O down the drain. Serve it to a plant instead. That liquid is chock-full of essential nutrients. So is the water that you've used to cook eggs, vegetables, or pasta, or to rinse out containers that held any of these popular libations: beer, coffee, juice, milk, soda pop, tea, whiskey, or wine.

Weeding Made Easy

Botanically speaking, there are no such things as weeds. But to gardeners, it's a different story. These interlopers crowd out other plants, use up essential nutrients in the soil, attract and shelter destructive insects—and make a whole lot of work for you! Like most problems in life, weed woes are a lot easier to prevent than they are to cope with after they've arrived. Try any of these weed-prevention procedures:

Smother 'em. If you're starting a new planting bed, or a whole series of them, use my super-soil sandwich recipe on page 316. For unpaved walkways or paths between beds, use a variation on the theme: Just lay cardboard, brown paper bags, or newspapers over the soil, then pile on whatever kind of topping suits your fancy. Shredded bark, pea gravel, and pine needles, for instance, are all easy on the feet and the eyes.

Procrastinate. Don't rush to get warmth-craving plants into the ground. When heat lovers have to struggle to grow in cold soil, weeds can crowd them out and do them in fast.

Seed heavily. Weeds pop up in any bare soil they find. When you're direct-sowing annual or perennial flowers, cover the space with the plants you want in your garden. Later, you can thin the seedlings to the right distance.

Use transplants. Young plants take off the minute you set them into the ground. That means they can start shading out weeds right from the get-go. Plus, when something green does pop up, you'll know it's a weed, and you

---

FAST FORMULA	**Flower Feeder Tonic**

For glorious color all season long, serve this tasty treat to all the flowers in your garden—annuals, perennials, *and* summer-blooming bulbs.

1 can of beer
2 tbsp. of fish emulsion
2 tbsp. of dishwashing liquid*
2 tbsp. of ammonia
2 tbsp. of hydrogen peroxide
2 tbsp. of whiskey
1 tbsp. of clear corn syrup
1 tbsp. of unflavored gelatin
4 tsp. of instant tea granules
2 gal. of warm water

Mix all of the ingredients in a large watering can. Water all your flowering plants with this mix every two weeks in the morning throughout the growing season.

* Do not use detergent or any product that contains antibacterial agents.

---

can pull it out without worrying that you're ousting a future friend.

Mulch early and often. A thick layer of organic mulch will stop weeds from popping up among your plants. It will also keep fungi in the soil from splashing up on plant stems and foliage.

Weed Whacker

Sometimes, in spite of your best efforts, you'll still find some tough customers popping up in your flower beds. This simple, four-step process will get rid of those intruders without hurting your plants' roots in the process:

Step 1. Cut each weed back to ground level.

Step 2. Slice the bottom off of a 1-quart plastic bottle that has a screw-on top. (You'll need a bottle for each troublesome weed.) Then set the bottle over the weed, and push it into the ground about 2 inches.

Step 3. Mix up a batch of my special weed killer (see Wild Weed Wipeout Tonic on page 270), stick your sprayer head into the top of the bottle, and squeeze the trigger. Drench that weed stub until the potion is running off in streams. Then screw the top on the bottle.

Step 4. Leave the bottle in place for a couple of weeks, then inspect your handiwork. Chances are, your weed woes will be history. But if any extra-tough guys are still showing signs of life, give them another dose of the potion. Before long, they, too, will go belly-up!

FOILING FLOWER FOULERS

Even with the best care in the world, your flower garden can come under attack from pesky pests and dastardly diseases. But never fear: With this collection of tricks at your beck and call, you can solve those small problems before they turn into big ones.

Stop Drips, Quick

If your flowers get wet from rain or your sprinklers, shake them gently to remove the water. Otherwise, the droplets can cause spotting on the petals (especially light-colored ones), and the moisture can encourage diseases on the buds and blooms.

The Early Bird Saves the Day

At least a good part of the time. I say that because no matter what kind of pest or disease has reared its ugly head in your garden, you can often stop trouble in its tracks—provided you catch the damage in its early stages *and* act fast. On the other hand, if the damage has gone very far, your only option may be to pull up the victim and destroy it. Follow this early-action plan:

Plant smart. I know I've said this before, but it bears repeating: Simply by selecting plants that naturally thrive where you live, you can head off mountains of trouble. That's because those plants will be stronger and better able to defend themselves against any pests or diseases that come their way.

Keep it clean. Get rid of dead plant debris the minute you spot it, especially at the base of plants, where fungal spores and many insect pests thrive.

Mulch often. A blanket of fresh organic mulch will keep fungi and insect eggs in the soil from splashing up on your plants when it rains or when you water. It will also help fend off disease-spreading weeds.

Aim low. When you water, point your hose at the ground. Better yet, install a drip irrigation system or a soaker hose. Wet foliage—especially after dark—is an open invitation to fungus.

Be careful. Both disease germs and pests zero in on plants with torn leaves, nicked stems, and damaged roots. So watch where you wheel carts, push mowers, and swing shovels—or hurl Frisbees!

Encourage allies. Good-guy bugs and other predators will polish off boatloads of disease-spreading insects. For the details on enlisting your own troops—and more on specific bad-guy bugs—see Chapter 16.

Search and destroy. Inspect your plants at least every couple of days, and if something doesn't look right, deal with it *now*. Tomorrow could be too late.

The Resistance Movement

One of the best garden-defense measures is to choose plants that are resistant to the pests and diseases that are most common in your area. Just bear in mind, though, that the word *resistant* does *not* mean that a plant is immune to trouble. It simply means that it is less likely to fall victim to a particular insect or disease organism than its nonresistant counterparts are. So whatever you do, don't get complacent and let your guard down!

A Pinch in Time

The simplest and most effective pest-control measure is right at your fingertips. In fact, it *is* your fingertips! Squashing a destructive insect with your fingers—or plucking it off the plant and dropping it into a pail of soapy water or rubbing alcohol—will stop the damage immediately. Plus, the little menace will have no chance to reproduce, so you'll reduce the chance of future problems. Best of all, by using this selective approach, you'll ensure the safety of beneficial insects and other predators.

If you're a tad squeamish about touching insects, even when you have gloves on, just clip off the infested flower, leaf, or shoot, and drop the whole shebang into the fatal drink.

Water Works

One of your best—and safest—methods for controlling some of the most troublesome flower-garden pests is none other than good old H_2O. A strong blast from the garden hose is especially effective against tiny terrors like aphids, flea beetles, spider mites, spittlebugs, and thrips.

Simple Solutions

When a pest situation calls for really tough measures, two of the most effective weapons I know of are also the simplest. My Grandma Putt's Simple Soap Spray (see page 330) will kill just about any soft-bodied bug you can name, including lace bugs, mealybugs, thrips, and aphids. And my "Instant Insecticide" (below) is just the ticket for beetles, weevils, and other insects that have hard or waxy shells.

Put Up Your Dukes

Or rather, your fences and other physical deterrents. When it comes to protecting your flower garden from uninvited, four-legged diners, the same defensive measures you use to protect your trees and shrubs will work just fine (see "Vamoose, Varmints!" on page 286).

Instant Insecticide

The strong smell of garlic apparently offends as many bugs as it does people. To put that odiferous power to work in your flower garden, just mince six cloves of garlic, and thoroughly mix 'em with 1 teaspoon of baby shampoo and 1 quart of water. Spray the potion on your plants, and any would-be munchers will beat a hasty retreat!

Stop Slimy Slugs and Snails

When slugs or snails have been slinking through your flowers, there's no mistaking the damage. They both chew ragged holes in leaves and flowers, often completely devouring seedlings and young transplants, and leaving behind disgusting trails of silvery slime. Slugs and snails

⌛ *Quick Fix*

When there's no time to fumble with fancy formulas—or if you prefer to keep things on the simple side—reach for this potent pest potion: Mix 1 cup of rubbing alcohol, 1 teaspoon of vegetable oil, and 1 quart of water in a handheld sprayer bottle. Then, take careful aim, and give each pest a direct hit. It's instant death to even hard- or waxy-shelled bugs. (The secret lies in the penetrating power of the alcohol.)

Just one note of caution: Before you use this or any other alcohol spray on an entire plant, test it on a few leaves. Then wait 24 hours and check for damage. Some plants are supersensitive to alcohol, and if you act too quickly, you could end up killing the pests <u>and</u> the victim!

are not insects; they're mollusks, closely related to shellfish like clams and oysters. The only real difference between the two is that a snail has a shell, and a slug does not. This dastardly duo can show up anywhere, but they appear most frequently and cause the most trouble in cool, damp, shady spots. Gardeners from coast to coast have come up with dozens of ways to get rid of these voracious villains, but for my money, you still can't beat these two time-honored tactics:

1. Stage a hunting expedition shortly after dusk, when the slimers come out to feed. Just rally some pals, or hire a few youngsters, and arm each one with a pair of tongs, a bucket filled with your choice of poisons (see "The Fatal Dose" below), and orders to snatch 'em up and drop 'em in the drink.

2. If a-hunting you'd rather not go, trap the slimy so-and-sos instead. In the evening, set citrus rinds, cabbage leaves, or potato chunks among your plants. In the morning, scoop up the traps, slugs and all, and send 'em to their doom.

The Fatal Dose

No matter what method you use to catch slugs and snails, you can send them to their just rewards by dropping them into a bucket of water laced with a cup or so of any of these lethal ingredients:

- Ammonia
- Baking soda
- Epsom salts
- Pine cleanser
- Rubbing alcohol
- Salt
- Soapy water
- Vinegar

If It Feels Bad, Use It

For centuries, gardeners have been keeping slugs and snails at bay by surrounding their plants with scratchy stuff that prickles, or even slices the slimers' skin when they slink over it. And that strategy still works today. Just choose your weapon, and spread it around. Some of the best and easiest to come by are ground-up eggshells, sharp sand, diatomaceous earth, wood ashes, shredded oak leaves, pine or hemlock needles, and coffee grounds.

CHAPTER 16

Mouthwatering Vegetables

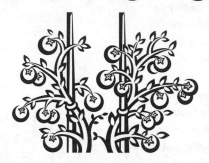

It's sad, but true, that vegetables tend to attract more
trouble than any other plants in your yard. Fortunately,
though, I've got a ton of terrific tips for solving your various
vegetable vexations. Read on for the cream of the crop
that guarantees a victorious vegetable garden!

PROBLEM PREVENTION BEGINS AT HOME

The first secret to growing a thriving
food garden is to remember one
simple fact: Most vegetables are
mighty picky about the place they call
home. If you can't provide just the right
kind of accommodations, the plants won't
give you the bountiful harvest you want.
In fact, they may not even survive the
summer. So pay attention to my real estate
primer, vegetable style.

Whether the Weather

Some vegetables, such as lettuce and potatoes,
prefer cool temperatures. Others, such as
peppers and tomatoes, want all the heat they

can get for as long as they can get it. That's
why two factors are crucial to vegetable-garden
success: how long your growing season lasts
and how much of it is cool or hot weather.
(For the full details, including where to find
the figures for your region, see "Doing the
Numbers" on page 293.) But when you plan your
garden, knowing season length and average
temperatures isn't enough. You also need to
consider a couple of other climatic conditions:

Humidity. Some plants can take the heat just
fine, but the combination of heat and muggy
air—and the damp soil that usually goes with
it—will do them in fast.

Day length. A few vegetables, including onions
and spinach, are sensitive to the number of
daylight hours they get. If it's not just right,
they won't produce well.

Take a Number

Although most vegetable plants are annuals, it's still useful to know your USDA Zone number because it's the number that gardeners—and garden writers—toss around more than any other. And it's essential information to have when you're growing perennial vegetables such as asparagus or rhubarb, or when you're planting a windbreak of trees or shrubs around your vegetable garden.

Let There Be Light!

And plenty of it! Most vegetables perform best when they can bask in sunshine all day long. But if your site doesn't command that much of Ol' Sol's time, don't worry—your garden will still produce well if it gets six to eight hours of sunlight a day.

If no place in your yard gets full sun, but you can choose between morning and afternoon sun, go with the morning. It's less intense, which encourages a higher rate of photosynthesis. (This is especially important if you live in the steamy South.)

A Breath of Fresh Air

Just like all other plants, vegetables need room to breathe. In fact, planting a garden where the air can't circulate freely is like throwing an open house for all kinds of diseases. So when you're looking for a good garden site, avoid any dips and hollows where cool (or damp) air hangs around. And also steer clear of tight spaces, especially ones between building walls and solid fences.

Beware of Wind

A nice, gentle breeze mixes together different pockets of air and helps keep both the temperature and humidity on the moderate side. Strong wind, however, is another matter altogether: It'll dry out leaves, rob moisture from the soil, and even break stems and send trellises flying off to who knows where. On a calm day, it's not always easy to know whether wind will be a problem in your garden site, but look for these clues:

- If you can stand there and see across the hills to the back of beyond, the area's almost guaranteed to be too windy.

- Any spot along the shore of an ocean or a big lake will get heavy gusts, at least from time to time.

- A site with western or northern exposure will leave your garden wide open to storm fronts moving through.

My Kingdom for a Slope

The very best place for a vegetable garden is on a gentle, easy slope, with no buildings, trees, or big shrubs nearby to block light or airflow.

Quick Fix

Put your vegetable garden as close to your house as you possibly can. That way, you'll have easy access to an outdoor water spigot, so you won't have to drag a heavy hose around or tote a watering can back and forth. You'll also be more likely to notice any small problems before they turn into big ones. Best of all, you'll know just when those new baby carrots, peas, and greens are ready for picking, and you won't waste a minute of their sweet, fresh flavor—and isn't that why you're taking the trouble to grow your own incredible edibles in the first place?

In the North, a south-facing incline is best. It'll warm up quickly in the spring and take its time welcoming Jack Frost in the fall. In the South, look for a slope that faces north; it won't get quite so hot during the dog days of summer.

Searching for Success

When you're looking for the ideal site for your garden, keep these two guidelines in mind:

1. Don't wait until it's almost planting time to start your search. Instead, explore your yard the year before you begin your garden, and do it in summer or early fall, when trees and shrubs are full, leafy, and casting their longest shadows. That way, you'll know which shady spots to avoid come spring.

2. Venture out early in the morning and look for the spot that feels the toastiest: A place that warms up early in the day will also warm up early in springtime, which will give you a jump on the growing season.

Making the Most of What You've Got

These days, not many folks have that perfect garden site: a big plot of rich, loamy soil on a gentle, sunny slope that's protected from harsh winds. There are plenty of other challenges for a backyard gardener to cope with, too, such as short growing seasons and harsh climates—not to mention the prolonged droughts that seem to hit more of the country every year. Well, as my Grandma Putt used to say, if there were such a thing as perfection on this earth, it would be pretty darn boring! So no matter what obstacles lie in your garden path, relax, smile, and reach for the following tricks:

Divide and conquer. No law says that your entire vegetable garden has to grow in the same place. If you don't have the right spot for a single garden—or if you can't bring yourself to dig up the kids' backyard soccer field—do what I do: Find all the sunny, sheltered spots in your yard, and plant whatever fits comfortably in 'em and grows well together. See "Perfect Pairings" at right for a few of my favorite mini gardens.

Mix and match. Some vegetable plants are so pretty, they'd be worth planting even if you didn't want to eat them. For instance, include rhubarb or asparagus (or both) in your perennial flower beds. Or put eggplant or salad greens right in with the cosmos and zinnias in your annual cutting garden.

Go with the flow. Although most vegetables do prefer a certain kind of climate (dry, wet, cool, or hot), there's a good chance you can grow whatever you're hankering for. Just adjust

HOME REMEDY

You can buy a terrific gadget specially designed to protect tender transplants from the cold. It's made of hollow, upright plastic cylinders that are fastened together to form a circle. You fill it with water and set it over a plant. It works like a charm, but if you've got a lot of heat lovers such as peppers, squash, and tomatoes, you could spend a small fortune trying to keep them warm! That's why I came up with a wonderful invention I call "wall-o'-bottles." All you do is tape quart-sized plastic pop bottles together in a circle and fill them with water. They work just as well as the store-bought product, and best of all—they're free!

your planting and harvesting times to suit your climate, and seek out varieties that are specifically bred to thrive in your particular growing conditions.

Use containers. You can grow a fine crop of lettuce or radishes in a window box. And if you pick the right variety, almost any veggie will feel right at home in a big pot or a wooden barrel sawed in half. What's more, a container holds whatever kind of soil and nutrients you put into it. That means, for instance, that you can grow potatoes in big barrels full of the sour soil they like, and use your garden space for crops that need sweeter surroundings.

Perfect Pairings

When you're ready to plant your mini garden (see above), keep these dynamic duos in mind:

- Cherry tomatoes surrounded by a border of basil

- A bed of mixed salad greens with a border of parsley

- Peas on a trellis with turnips underneath

- Beets intermingled with bush beans

Too Darn Cold

A lot of folks tell me that the vegetables they love best need higher temperatures for a longer period of time than their climate can deliver. Well, if that's on your list of gardening woes, take heart: While it is true that some veggies are natural heat lovers, some varieties take to cool territory better than others. Here's a sampling of those that like it hot, but can bend a little. They can handle lower temperatures than usual or they mature fast, so you can plant 'em and harvest 'em before the mercury plummets:

Beans (dry): 'Soldier' (bred to perform in cool climates)

Beans (snap): 'Black Valentine' (green, 50 days to maturity); 'Pencil Pod' (yellow, 53 days)

Corn: 'Early Sunglow' (yellow, 65 days); 'Trinity' (bicolor, 68 days); 'Sugar Snow' (white, 70 days)

Eggplant: 'Baby Bell', a.k.a. 'Bambino' (45 days)

Peppers: 'Yankee Bell' (sweet, green to red, 65 to 85 days); 'Early Jalapeño' (hot, 70 to 90 days)

Tomatoes: 'Oregon Spring' (red vining type bred to thrive in places with cool, short summers)

PUTTING DOWN ROOTS: THE SEARCH FOR PERFECT SOIL

One of the most important keys to a happy, healthy, and productive vegetable garden is strong, fertile soil that's teeming with life. So why am I talking about it after discussing such factors as sunlight, fresh air, protection from harsh winds, and having a handy water supply? Simply because those things are hard, and sometimes impossible to change. But you can always improve your soil—and it's fun to do, besides. In this section, I'll let you in on some of my favorite soil-building tricks.

Loam on the Range

When it comes to soil, a vegetable's dream-come-true is a nicely balanced mix of sand, silt, clay, and organic matter (a.k.a. loam). It holds a

315

good supply of nutrients, doesn't dry out too fast, and doesn't stay soggy. A thorough, professional soil test will tell you how close your soil texture comes to that level of excellence—as well as its pH and nutrient content. See "The Root(s) of the Matter" on page 292.

Anybody Home?

In our grandparents' day, fancy lab tests didn't exist. But folks knew how to find out whether their soil was healthy by taking a worm count. This method still works today. That's because for earthworms to call a chunk of ground "home," it has to be well drained and well aerated, with a pH between 6.0 and 7.0, and chock-full of organic matter. In other words, it's just the kind of soil vegetables need to grow up big, juicy, and tasty.

To take your own census, wait for a nice spring or fall day, when the soil temperature is about 60°F. (When it's warmer than that, worms have to head for deeper territory.) Dig up a block of soil that's about 1 foot square and 7 inches deep, and ease it onto a board. Very gently break up the clumps with your fingers and lift out the worms. Then count them as quickly as you can and send them home again before they dry out.

What the Numbers Mean

If your census counts more than 10 worms, congratulations! That means your garden has laid out a welcome mat for them and other tiny critters that'll keep the soil healthy and productive. The higher the head count (so to speak), the better. When it comes to earthworms, there's no such thing as overpopulation.

On the other hand, a count of fewer than 10 means that there's work to do. You'll need fancier tests than this one to figure out exactly

---

FAST FORMULA

Super-Soil Sandwich Dressing

If you're following the "Rocks to Riches" routine below, top off your "super-soil sandwich" with this zesty condiment. It'll kick-start the cooking process, and by the following spring, your super soil will be rarin' to grow!

1 can of beer
1 can of regular cola (not diet)
$1/2$ cup of ammonia
$1/4$ cup of instant tea granules

Mix all of these ingredients in a bucket, and pour the solution into a 20 gallon hose-end sprayer. Then spray your "sandwich" until all the layers are saturated.

---

what the problem is, but one thing is almost certain: You can make any soil healthier immediately by adding big helpings of organic matter to it.

From Rocks to Riches

Nothing's more frustrating than getting all fired up to grow your own garden-fresh vegetables, and then finding out that your soil is worthless. But, believe it or not, you can turn that no-good ground into fertile, fluffy beds without lifting a shovel—or renting a tiller. It's best to start in the spring, a year before you intend to plant your garden. Here's what you should do:

Step 1. Mark off your planting beds. If you want straight-sided plots, use stakes and string. For curvy shapes, outline the space with flour or bread crumbs, or by laying a rope or garden hose on the ground.

Step 2. If you have hardpan (a rock-hard layer of compacted soil), puncture the layer in a few places, using a garden fork or even a hammer and metal rod. That way, earthworms can penetrate the nasty stuff and eventually soften it.

Step 3. Lay a 1- to 2-inch-thick layer of newspapers over the bed, overlapping the edges as you go, and trampling any tall weeds down. (Just ignore turf grass and short weeds.) Then soak the papers thoroughly with water.

Step 4. Spread 1 to 2 inches of compost over the papers. Then cover the compost with 4 to 6 inches of whatever organic matter you can come by easily. Leaves, pine needles, dried grass clippings, seaweed, and shredded paper will all work well.

Step 5. Add alternate layers of compost and organic matter until the stack reaches 12 to 24 inches high.

Step 6. Saturate the bed-to-be with my Super-Soil Sandwich Dressing (at left), then go about your business. Meanwhile, the "sandwich" will cook, and by the following spring, you'll have 6 or 8 inches of loose, rich, super soil, all ready for planting.

Step 7. Set in your seedlings, or sow your seeds, and mulch with compost, dried grass clippings, or finely shredded pine bark. As the plants grow, keep mulching. As time goes by and the mulch breaks down, the layer of super soil will reach deeper and deeper into the ground (thanks to the earthworms, beneficial bacteria, and other helpful soil dwellers).

I Want to Plant *Now*!

But what if spring has sprung, and you don't want to wait months for the soil sandwich to cook—you want to get some plants in the ground pronto? No problem! Just make the top layer 4 to 6 inches of good-quality topsoil, or a half-and-half mix of compost and topsoil. Then saturate it with my Super-Soil Sandwich Dressing (at left), wait two weeks, and plant to your heart's content.

READY, SET, GROW!

Even when your soil is the answer to any vegetable's dream, *your* dreams of a happy harvest could go right down the drain if you don't get your plants off to a good, healthy start in life. Fortunately, there's no great mystery to the process—in this section, you'll find everything you need to know, from choosing the right plants to setting them into the ground.

Transplants or Seeds?

If you walk into any big garden center in the spring, you'll see table after table covered with vegetable seedlings. Except for root crops and a few others that are almost never sold as started plants, you can find just about any veggie your little heart desires. So doesn't it make sense to buy a few cell packs, take them home, and tuck them into your garden? Well, sometimes yes, and sometimes no:

Buy started plants when:

- The vegetables you want to grow need an early start indoors, and you don't have the time, the space, or the inclination to do the job.

- You want to be certain of getting varieties that will grow well in your climate.

317

- You want instant results for a container garden or an ornamental-edible planting.

- You're happy with whatever varieties the garden center has for sale.

Start from seed when:

- You want varieties you can't find at the garden center. Many vegetables come in hundreds—some, in thousands—of varieties, and even the biggest garden center in the world can't carry all of them. If you want something extra special in the way of flavor, giant size, color, or history that's worth bragging about, you'll have a whole lot more options if you start from seed.

- The vegetables you want to grow don't like to be transplanted. Root crops aren't the only edibles that resent having their underground parts disturbed. Cucumbers, squash, and melons don't like it any better. As for corn and beans, their seeds all but carry signs saying "Just plant me and let me settle down!"

Let Your Fingers Do the Driving

To avoid disappointment—and save a whole lot of time—do yourself a favor. Before the busy spring shopping season starts, call a few garden centers and ask these questions:

- What kinds of vegetable plants are they planning to carry this year, and will they have the particular varieties you want?

- When will their shipments start arriving, how often do they resupply, on what days of the week do shipments arrive, and for how long will they continue to arrive?

- What are the best days and times to find the freshest plants and the best selection?

On Shopping Day

Try to get up with the birds and be at the garden center when it opens the day a new shipment has been put on display. That way, you'll have the best selection of plants to choose from, and the staff will have time to answer your questions before the crowds descend. Once you're face-to-face with the vegetables (so to speak), follow the same inspection procedures I recommended for flowers in Chapter 15 (see "Shop Smart" on page 299). In particular, look for young, sturdy, stocky specimens without blossoms. A plant that's leggy, lanky, or already in bloom is too old and stressed to perform well in your garden.

The Great Indoors

If you live in a nice, balmy climate, you can start just about any kind of vegetable seed right in the garden and it should take off like a superstar. But in cooler climes, most crops perform best if you give them a head start indoors. Don't worry—the process isn't nearly as hard as some folks make it out to be. First, find the ideal starting date on your seed packet (generally, it's from three to six weeks before the last expected frost in your area). Then proceed as follows:

1. Fill clean, well-draining containers with fresh, sterilized seed-starting mix (available in garden centers), and dampen, but don't soak it. Then plant your seeds according to the depth and spacing instructions on the packet.

2. Cover the seeds with a sprinkling of milled sphagnum moss (also available at garden centers). It has an antibiotic quality that will kill the damping-off fungus, which is seedlings' Public Enemy No. 1. (For more on this nasty stuff, see "Stamping Out Damping-Off" at right.)

3. Set the containers on a tray, wrap the whole thing loosely in a clear plastic bag to hold in moisture, and put the tray in a warm spot—the top of your refrigerator is perfect! Check it every day, and mist the soil with water if it feels dry.

4. When the first bits of green appear above the soil mix, take off the cover, and move the tray to a spot where it will get at least 12 hours of light a day from the sun, grow lights, or a combination of both. Then spray the infant plants with my Damping-Off Prevention Potion (see the Home Remedy box below).

5. When the first two real leaves appear, move each seedling to its own pot filled with pasteurized commercial potting mix. Don't touch the fragile stems; instead, use a spoon to lift out the little root-ball, taking as much of the starter mix with it as you can. Then just look after the tiny tykes as you would any houseplant until it's time to move them to their permanent home outdoors.

Stamping Out Damping-Off

It happens to every new gardener (and even not-so-new ones). One night, when you turn out the lights and go to bed, you've got trays of fine-lookin' young seedlings. But the next morning, when you go to admire your handiwork, you find the plants dead in their tracks. The problem: damping-off. It's a fungus that shoots like lightning through a seedling tray. The prime cause: nonsterilized soil, stagnant air, or dirt from hands, pots, or tools.

If the disease has felled only a few seedlings in a flat, you can probably stop it before it does any more damage—but you need to act fast! Just mix up a half-and-half solution of hydrogen peroxide and water, and saturate the affected soil. To head off future attacks, follow these guidelines:

- Never use regular soil to start seeds. Always use a sterile, soilless potting mix that's made especially for starting seeds.

- If your containers have been used before, soak them for 15 minutes or so in a solution of 1 part household bleach to 8 parts hot water. Also, use this solution to clean any tools that could come into contact with your seeds or starting mix (such as tweezers, soil scoops, or spoons).

- Keep the air moving. Poor air circulation is an open invitation to damping-off (or any other) fungus. If necessary, use a fan or two, turned on low. Don't aim them directly at the seedling flats—just a soft breeze in the general vicinity will do nicely.

- Water from the bottom. Seedlings with wet leaves are prime candidates for damping-off. Set your starter pots into a tray that has no

HOME REMEDY

This simple potion will say a loud and clear "No way!" to damping-off fungus. Mix 4 teaspoons of chamomile tea and 1/2 teaspoon of mild liquid soap in 1 quart of boiling water. Let the mixture steep for at least an hour (the longer, the better). Cool it to room temperature, then mist-spray your seedlings as soon as their little heads appear above the starter mix. Just be *sure* to do this early in the morning, so the leaves have plenty of time to dry off before nightfall.

holes, then pour water into the tray. The roots will take up the moisture they need, and the baby foliage will stay nice and dry.

Reluctant Travelers

Most vegetable plants will sail through their early days in a group flat, move right along to bigger pots of their own, then settle into the garden without a care in the world. But some veggies want to sink their first little roots into a good home and settle in for the long haul. And if they can't do it, they're likely to give you nothing but trouble. These not-so-rugged individualists fall into that category:

- Beans
- Carrots
- Corn
- Cucumbers
- Melons
- Okra
- Parsnips
- Peas
- Radishes
- Rutabagas
- Squash

A Single Room to Go

So what do you do if your growing season is too short for stay-at-home crops to begin life in your garden? It's simple: Start your seeds in individual pots that can be put right into the ground at planting time (what I call travelin' pots). That way, you won't disturb their roots when you move them outdoors. Use pots that are 2 to $2^1/_2$ inches wide, and sow several seeds in each one. When the youngsters have two sets of true leaves, snip out all but the strongest seedling. In

garden centers and catalogs, you can buy tiny, degradable containers, but I've found that my homemade versions perform better—and they're free, besides! The two types I like best:

Newspaper pots. Gather up some newspaper and a tin can (a soft-drink can is just the right size). Then, for each pot, cut a strip of newspaper about 12 inches long and 6 inches wide. Wrap the paper around the can lengthwise, with about 4 inches covering the side of the can and 2 inches hanging over the bottom. Fold that extra piece onto the bottom of the can, press it tight with your fingers, and bingo! Take away the can and you've got yourself a pot. Make as many as you need, fill them with seed-starting mix, and put them into flats with holes in the bottom for drainage. Be sure to pack 'em in tight so they don't unravel.

Sod-buster pots. I use this kind for big seeds like melons and cucumbers. First, dig up slabs of turf that are about 3 inches deep, and cut them into 2-inch-square chunks. (Just make sure the grass hasn't been treated with an herbicide—that'll do in your seeds almost before they're in the soil.) Turn the sod pieces upside down, and set them into a flat that has drainage holes in the bottom. That's all there is to it!

No matter which kind of travelin' pots you make (or buy), be sure to set the draining flats into other, larger trays that have no holes. That way, you can water your seedlings from the bottom (see "Stamping Out Damping-Off" on page 319).

Don't Rush the Season

A lot of folks say that no matter how well they nurse their seedlings, the little guys never seem to grow up right in the garden. More often than not, the problem is that these folks started their seeds too soon. If you do that, your seedlings will get tall, weak, and spindly before transplanting time rolls around. And that means they'll never perform their best when they get to the great outdoors—and they might not even survive. To make sure your seedlings make the grade, sow them according to this weeks-before-transplanting schedule:

- **Celery:** 10 weeks

- **Peppers:** 7–8 weeks

- **Eggplant:** 6–7 weeks

- **Broccoli, Brussels sprouts, and tomatoes:** 4–5 weeks

- **Cauliflower:** 4 weeks

- **Cucumbers, lettuce, and melons:** 3–4 weeks

- **Pumpkins and squash:** 3 weeks

Toughen 'Em Up!

A premature start isn't the only reason for seedling-transplant failure. Baby plants can—and often do—die if you move them to the garden without taking them through a process

HOME REMEDY

While your seedlings are growing up indoors, give them a boost—brush 'em lightly with your hand a couple of times a day, or aim a slow-turning fan in their direction for a few minutes so they get a nice, gentle breeze. The motion helps the plants produce a hormone called cytokinin, which makes for thicker, sturdier stems.

called hardening off. (This goes for most greenhouse-grown transplants, as well as ones you've raised yourself.) The routine is easy, and it can mean the difference between life and death for your crop. Here's all you need to do:

Step 1. A week before transplanting time, stop feeding the seedlings and cut back on watering.

Step 2. Take your seedlings outside to a partly shady spot for part of each day. A covered porch works great; so does the area under a big shade tree.

Step 3. Start with a couple of hours in the afternoon, and gradually work up to a full day. But the minute a heavy rain starts, or a strong wind comes up, rush the little guys back indoors.

Step 4. Just before you're ready to set your seedlings in the garden, water them with a solution of 2 ounces of salt or baking soda per gallon of water. This mix will temporarily stop their growth and increase the plants' strength.

Step 5. Tuck your plants into the soil at the same depth they were growing in their pots, then spray them with my Seedling Transplant Recovery Tonic (see page 322). It'll ease the stress of moving day and make 'em feel right at home.

The Direct Approach

In theory, sowing vegetable seeds directly in the garden couldn't be simpler: Once you've prepared the seedbed (see "From Rocks to Riches" on page 316), you just pop them into the soil according to the planting time, depth, and spacing guidelines on the seed packet. I say "in theory" because tiny seeds, like those of lettuce and carrots, can be all but impossible to work

---

FAST FORMULA

Seedling Transplant Recovery Tonic

Give your transplants a break on moving day by serving them a sip of this soothing drink. It'll help them recover more quickly from the shock of transplanting.

1 tbsp. of fish emulsion
1 tsp. of instant tea granules
¼ tsp. of Murphy® Oil Soap
1 qt. of warm water

Mix all of these ingredients together, and pour the solution into a handheld sprayer. Then mist-spray your little plants several times a day until they're off and growing on the right root. And always do the job early in the day, so the leaves can dry off before nightfall.

---

with. It seems either they fall out of the packet in one big glob, or a breeze comes up and they sail off. So how do you get the little rascals into the ground? Simple: When you go out to the garden to plant your seeds, take along a shallow bowl, a bucket of water, and some cotton string. Pour your seeds into the bowl (one kind of seed at a time). Next, dip a piece of string in the water and press it into the seeds. Then lay the string on the ground, and cover it lightly with soil. The seeds will stay put, right where they belong.

Help for Budding Gardeners

If you have children or grandchildren who like to help you garden, but the seeds they plant seem to wind up everywhere but in the holes where they belong, here's a simple solution: seed tapes. These are long strips of laminated paper coated with water-soluble material, and

the seeds are already spaced the right distance apart. All you—or the youngsters—need to do is prepare the soil, place the seed tape on top, cover it lightly with soil, firm it down with your hand, and water. The seeds sprout, and the paper dissolves from the moisture in the soil. Your future gardeners get a kick out of planting, and you'll know that the seeds have been sown right where you want them, not scattered across the yard to kingdom come!

Clip, Don't Pull

When it comes time to thin your seedlings— whether you've planted them in the ground or in starter pots—don't even think of pulling them up. If you do, you'll disturb the roots of the ones you leave behind, and that can spell trouble! Instead, snip the stems off at soil level with a pair of small scissors.

Plant on the Up and Up

Plants that sprawl across the ground are disasters waiting to happen: Pests and diseases of all kinds can stroll out of the soil and right into the stems, leaves, and fruit. So what do you do to head off trouble? Support those stems with stakes or trellises that are made of metal— especially copper. The reason has to do with an old-time kind of gardening called electroculture. To see it in action, just notice how much greener your lawn is after a thunderstorm. That's because the electricity in the air combines with oxygen and nitrogen to form nitric oxide—a real wonder drug for plants. To put electroculture to work in your garden, here's all you have to do:

- Use only metal poles for staking your plants.

- Grow cucumbers, indeterminate tomatoes, and other vining crops on metal fences, guide wires, or trellises.

- If you normally grow peas or other lightweight vines on string trellises, use wire instead.

- Tie up your plants with old pantyhose, or strips of other nylon fabric (it attracts electricity).

Give 'Em a Lift

What if you're growing crops such as winter squash or pumpkins that are just too heavy to tie to a trellis? No problem: Just get some hardware cloth or construction-grade wire mesh (you can find both at hardware or building-supply stores). Cut the mesh into pieces about 3 by 5 feet, bend each one into an arch, and set it in place on your planting bed. Then, plant your seeds along the sides, and train the young plants up the sides. If you think your crops' mature weight will be too much for the structure to bear, support the center with bricks or blocks of wood. Better yet, use pieces of metal drainpipe—they'll attract even more electricity!

A LITTLE TIMELY TLC

Just like any other plants, vegetables need good, consistent care if they're going to perform the way you want them to—which in this case, of course, means offering up a big, tasty harvest. Read on to discover how to deliver basic TLC in a nutshell.

Feed Them—and They'll Feed You

For a vegetable plant (or any other kind), dinnertime means chowing down on many nutrients in the soil. The most important of these are what gardeners call "The Big Three": nitrogen, phosphorus, and potassium (sometimes referred to as potash). Here's what each one does for your plants, and how to tell when they're getting too little or too much of these good things:

Nitrogen (N)

This is the first number you'll see on a fertilizer package. It keeps plants green and promotes good leaf and stem growth. As you might expect, the biggest consumers of nitrogen are leafy crops, such as lettuce, cabbage, and spinach.

Signs of deficiency:

- Stunted growth

- Small leaves and/or vegetables

- Pale green or yellow foliage

Signs of an overdose:

- Too much leafy growth

- Foliage that's too dark

- Plants that are slow to mature

- Lush foliage with reduced flowering and (therefore) fruiting

- Problems with aphids and other sap-sucking insects

Phosphorus (P)

The second element on the plant-food label promotes good, strong root development, encourages fruit production, and helps plants resist disease. It's especially important for root crops, such as potatoes, beets, and carrots, and for fruiting vegetables, such as tomatoes, peppers, and squash.

Signs of deficiency:

- Red, purplish, or bronzed leaves

- Few blossoms or vegetables

Signs of an overdose:

- Other essential nutrients get tied up, so plants exhibit signs of other deficiencies.

Potassium (K)

Sometimes referred to in gardening circles as "potash," the Big K makes plants grow and, like phosphorus, helps fend off diseases. All plants need a plentiful supply of this essential element.

Signs of deficiency:

- Reduced vigor

- Thin stems

- Small, misshapen vegetables with thin skins

- Curling, scorched-looking leaves with brown edges

- Plants that become diseased easily

Signs of an overdose:

- Poorly colored, coarse-looking vegetables

Ask the Experts

A diet that's too low or too high in other nutrients, such as iron, calcium, and magnesium, can cause problems, too, but they're trickier to diagnose. If your plants start showing signs that don't match anything in the above list, such as yellow leaves with green veins, just give them a good dose of an all-purpose organic fertilizer that also contains trace minerals. If that doesn't perk them up, call your local Cooperative Extension Service and ask for help.

The Diet of Champions

At any garden center, you can buy some excellent organic fertilizers that are formulated especially for vegetables. And my All-Season Green-Up Tonic (see page 256) makes for some great summer snacking. Hands down, though, the healthiest diet you can feed your food crops is compost—what gardeners call "black gold." It delivers a well-balanced supply of all the important nutrients, both major and minor, and helps fend off diseases at the same time. What's more, creating this miracle chow is a whole lot easier than some folks make it out to be. Just get yourself a commercial compost bin. I like the ones that look like big, fat, black wheels, mounted on a turning mechanism. Then simply throw in your raw ingredients, and give the wheel a spin every week or two, so that air can get into the mixture (the sides are perforated, so the more you twirl the wheel, the more oxygen gets in, and the faster the stuff inside breaks down). Every month or so, open the door and spritz your future treasure with my Compost Booster (at right).

As for what to put inside your bin, you want roughly three high-carbon ingredients ("browns") for every one that's high in nitrogen ("greens"). That's important, because if you have too much carbon, the compost could take years to cook. Too much nitrogen, and it'll give off an odor that would make a skunk turn green with envy. Here's the menu:

The Browns

- Chipped twigs and branches

- Dead flower and vegetable stalks

- Dry leaves and plant stalks

- Hay

- Pine needles

- Sawdust

- Shredded paper

- Straw

The Greens

- Coffee grounds
- Eggshells
- Feathers
- Flowers
- Fruit and vegetable scraps
- Grass clippings
- Green leaves or stems
- Hair (pet or human)
- Manure
- Seaweed
- Tea bags

Cool and Easy Composting

You say that balancing ingredients and spinning a compost bin is not your idea of fun, even if the end product is worth its weight in gold, silver, *and* platinum? Then try cold composting. In this method, anaerobic bacteria break down the organic material without the help of oxygen, so there's no turning required. And there's no need to worry about the ratio of browns to greens. Just one word of warning: When you open the bags, you'll be hit with a potent odor, but it will disappear as soon as the compost is exposed to the open air. Follow my three-step method:

Step 1. Fill a large plastic garbage bag with a mixture of chopped leaves, grass clippings, and vegetable scraps. For every couple of shovelfuls of bulky, carbon-rich material, add a few cupfuls of my Compost Booster (above).

Step 2. When the bag is nearly full, sprinkle a couple of quarts of water over the contents, and mix until all the ingredients are moist.

| FAST FORMULA | **Compost Booster** |

Just like your plants, your compost needs a boost every now and then. So once a month, spray it with this energizing elixir.

1 cup of beer
1 cup of regular cola (not diet)
1 cup of ammonia
$\frac{1}{2}$ cup of weak tea
2 tbsp. of baby shampoo

Mix all of these ingredients together in a 20 gallon hose-end sprayer, and saturate your compost with the solution every month or so. This'll really keep things cookin'!

To do that, just shake small or light bags; roll large or heavy ones.

Step 3. Tie the bag shut, and leave it in an out-of-the-way place where the temperature will stay above 45°F for a few months. For faster results, roll or shake the bag every few days. That's all there is to it!

Teatime

No matter how you make your compost—or even if you buy it at the garden center—you have the makings of a genuine wonder drink for your vegetables (and all your other plants, too). And the recipe couldn't be simpler. First, pour 4 gallons of warm water into a big bucket. Then scoop 1 gallon of fresh compost into a cotton, burlap, or pantyhose sack, tie it closed, and put it in the water. Cover the bucket, and let the mixture steep for three to seven days. Pour the solution into a watering can or misting bottle, and give your plants a good spritzing with it every two to three weeks. They'll grow up healthy, happy, and mighty tasty.

Weed It and Reap

To hear a lot of folks talk, you might think that keeping a vegetable garden free of weeds was a summer-long, backbreaking nightmare. Well, friends, it just ain't so! If you're starting a brand-new garden on a site that's currently occupied by weeds or turf grass, you can get rid of those interlopers—and build nutritious, healthy soil at the same time—simply by cooking up a super-soil sandwich (see "From Rocks to Riches" on page 316).

It's All in the Timing

The weeding guidelines described in Chapter 15 apply just as much to a vegetable garden as they do to flower beds (see "Weeding Made Easy" on page 308). But here are a couple more secrets that are tailor-made for keeping your harvest safe from nutrient-robbing invaders:

Weed early. Even if you keep on top of your weeds for only a month in late spring, you'll still be way ahead of the game. The people who study these things have found that the most critical period of weed control is the four weeks after the seeds germinate.

Weed often. Every two weeks, to be precise. Those same studious folks pondered bell peppers for a while and discovered that if you weed every two weeks all summer long, you'll get twice as many peppers as you will if you weed just twice a season.

It's Thirsty Work Being a Vegetable

Some vegetable plants get thirstier than others, but most of them need about an inch of

moisture every week. That's about 62 gallons for every 100 square feet of garden—and that's a lot of H_2O! To make your chores easier and lower your water bill, follow the same basic guidelines we discussed for watering flowers (see "Weather-Wise Watering" on page 306). In addition, follow these guidelines:

- Water your plants only when they're thirsty. After a while, you'll learn to tell just by looking at them whether they need a drink. But to play it safe, keep a rain gauge handy. That way, you'll always know just how much water is falling from the sky and how much you have to supply.

- Cultivate before you water. Soil that's nice and loose lets the water filter right down to the plants' roots. If you don't at least scratch up the surface, a crust will form, and the water will just sit there on top or run off to who knows where.

- Water in the morning. That's when your plants make the most efficient use of the water you give them, because at that time of day, temperatures are lowest and humidity is

Quick Fix

One of the simplest ways to cut back on watering is to plant drought-tolerant vegetable varieties. Garden centers and catalogs have more of them in stock every year. In particular, many heirloom types tend to need much less water than do newer hybrids. To find the best old-timers for your region, just search the Internet for "heirloom vegetables."

usually at its highest. Therefore, evaporation is slow, and the water seeps into the soil, instead of vanishing into thin air.

TROUBLESHOOTING TIPS AND TRICKS

At the beginning of this chapter, I told you that vegetables can be the most trouble-prone plants under the sun. Unfortunately, I can't tell you how to handle every problem that could possibly plague your crops, but I can—and will—share my best secrets for solving some of the most vexing veggie dilemmas that are likely to come your way.

Welcome, Friends!

Believe it or not, you can solve a whole lot of garden-variety woes without even lifting a finger. How? By inviting over an army of beneficial bugs and other insect predators, such as birds, bats, toads, and lizards, to eat in your yard and garden. Simply by going about life as they know it, these priceless allies will polish off hordes of plant-munching and disease-spreading insects. (For more specific guidelines on fending off diseases, see "The Early Bird Saves the Day" on page 309.) Take a look at my surefire recruitment policy:

Lay off pesticides. I know that's a frightening thought if you've been using them for a long time, but you can bet your sweet bippy that a couple of weeks after you quit cold turkey, throngs of good guys will show up and start chowing down on the bad guys.

Give 'em a drink. All living things need water, but you don't need to install a fancy pond. Just sink some nonporous plant saucers into the ground, set some pebbles inside, and add water, letting a few of the stones stick up above the surface. It gives insects—and insect eaters such as toads, frogs, birds, and bats—a bar to belly up to.

Mix it up. Don't just plop your vegetable garden down in the middle of your lawn. Instead, give your crops good companions in the form of flowers, herbs, trees, and shrubs. The more menu and shelter options you offer up, the more kinds of helpers will come calling—and the more kinds of pests they'll polish off. To invite a genuine dream team to your yard, look for plants that are native to your neck of the woods. Believe you me, local heroes will flock to your doorstep!

Don't panic. Or, as my Grandma Putt always said, "Live and let live." The good guys can't stay around unless they have some bad guys to dine on. So don't reach for your spray gun—or even your blast-'em-off water hose—at the first sign of a slug or an aphid. Instead, just think of the little thug as lunch for your heroes. And don't worry: Even if you lose a tomato or a pepper here and there, you'll still have a garden full of great things to eat.

They're Here Anyway!

It's gone and happened: In spite of your best efforts, the good-guy/bad-guy balance has gotten out of whack, and your crops are under attack. So what do you do now? Well, for starters, follow the simple good-riddance methods in Chapter 15 (see "Foiling Flower Foulers" on page 309). Beyond that, there are specific tricks you can use to vanquish some of the most voracious vegetable villains like the ones that follow.

Out-Craft Cabbage Loopers

Don't let the name fool you; these caterpillars munch on the foliage, buds, and flowers of a great many plants, including all members of the brassica family, as well as beans, beets, celery, lettuce, peas, potatoes, spinach, and tomatoes. They leave behind ragged holes and masses of brown or green excrement pellets. One or two loopers won't do fatal damage, but in large numbers, they can demolish even mature plants. These gluttons are pale green caterpillars with wavy, lighter green or yellow stripes on their backs and sides. The best control measures for these nasties:

- Keep a close watch on your plants, and pluck off adults or egg cases (silk cocoons attached to leaves or stems) the minute you see them. Then crush them or toss them into a pail of soapy water.

- Go after them with this potent weapon: Put 1 cup of chopped citrus peels (any kind will do) in a blender or food processor, and pour ¼ cup of boiling water over them. Liquefy, then let the mixture sit overnight at room temperature. Strain the slurry through cheesecloth, and pour the liquid into a handheld sprayer bottle. Fill the balance of the bottle with water, then take aim, and let 'er rip. (*Note:* This spray will kill any kind of caterpillar on contact, and the potent aroma will discourage more from moving in.)

- After you've harvested your crops, bury whatever remains of the plants. That way, you'll polish off next spring's egg layers while they're still asleep in their cocoons. Don't try

HOME REMEDY

Of course, insects aren't the only pests that are out gunnin' for your crops. Plenty of multilegged diners would love to help themselves to your harvest, too. Well, never fear: You can protect your vegetable garden using the same tried-and-true remedies I recommended for trees and shrubs in Chapter 14 on pages 286–290.

to compost the stuff unless your bin or pile is *very* hot.

Clobber Colorado Potato Beetles

Both adults and larvae mainly plague members of the *Solanaceae* family, which includes the beetles' namesake crop, as well as tomatoes, peppers, and eggplant. In large numbers, the pests commonly kill young plants, and reduce the yield of mature ones. The adults are rounded, shiny, yellowish orange beetles with 10 black stripes running the length of their back, and black spots on the thorax. The larvae are dark orange, humpbacked grubs with a double row of spots along each side. Best control measures:

- In fall or very early spring (before the soil temperature hits the mid-50°F mark), dig a trench around your garden, with the sides vertical or sloping at least 45 degrees. Then line it with plastic. When the beetles awaken from hibernation in the soil, they'll be too weak to fly, so they'll start walking toward breakfast and fall right into the ditch. And thanks to the slippery plastic, they won't get out.

- When it's too late for prevention, sprinkle cornmeal or wheat bran on the leaves of your plants. When the beetles eat the stuff, it'll expand inside their tummies, and they'll explode.

- If you'd rather spray than sprinkle, mix up a batch of my garlic-based insecticide (see "Instant Insecticide" on page 310) and let 'em have it.

Cast Out Cucumber Beetles

These menaces chew ragged holes in the foliage, flowers, stems, and fruits of many vegetables, including their namesake crop and the rest of the cucurbit clan, as well as beans, peas, tomatoes, and ornamental flowers. In the process of feeding, they infect their victims with two fatal garden plant diseases: fusarium wilt and cucumber mosaic virus. These beetles come in two basic types: striped (orange- to cream-colored with three broad, black stripes) and spotted (yellow with black spots). The larvae of both types (thin, whitish grubs with a black or reddish brown head) eat plants' roots and, sometimes, fallen fruit. Get 'em under control with these techniques:

- Handpick and drown them in soapy water, or vacuum them off of your plants.

- Trap them by setting out shallow bowls of soapy water with strips of melon rind or cucumber peel added to it. The beetles will dive in for dinner and never get up from the table.

- To repel them, mix 2 tablespoons of artificial vanilla flavoring per quart of water in a handheld sprayer bottle, and spray your plants thoroughly. (Real vanilla extract works just as well, but why waste it?)

Banish Squash Beetles

These ladybug look-alikes (both adults and larvae) munch on plants of the cucurbit clan, filling the leaves with holes and sometimes turning them to mere skeletons. The two generations work as a team: The youngsters feed on the undersides of leaves, while the grown-ups dine on top. The beetles look like pale, orange-yellow ladybugs, with seven black spots on each wing cover. The larvae are plain yellow and covered with spines. Send them packing this way:

- Get some shallow, yellow plastic bowls (like the kind margarine and soft butter come in), fill them with soapy water, and set them on the ground near your plagued plants. Like many other insects, squash beetles are attracted to the color yellow, so they'll make a beeline for the bowls, fall in, and drown.

- As soon as the weather allows, plant an early crop of squash, and cover the ground under the plants with yellow plastic mulch (available at garden centers). The minute you see the beetles descend on the plants—and will they ever!—throw a sheet over them, pull 'em up by the roots, and dump 'em into soapy water. Just be sure to use the yellow mulch *only* on the lure crop, and put it as far away as possible from the cukes and squash that you intend to eat.

- To send the beetles scurryin' away (at least most of the time), plant tansy or nasturtiums among their target plants.

Give the Heave-Ho to Terrible Tomato Hornworms

These giant caterpillars target every member of the tomato family, as well as peas, okra, squash, grapes, dill, and many flowers. Even a few of them can demolish a plant in no time flat. In spite of their size and appearance (up to 5 inches long, with a nasty-looking horn on their rear end), they can be tricky to spot, because they usually hang out on the undersides of leaves, and their color—green with white diagonal stripes—blends right into the foliage. But you can track them down by looking on the ground for dark green or black droppings that are almost the size of rabbit pellets. Here's the best way to get rid of these pests:

- Spray young worms (2 inches long or less) with Btk *(Bacillus thuringiensis kurstaki)*, which is available in catalogs and some garden centers.

- Handpick any worms that are longer than 2 inches, and drop 'em into a bucket of soapy water with about half a cup of alcohol added to it for extra penetrating power.

- Repel them (and a lot of other bad bugs besides) by planting bunches of pot marigolds *(Calendula officinalis)* throughout your vegetable garden.

FAST FORMULA

Grandma Putt's Simple Soap Spray

This old-fashioned solution kills off just about any soft-bodied insect you can name, including mealybugs, thrips, and aphids.

1/4 bar of Fels Naptha® or Octagon® soap, shredded*
3 gal. of water

Add the soap to the water and heat, stirring, until the soap dissolves completely. Let the solution cool, then pour it into a handheld sprayer bottle, and let 'er rip. Test it on one plant first, though—and be sure to rinse it off of the plants after the bugs have bitten the dust, because lingering soap film can damage leaves.

You'll find Fels Naptha and Octagon in either the bath soap or laundry section of your local supermarket.

CHAPTER 17

Healthy, Helpful Herbs

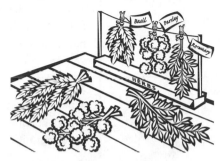

It's no secret that herbs can help you solve a lot of problems
around the old homestead. But even these wonder workers
can attract their fair share of trouble every now and again.
In this chapter, you'll find a passel of pointers for helping
your herbs through tough times—and using them to
overcome your biggest yard and garden problems.

HOMEGROWN HELP

In the days before commercial
fertilizers and pesticides came on the
scene, folks had to rely on homemade
concoctions to solve their garden-variety
woes. And at the heart of many, if not
most, of those remedies were—you
guessed it—herbs. I've gathered just a
small sampling of their problem-solving
repertoire to share with you.

Super Bulb to the Rescue

For some of the most annoying pest and disease
problems you can imagine, quick relief is spelled
g-a-r-l-i-c. Here are just a few of the feats this
easy-to-grow bulb can perform:

Prevents mildew. If you grow such "mildew
magnets" as garden phlox, asters, and mums,
protect them with this ultra-easy spray that
fends off both downy and powdery mildew.
Just boil 10 cloves of garlic in 1 quart of water
for half an hour. Strain, let the liquid cool to
room temperature, and pour it into a handheld
sprayer. Then, when you get a spell of warm
days and cool, humid nights—which is prime
mildew weather—spray your trouble-prone
plants from stem to stern every four or five days.

Stamps out damping-off. The same garlic tea
recipe (above) will protect seedlings from
the dreaded damping-off fungus. Start mist-
spraying your baby plants with the brew as
soon as their little heads appear above the
starter mix.

Kills insect pests. Mince 1 whole bulb of garlic, mix it with 1 cup of vegetable oil, and put it in a glass jar with a tight lid. Set it in the refrigerator, and let it steep for a day or two. To test it for "doneness," remove the lid and take a whiff. If the aroma is so strong that you want to drop the jar and run, it's ready. If the scent isn't so strong, add half a garlic bulb, and wait another day. Then strain out the solids, pour the oil into a fresh jar, and store it in the refrigerator. Turn your "condiment" into a potent pesticide by whirling 1 tablespoon of the oil in a blender with 1 quart of water and 3 drops of dishwashing liquid added. Pour the mixture into a handheld sprayer, then take aim and fire. The potion will deal a death blow to any soft-bodied insects including aphids, whiteflies, and destructive caterpillars. *Note:* Anytime a recipe calls for dishwashing liquid, do not use detergent or any product that contains antibacterial agents.

Repels pests. In this case, there's no mixing required. All you need to do is plant garlic throughout your flower, vegetable, and herb gardens. The pungent bulbs will say a loud "Keep out!" to deer, rabbits, and hordes of destructive insects, including aphids, cabbage loopers, Japanese beetles, plum curculios, and borers of all kinds.

Scat!

Garlic isn't the only herb that can keep your garden safe from plant-eating pests. Check out these other glorious green repellents:

- Basil deters aphids, asparagus beetles, spider mites, and tomato hornworms.

- Catnip sends black vine weevils scurrying, along with squash bugs and Colorado potato beetles.

FAST FORMULA	**Lavender Bath Blend**

When a day of working in the garden (or playing on the golf course) leaves you with tired, achy muscles, this simple concoction will put you back in action fast.

1 part lavender blossoms
1 part comfrey leaves
1 part Epsom salts
Lavender oil

Mix the blossoms, leaves, and salts in a bowl. Add a few drops of the oil (let your nose be your guide), and blend the ingredients well with your hands or a wooden spoon. Store in a decorative jar or other lidded container. Then whenever the need arises, toss a handful of the mix into a tub of hot water, ease in, and relax.

- Mint says "Scram!" to ants, flea beetles, and mice.

- Rosemary fends off cabbage moths, carrot rust flies, and Mexican bean beetles. The creeping variety, *Rosmarinus officinalis* 'Prostratus', also sends slugs and snails packing.

- Rue acts like a stop sign for both cats and Japanese beetles.

Toodle-oo, Ticks

In my Grandma Putt's day, ticks could put a damper on your fun at a picnic, a backyard barbecue, or a walk in the woods. Nowadays— as we all know too well—they can do a lot worse than that. These vile villains can also spread dreaded diseases to you and your four-footed pals. Fortunately, two of Grandma's most effective tick repellents still do a first-class job. (They repel fleas, too.) Here's the dynamic duo:

Pennyroyal. This small-leaved, low-growing perennial herb makes a terrific groundcover for shady spots. What's more, it has spikes of fragrant lavender flowers, it's a snap to grow, and it's hardy in Zones 4 to 10.

Rosemary. It's an evergreen shrub with pale blue flowers and aromatic, grayish foliage. It's hardy only in Zones 8 to 10, but in colder territory, you can grow it in a pot outside, then bring it indoors at the first sign of frost. It'll sail right through the winter in a sunny window.

To use either herb in your war against fleas and ticks, just dry the leaves and grind them up in a blender or coffee grinder. Then rub the powder into your pets' fur and sprinkle it around in their (and your) outdoor play spaces.

Vamoose, Vampires!

Fleas and ticks aren't the only blood-sucking villains lurking in your lovely landscape. Mosquitoes are also eager to sink their choppers into your unsuspecting skin. Fortunately, a number of herbs repel these vampires. There's just one minor catch: Contrary to what you see in some magazine ads, you can't just plant them and expect the skeeters to flee in horror. You need to crush the leaves to release their volatile oils, then rub them on your skin. When you do that, you can expect to stay bite-free for a couple of hours. The most effective bug-control herbs have one thing in common: a strong, citrusy scent that's very pleasant to humans, but repugnant to mosquitoes and many other insects. Here are some of my favorite anti-mosquito plants:

Lemon balm (*Melissa officinalis*)

Lemon basil (*Ocimum basilicum* 'Citriodorum')

Lemon-scented thyme (*Thymus* × *citriodorus*)

Scented geraniums (*Pelargonium* 'Citrosa' and *P.* 'Citronella')

Don't Give Blood

When you invite friends to a barbecue, you want 'em to *have* dinner, not *be* dinner. Here's a simple (and simply delicious) way to tell the skeeters you're throwing a party—not a blood drive. Just toss a handful of sage or rosemary sprigs onto the coals. You'll keep the biters at bay and spice up your chow at the same time!

START 'EM OFF RIGHT

While it is true that mature herbs tend to be as easygoing as plants can be, they can be mighty particular about how and where they get their start in life. If they don't get just the right kind of growing-up conditions, they'll do a less than stellar job. In fact, they may even refuse to perform at all. In this section, you'll find my surefire tips for launching your worker plants on brilliant careers.

Nothing Happened!

You say you carefully planted your herb seeds, but they never came up? The blame could lie with any number of factors. Fortunately, if it's early enough in the growing season, you can get a fresh start. Here are some things that might have gone wrong—and how to get it right the second time around. (By the way, these tips also apply to flower and vegetable seeds.)

They froze to death. If you tried to rush the season, this is the most likely culprit. Some seeds can hold their own in cold, wet ground; others will freeze or rot. The next time, wait until the soil is warm enough to suit your plants. (Check the time and temperature guidelines on the seed packet.)

They floated off. Heavy rains could have washed the seeds away. Or, perhaps you went overboard with the garden hose. When you water a seedbed, you must use a fine mist. You want to keep the soil evenly moist, but never sopping wet. And if the weather forecaster predicts a downpour, cover your planting site.

They were eaten. Birds and squirrels could have gobbled up your future plants. To put a halt to their dining pleasure, push twigs into the ground throughout the planting bed, and lay an old, sheer curtain panel on top. Be sure the twigs are short enough so the critters can't sneak in under the big top. Then remove the covering when the seedlings are large enough to fend for themselves.

They were planted too deep. Or maybe not deep enough. Some seeds need light to germinate—press them into the soil just enough to keep them from blowing away. Other seeds must be completely covered. The depth varies, but my rule of thumb is to set a seed into the ground at a depth equal to two times its diameter.

They needed a head start. Some herbs are easy as pie to grow from seed sown directly in the garden. Many, though, prefer a little coddling before they face life in the great

outdoors. With the latter, you have two choices: Start your seeds indoors, anywhere from 4 to 12 weeks before planting time (depending on the type of plant), or buy started plants at the garden center, and set them into the ground as you would any other transplants (see "Timely Transplanting" on page 303).

Another Possibility

If your seeds didn't come up at all, they could have fallen victim to one of the disasters at left. Or, the problem could lie with your choice of planting methods. Some herbs either don't come true from seed, or take forever to germinate. My advice: Get out there and try again. And this time, handle your growing stock according to the lists below:

Sensational Seeders

These herbs will start right off from seed sown directly in the garden. Or, if you want to get a jump on the growing season, start 'em indoors according to the simple guidelines in Chapter 16 (see "The Great Indoors" on page 318).

Basil (*Ocimum basilicum*), annual

Chervil, a.k.a. French parsley (*Anthriscus cerefolium*), annual*

Chives (*Allium schoenoprasum*), perennial, Zones 3 to 10

Cilantro, a.k.a. coriander (*Coriandrum sativum*), annual*

Dill (*Anethum graveolens*), annual*

Fennel (*Foeniculum vulgare*), perennial, Zones 4 to 10*

Garlic (*Allium sativum*), grown from bulbs

Marjoram (*Origanum majorana*), perennial, Zones 5 to 10

Parsley (*Petroselinum crispum*), perennial, Zones 6 to 10*

* These herbs resent having their roots disturbed. Sow the seeds directly in the garden when the soil has warmed up, or start them in individual travelin' pots (for how to make your own supply, see "A Single Room to Go" on page 320).

Potted Perfectionists

Don't even bother trying to start the following perennials from seed. Buy started plants from a garden center or catalog, and you'll be off to the races. If some of the zone numbers below don't match up with your climate, don't fret: Just treat the plants as annuals, and replace them every year. Better yet, grow them in containers and let them bask in a sunny window all winter long.

Bay (*Laurus nobilis*), Zones 8 to 10

French tarragon (*Artemisia dracunculus*), Zones 4 to 8

Garden sage (*Salvia officinalis*), Zones 5 to 9

Lavender (*Lavandula*), Zones 5 to 9

Mint (*Mentha*), Zones 4 to 10

Oregano (*Origanum heracleoticum*), Zones 5 to 10

Rosemary (*Rosmarinus officinalis*), Zones 7 to 10

Thyme (*Thymus*), Zones 4 to 9

What You Smell Is What You Get

Many herbs—including lavender, oregano, and French tarragon—don't come true from seed. Yet, the baby plants you find in a garden center or big home-store chain were probably started from seed. The result: Those seedlings may have no fragrance at all, or the aroma may be

---

HOME REMEDY

Whether you're starting herbs from transplants or direct-sown seed, spur them into action with this soil-building booster "shot": Mix together 5 pounds each of lime and gypsum; 1 pound of 5–10–5 dry, organic fertilizer; and 1/2 cup of Epsom salts. Work the formula into each 50-square-foot area of your herb garden to a depth of 12 to 18 inches. Then let it sit for 7 to 10 days before you plant. Your young herbs will get off to a rip-roarin' start!

---

only a faint shadow of the right stuff. So, to avoid disappointment, shop with your nose—and shop carefully. You *could* find a winner. Rub a leaf between your fingers, then bring it up to your nose and smell it. If you don't get a concentrated whiff of scent, put that plant right back where you got it. Don't take it home, thinking that it'll somehow develop fragrance and flavor as it grows, because it won't. What you smell and taste now is as good as it gets.

If you want to be sure of getting the biggest bang for your buck, buy your plants from small growers who specialize in herbs. And always ask how the stock was propagated. The good growers will be more than happy to tell you!

The Usual Suspects

Once your baby herbs sprout, remember that like all other seedlings, they have two big-time enemies: cutworms and damping-off fungi. Fortunately, your mission is clear. To foil cutworms, give each of your outdoor seedlings a protective collar that reaches about 2 inches into the ground and 3 inches above. Cardboard tubes from paper towel roles are perfect; so are old aluminum cans with both ends cut off. Indoors, fend off foul fungi by following my damping-off prevention guidelines in Chapter 16 (see "Stamping Out Damping-Off" on page 319).

Cool It!

Most grown-up herbs are real sun worshippers. With seedlings, though, it's a different story. Even in cool climates, they do better with a little shade. Out West or down South, Ol' Sol can make them go belly-up faster than you can say "Please pass the sunscreen." If your direct-sown herbs are keeling over, the reason is probably sunstroke.

Here's a simple way to give them shelter: When you sow your seeds, cut some fresh, feathery fern fronds, and stick them in the soil so they shade the bed. (Bracken or wood ferns are perfect; steer clear of heavier-leaved plants such as sword ferns.) When the seedlings germinate and stick their heads aboveground, they'll bask in the shade. But as those young plants grow bigger and tougher, the ferns will keep pace, dying back and gradually letting in more of the sun's rays.

Translation, Please

To perform their best, most of the herbs folks grow for kitchen use need 8 to 10 hours of direct sun a day—what the garden books and catalogs call "full sun." But in a hot climate, that much sun will cook your herbs before you ever get them into the kitchen. So if you live in the South or Southwest, or at a high altitude, remember that full sun generally means a maximum of four hours—preferably in the morning.

Exceptions to the Rule

If you think your yard doesn't get enough

sunshine to keep herbs happy, think again: Even up North, not all herbs demand a full day of Ol' Sol's time. In fact, mint will thrive in just three to four hours of sun a day. And these popular winners will all perform well in four to six hours of sunlight (what gardening books generally describe as either "partial shade" or "partial sun"). But be aware that the flavor and aroma won't be as intense as they would be if the plants grew in full sun.

Basil (*Ocimum basilicum*)

Chives (*Allium schoenoprasum*)

Cilantro, a.k.a. coriander (*Coriandrum sativum*)

Parsley (*Petroselinum crispum*)

MERRY MATURITY

Once your herbs have passed their infancy, they need the same basic feedin', weedin', waterin', and pest-control tactics as flowers and vegetables do. But, as the old saying goes, the devil is in the details. And the details we'll talk about include special kinds of TLC you need to give your herbs if you want to avoid problems—and how to respond if trouble does strike.

Look Out Below!

If your herbs are looking a tad too soft and lush aboveground, and pests are traveling from near and far, the trouble lies below the soil. In other words, the roots are getting too much to eat. In particular, they're getting an overdose of nitrogen, which encourages mountains of leafy

FAST FORMULA

Herb Booster Tonic

Even herbs enjoy a nice, cool drink when the going gets hot. Quench their thirst with this super summertime pick-me-up.

1 can of beer
1 cup of ammonia
$^1/_2$ cup of Murphy® Oil Soap
$^1/_2$ cup of corn syrup

Mix all of these ingredients in a 20 gallon hose-end sprayer. Then spray your herbs to the point of runoff every six weeks during the growing season.

growth. That, in turn, makes the plants sitting ducks for slugs and snails, as well as rot and other diseases. But you can save the day. First, clip away the lush foliage, and spread an inch or two of compost over the planting bed. It'll help balance the nitrogen overload, and fight off pests and diseases. Then put those plants on a diet and always remember: Most herbs are light to moderate feeders.

Herbal Meal Planning

Once you've administered dietary first aid, follow these feeding guidelines for the rest of the growing season:

- Give your herbs a light meal two or three times during the growing season, but stop feeding your perennials at least a month before you expect the first fall frost. Feeding too late in the fall tends to weaken perennials and makes them more susceptible to winter's harsh cold.

- As for what kind of chow to serve up, most herbs perform their best on what my Grandma Putt called punched-up compost. By that, she meant a mixture of good-quality compost and either rabbit, chicken, or sheep manure. Why those three? Because those critters' waste material has a higher concentration of the nutrients that herbs need than either horse or cow manure has. To make this super health food, use about 2 parts compost to 1 part manure. Let it sit for about a week so the hot compost can kill any lingering weed seeds, then spread it around your plants, and gently work it into the top inch or so of soil. If you listen closely, you'll almost hear those herbs say "Yum, yum."

So Long, Slugger!

Slugs and snails zero in on unhealthy herbs like ants throng to a picnic. Of course, there are a jillion good baits you can use, but what if you've got kids or pets on the scene? Even if your bait is harmless to the good guys, you don't want it disappearing into the mouths of your family and friends. Fortunately, I've got a nifty trick for serving up bait in a way that *only* slugs and snails can get to it: First, find some wide-mouthed pint bottles, such as the kind many juices come in. Pour about an inch of my Slugweiser into each bottle (see the Quick Fix box on page 339), then sink the traps in the ground so that the top of the bottle is just at ground level. The slimers will slither up to the edge and dive right in, but the beverage at the bottom will be beyond the reach of small human hands and long canine tongues.

Unwanted Houseguests

Healthy herbs suffer from very few pest problems, but if you bring your plants indoors for the winter, there are two mischief makers you're quite likely to see: spider mites and whiteflies. Bid them good-bye this way:

Spider mites. For some reason, dry indoor air seems to call out to these terrible tykes. But you can strike back. First, spray your herbs with water or, if the plants are small enough, set them in the bathtub, and turn on the shower. Just be sure to cover the pot with a plastic bag first, so the soil doesn't wash out. Then fend off future attacks by adding humidity to the air with this simple trick: Fill some trays with pebbles, and set your pots on top. Then pour in water to within about $1/2$ inch of the stones' surface. Add more water as the level goes down, but don't let it touch the bottom of the pots—you want your plants to be sitting *over*, not *in* the water.

Whiteflies. Just grab your vacuum cleaner, and sweep those pests right up. To make the job even easier, wrap some yellow electrical tape around the vacuum hose nozzle. The tiny terrors will flock to the scene. When you've made a clean sweep, tuck the vacuum cleaner bag into the freezer to kill the flies. Then dump the whole shebang on the compost pile.

If your indoor herbs live in their own sunroom or greenhouse, you're in luck: A teeny hired gun can stand guard over your flock. An almost invisible parasitic wasp, *Encarsia formosa*, a.k.a. whitefly parasite, lays its eggs in whitefly nymphs—thereby keeping the population to a minimum. You can order up your own posse from catalogs or on the Internet.

But They're in the Garden!

When either spider mites or whiteflies get out of hand outdoors, there's a definite reason—and some simple remedies.

Spider mites

Nearly all of the plants that suffer from severe spider mite attacks have one thing in common: They've been repeatedly sprayed with chemical pesticides of one kind or another. There are a couple of reasons for this. First, these potent potions kill off the mites' natural enemies, of which they have many. Second (and this is sobering, folks), scientific studies show that not only have mites become immune to many pesticides, but when they're exposed to some of these chemicals, namely carbaryl and parathion, they reproduce even faster than usual!

Best control measures:

- Blast the mites with cold water from the garden hose. (Do the job early in the morning, before the sun has a chance to heat up the hose.) Or, if your plants are small, fill a handheld sprayer with ice water, and let 'em have it.

- During dry spells, or if you live in an arid part of the country, sprinkle dirt pathways and other bare ground with water to keep dust to a minimum. There's nothing spider mites love more than dry, dusty spots.

- Invite the mites' natural predators into your yard. Many birds and hordes of beneficial insects, including ladybugs, damsel bugs, big-eyed bugs, and firefly larvae (a.k.a. glowworms) eat spider mites (see "Welcome, Friends!" on page 327).

Whiteflies

Just like spider mites, these minute marauders rarely cause real trouble if you've laid out the welcome mat for their predators. But they're most attracted to plants that aren't getting enough phosphorus or magnesium in their diet.

Best control measures:

- Test your soil. Then, if the results show a deficiency of phosphorus, add bonemeal, fish emulsion, poultry manure, or seaweed to the soil. If magnesium is lacking, add dolomitic limestone or Epsom salts.

- Staple a 24- by 36-inch sheet of yellow poster board to a wooden stake, and coat the paper with Tanglefoot® or another commercial stickum. Shove the stake into the ground so that the sticky trap is behind your stricken plants. Then spray your plants' foliage with water from the garden hose. You'll blast the flies off of the leaves and right onto your clever trap.

- Include plenty of lemon basil in your herb garden. Whiteflies hate the stuff, but you'll love it! It's a tender annual with small, pretty flowers, a lemony fragrance, and a flavor that's tailor-made for salads, stir-fries, and cream-based sauces. Plus, it's a snap to grow from seed anyplace in the country.

⧗ *Quick Fix*

Beer is a classic bait for slug and snail traps. But what attracts the slimy thugs is not the alcohol in the beer, or even the hops and malt—it's the yeast. So why waste a good brewski on the enemy? Instead, make a batch of my Slugweiser: Pour 1 pound of brown sugar and $^1/_2$ package (1$^1/_2$ teaspoons) of dry yeast into a 1-gallon jug, fill it with warm water, and let it sit for two days, uncovered. The pour it into your slug traps, and watch the culprits belly up to the bar!

Foul Fungi

When herbs fall prey to a root rot fungus, it's all but guaranteed that you have one of two problems: Either your plants are getting too much water, or they're sitting in poorly drained soil. Here are your best responses:

- If you catch the problem when the plants are just turning yellow—a sure sign of overwatering—ease off on the hose trigger. How do you know when to water again? Stick your index finger in the ground. If it's dry from the tip up, then you can reach for the hose.

- When drainage is poor, even if you're keeping a tight rein on the water supply, moisture will hang around the roots too long and cause trouble. In that case, you need to improve the soil pronto, or grow your herbs in containers.

Rhizoctonia Rides Again

There is one exception to the good-drainage-eliminates-fungus rule. That's rhizoctonia root and stem rot, a disease that can plague a number of herbs, even in loose, well-drained soil. Prime targets include oregano, marjoram, rosemary, sage, tarragon, thyme, and savory—both winter (*Satureja montana*) and summer (*S. hortensis*) types. In later stages, the stems, lower leaves, and roots turn to black, rotten messes. If that happens, your only option is to pull up the plants and destroy them. But don't panic! If you reach the scene early, you can still save the day: Just cut off the droopy leaves and saturate the soil with my Fungus-Fighter Soil Drench (see page 340). Then mulch the soil with compost or shredded pine bark (a.k.a. pine bark fines) to fend off further attacks.

A Pinch in Time

You say your herbs are pest-free and as healthy

as can be, but they're not giving you the full, leafy growth that you'd like? That's an easy problem to solve: Just pinch 'em. Then pinch 'em again. Every week throughout the growing season, pluck or cut off the growing tip of every single shoot. If you can't do the job every week, just do the best you can. The more you pinch, the more new leaves (or fresh flowers) the plants will churn out.

Besides giving you beautiful plants, this maneuver will leave you with mountains of little growing tips. And, take it from me—there's gold in them thar tips! Depending on what kind of herbs they are, here are some great ways to use your bonus leaves (or flowers):

- Toss basil, parsley, rosemary, or salad burnet into salads, casseroles, or stir-fries.

- Dry santolina, lavender, or artemisia to use in craft projects.

- Freeze mint, lemon balm, or scented geraniums in ice cube trays, and then use the cubes in drinks.

- Scatter rue, tansy, or mint wherever you need to repel pesky pests, such as mice, moths, or fleas.

- Add yarrow, valerian, or comfrey to your compost bin. They all deliver a kick that jump-starts the breakdown process for other plant material.

It's Too Darn Hot

Even the healthiest, heat-loving herbs call it quits when both temperature and humidity skyrocket. Especially in the steamy South, plants' stems, leaves, and roots are all sitting ducks for fungal diseases—not to mention simple heatstroke. So how do you save your crops? Just learn to cope! These simple tricks will keep your herbs fit as a

---

FAST FORMULA

Fungus-Fighter Soil Drench

When soil-borne fungi are making trouble in your lawn or gardens, fight back with this potent potion that packs a powerful punch.

4 garlic bulbs, crushed
1/2 cup of baking soda
1 gal. of water

Mix these ingredients in a big pot and bring to a boil. Then turn off the heat, and let the mixture cool to room temperature. Strain the liquid into a watering can, and soak the ground in the problem areas (remove any dead grass first). Go VERY slowly, so the elixir penetrates deep into the soil. Then dump the strained-out garlic bits onto the soil, and gently work them in.

---

fiddle down South, or anywhere else that Mother Nature opens up the steam vents.

Grow your herbs in raised beds or containers. This will improve both drainage and air circulation—and that's crucial for fending off fungal diseases.

Add manure and compost to the soil. In addition to giving off chemicals that destroy fungi, this duo provides steady, balanced nutrition that keeps plants free of stress. And in brutal heat, a stressed plant can become a dead plant mighty fast.

Cast shade on the scene. Down South, all herbs need shade from 2 p.m. on, and some— including chives, parsley, sorrel, and the mint clan—require permanent shelter. If you can't grow them in the shade of taller plants, cover their raised bed with a lattice roof, or an awning made of greenhouse shade cloth (available in catalogs and many garden centers).

Juggle your calendar. Some herbs won't survive a southern summer no matter how much you baby them. If you're not sure what to grow in your neck of the woods, check with gardening friends, your local garden club or herb society, or the closest Cooperative Extension Service.

HAPPY HARVESTING

As we've seen, herbs can perform a yeoman's work throughout your outdoor green scene (and indoors, too). But if you want to employ the leaves or flowers *after* you've plucked them from the plants, it's crucial to harvest and preserve them at just the right time and in just the right way. Follow these helpful hints and you'll know what to do and when to do it.

Less Than Gorgeous Garlic

There aren't many plants that are easier to please than garlic, but there are a couple of problems you may notice at harvest time: split husks or undersized cloves. Well, you can't send the bulbs back and exchange them for new ones, but you can head off trouble the next time around:

Split husks. This condition indicates that you waited too long to harvest your crop, and the cloves outgrew their skin. Next year, dig up the bulbs when most of the leaves have yellowed. That's generally by late August.

Undersized cloves. Garlic bulbs grow smaller than they should when their home ground is compacted. When you plant your next crop, work at least an inch of compost into the soil to make it nice and loose—and don't let anybody step on the bed!

It's All in the Timing

If you're anything like me, harvesting herbs is an ongoing process—you just clip whatever you're planning to cook with that day, or whatever strikes your fancy as you're strolling through the garden. It's another matter, though, when you want larger quantities, either to use fresh or to store for the winter. At those times, make sure you get the biggest flavor bang for your buck by following these guidelines:

- Keep a close watch on your plants, and clip the leaves just before the flower buds open. That's when most herbs reach their peak of flavor, fragrance, and quantity. If you cut them way back then, the plants will often regrow and give you a second harvest.

- Try to harvest your herbs early, after the dew has dried, but before the sun gets hot. That's when the volatile oils that give herbs their flavor and aroma reach their highest levels. The plants are also cool then, so they'll stay fresh longer. If early morning isn't possible, aim for an overcast day.

- Once they're cut, herbs go downhill fast, so harvest only as many as you're sure you can handle before the cuttings start to wilt. (You can always go back for more the next day.)

- About an hour before you plan to harvest your herbs, hose them off with a light spray to remove any lingering soil, bugs, or film from any soap sprays you may have used. The leaves and stems will retain more of their fresh color and fragrance if you perform this necessary chore before cutting the plants (and you won't have the mess indoors, either). Then as soon as the leaves are dry, grab your shears, and start clippin'.

Oops! I Missed

So what happens if you go away on vacation and miss the peak harvest season? Do you just have to pack it in for the year? Not at all—just shift your sights. You have three excellent options:

1. Instead of leaves, harvest the seeds.

2. Clip the flowers. Then toss them into salads or desserts, add them to homemade herbal vinegars, or dry them for use in craft projects later in the year.

3. Let some of the seeds self-sow and give you plants for next year.

How Dry They Are

When you dry herbs—no matter how you intend to use them—it's important to do the job in a place that has low humidity, good air circulation, and near-total darkness. Otherwise, the plants won't retain their volatile oils (the secret of their health-giving, food-flavoring, pest-defying power). Many attics fill the bill perfectly. But if yours

doesn't—or if you don't have an attic—you still have several simple alternatives, such as these:

In a dark room. Set old window screens or hardware cloth on bricks or other supports, and spread the herb stalks on top. Leave a door or window cracked open, and unless you live in a dry climate, turn on a fan or two for air circulation.

In a room where light penetrates. Gather the sprays into bunches of five or six stems each, and tie the stems together with twine. Then put each bunch upside down in a brown paper bag (making sure the herbs clear the bottom), fasten the top with a rubber band, and hang the bundles from anything that'll hold them.

In a microwave oven. Put a single layer of herbs between two paper towels, and nuke 'em for two to three minutes. Give them additional 30-second jolts as necessary until they're crisp.

In a gas oven. Spread your herbs in a single layer on a baking sheet. Then turn the oven to its lowest setting, and heat, with the door open, for two to three minutes at the lowest temperature that will keep the pilot light on. (This will get rid of any moisture.) Turn off the oven, set the herbs inside, and close the door.

In a food dehydrator. Set the temperature between 95 and 100°F. Spread your herbs in a single layer on a tray, and put them in the dehydrator. Then be prepared to wait. Depending on the fleshiness of the leaves, the drying process can take anywhere from 4 to 18 hours. So be patient, and keep checking!

Note: If you use one of the last three options, dry only one type of herb at a time. That way, you'll keep the flavors and scents from mixing and mingling.

Quick Fix

Want sweeter flavor from your garlic? Then try this simple trick: When you plant it, crush the cloves a little to bruise them, and tuck a couple of olive pits into each planting hole. Talk about sweet! When you harvest those bulbs, roast 'em and spread 'em on toasted Italian bread—your taste buds will think they've died and gone to heaven!

Dried Is Dandy, But Frozen Is Finer

That is, if you plan to use your herbs in cooking, rather than in craft projects or garden tonics. The reason: Most culinary herbs retain a lot more of their fresh-from-the-garden flavor when they're frozen rather than dried (although, of course, they won't keep their good looks). There are several easy-as-pie freezing methods. Whichever one you use, just pull out whatever quantity you want to cook with, and put the rest back in the freezer. Your choices are:

- Wrap bunches of herb sprigs (one kind per bunch) in aluminum foil.

- Chop fresh herbs, and freeze them in plastic containers.

- Puree chopped herbs with water, butter, or olive oil. Then pour the mixture into ice cube trays. When the cubes are frozen, pop them out of the trays and store them in plastic containers or freezer bags.

We're Buried in Herbs!

You know the old saying, "When life hands you lemons, make lemonade"? Well, what do you do when Mother Nature (or your own misjudgment at seed-shopping time) hands you more herbs than you can possibly use? Make herbal vinegar, that's what! It packs a flavor punch you'll never find in store-bought vinegars, and it's as easy to make as a pot of tea. Why, in just a few hours, you can whip up a year's worth of Christmas, birthday, and hostess gifts. What's more, the final product looks as elegant as anything you'd pay megabucks for at a fancy-food boutique. For each batch, you'll need six to eight fresh herb sprigs and 1 quart of good-quality vinegar. Here's the procedure:

Step 1. Wash and dry the herbs, then pack them into a clean, quart-sized glass canning jar. Heat the vinegar until it's warm (don't let it boil!), and pour it over the herbs. Cover the jar opening with plastic wrap or wax paper, and screw on the top. (If the jar lid is plastic, you can dispense with the inner wrap; it simply keeps any metal in the lid from reacting with the vinegar.)

Step 2. Put the jar in a dark place at normal room temperature, and let it sit for a couple of weeks. Then open the lid and sniff. You'll know the vinegar is ready when you get a strong fragrance of herbs.

Step 3. Strain out the solids, pour the flavored vinegar into a pretty bottle, and tuck in a fresh herb sprig or two. Then get ready for all the oohs and aahs!

Tips for Terrific Vinegar

These pointers will put you on the high road to herbal vinegar victory:

- Don't try to economize by using bargain-priced vinegars. If the vinegar you start with doesn't taste good, the finished product won't either—no matter how much herbal flavoring you pack into it.

- Use any kind of vinegar, and any kind of herbs that appeal to you. If you need inspiration, check some herbal cooking and craft books. There are many good ones, including some devoted entirely to making and using herbal vinegars.

- Don't put your handiwork on display. Fancy bottles filled with herbal vinegar look great on a windowsill, with sunlight streaming through them. But that light will make the flavor fade fast. Make up a few just-for-show batches if you want to, but keep your cooking and gift-giving supply in a dark place at room temperature.

Think Outside the Kitchen

It goes without saying that your homemade vinegar will make a fine addition to salad dressings, marinades, and other culinary delights. But herbal vinegars belong in your medicine chest, too. Here are some examples of flavors that can do wonders for your health and well-being—and your good looks. (Except where noted, simply dab the vinegar onto your skin with a cotton ball or pad.)

Bay leaves: Antiseptic; soothes and refreshes all types of skin.

Marjoram or oregano: Antiseptic; soothes sore throats (use as a gargle); relieves aching joints and muscles (rub it into your ailing body parts).

Mint: Relieves headaches; cools and refreshes (either spray it onto your skin, or pour $1/2$ cup or so into a tub of lukewarm water and settle in for a good soak).

Parsley: Cleanses and balances oily skin; lightens freckles; adds shine to dark hair (use it as a rinse after shampooing).

Rosemary: Repels insects; antiseptic; helps normalize oily skin.

Thyme: Antiseptic; deodorizes.

HOME REMEDY

When it comes to taste, dried basil is a pale ghost of the fresh version. But when you freeze it, it retains nearly all of its fresh-from-the-garden flavor and aroma. Problem solved, right? Wrong. Unfortunately, popping it into the freezer presents it's own conundrum: When basil is frozen, it turns black. The color change doesn't affect the flavor, but who wants to eat black leaves? Not me. So to keep them green, do what I do: Blanch them before freezing. Just put the leaves in a strainer and pour boiling water over them for a second. Then lay the leaves on paper towels and let them cool naturally. Don't dip them into ice water, as you do when you blanch vegetables—that will only dilute the flavor.

CHAPTER 18

Fine-Feathered Friends

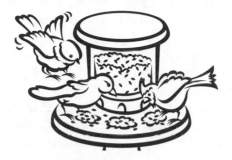

As we've discussed throughout this section, birds are some of the best pest-control helpers you could ever ask for. But their problem-solving talent extends far beyond your yard and gardens. Believe it or not, simply watching your fine-feathered friends in action can solve or head off some of your own health problems. Get ready to discover my best secrets for welcoming birds into your yard—and helping them overcome some challenges of their own.

CALLING DR. BIRD!

The folks who study social trends tell us that bird-watching is one of the most popular and fastest-growing pastimes in the country for a couple of reasons: First, it's a whole lot of fun—and, second, it's good for you, too! I love watching the birds in my yard. In this section, I'll let you in on some of the ways backyard birding can lead to better physical *and* mental health for you and your family.

Stress Be Gone

Look, right there—see that chickadee? Oops, there he goes. Well, he'll be right back. See? There he is again! And now look—a whole flock of goldfinches just flew in!

That's the way bird-watching works, whether you're sharing the view with family or friends, or talking to yourself. And that's exactly why health experts say it's so good for us. We forget all about our busy lives and workaday worries, and get lost in the action that's happening right in front of us. Try it yourself: Ten minutes with the towhees, and you might even have the peace of mind you need to balance the checkbook!

Just Say "Om"

If your blood pressure is higher than it should be, you *could* sign up for a meditation class, or even get yourself a personal guru. Or you could just put up a bird feeder or two in your yard, and then sit back and enjoy the show for a little while each day. I say that because scientists have found that watching birds at a feeder can lower your blood pressure *and* decrease your heart rate just as well as meditation can. Both of these activities perform their magic in the same way: by shifting our conscious focus away from ourselves, thus calming the chaos in our busy brains.

Memories Are Made of This

Speaking of brains, have you found that yours isn't quite as good at remembering things as it used to be? If so, then chalk up another proven benefit you can gain from bird-watching: It actually improves both long- and short-term memory. That's because you have to pay attention to all the little details that set one bird apart from another. Then you have to remember those identifying marks and shapes, so you can look up your "trophy" in a field guide and maybe write it down on your list of sightings. Finally, you really stretch the old gray cells when you relive the experience by describing it to another person.

To me, though, the reason for this mental improvement isn't important. I just know that since I've taken up bird-watching, I spend a lot less time trying to remember the names of old boyhood pals—or where I put the car keys last night!

Beat the Winter Blahs

Except for folks who live deep down in the Sunbelt, winter brings a steady stream of gray skies, drab landscapes, and long, dark nights. Even if you're a cheery soul by nature, the moody blues can really get a grip on you—especially during that long stretch after the holidays, when it starts to seem as though spring will never arrive. One solution: Put up a bird feeder or two where you can easily see them from the house. It's hard to stay down in the dumps when you look out the window and see a colorful crowd of cavorting cardinals or chirping chickadees. If you already have a feeder, expand your offerings to attract more kinds of birds. You'll get so distracted by watching to see who'll be the first to spy your new concoction that, before you know it, the days will be getting longer again and the air will be all but shouting "Spring is here!"

THIS GARDEN IS FOR THE BIRDS!

There's a simple secret to having a yard that looks great to you and encourages birds to set up housekeeping. What is it? Just choose a variety of plants—including trees, shrubs, annuals, and perennials—that hold their good looks over a long period of time. Of course, it's not the plants' attractive appearance that keeps the frequent fliers hanging around. It's the food, shelter, and nesting nooks provided by the flowers, fruits, foliage, and branches. The best plants for you depend upon your climate and other growing conditions, as well as your personal taste. So read on for my hospitality primer, avian style.

Three for the Show

The first step in planning a bird-pleasing yard

and gardens is to keep these three bird-friendly guidelines in mind:

1. Flowers don't matter much. That is, not the flowers themselves. What songbirds want (and need) are the insects that may be on those pretty posies, or the seeds, berries, or other fruits that follow. In terms of annuals and perennials, birds are especially fond of anything with daisylike blooms, including asters, black-eyed Susans, cosmos, marigolds, and zinnias.

2. Although birds will eat such sweet treats as cherries, raspberries, and blueberries, they actually prefer tangy fruits, including barberry, chokecherry, dogwood, Russian olive, and wild honeysuckle. And planting bitter berries like these can go a long way toward ensuring that you get a bountiful harvest of the goodies *you* want! (For more on protecting fruits from birds, see "Bye-Bye, Birdies" on page 287.)

3. Birds flock to evergreen trees and shrubs, and for good reason: Their year-round foliage and dense, twiggy growth provide shelter from the cold, safe nesting sites, and protection from predators.

I'll Drink to That!

Don't be surprised if birds ignore your berried shrubs for a long time, then suddenly feast on them in mid- to late winter. The berries of some plants, such as hollies *(Ilex)* and junipers *(Juniperus)*, are simply not pleasing to avian taste buds until they've been frozen and thawed several times, and actually begin to ferment. Some wildlife experts suspect that birds enjoy the alcohol the well-aged berries contain—most likely because it helps keep their little bodies warm in the cold weather.

Let 'Em Eat Seeds

When you're making out your plant list for your bird-friendly garden, be sure to include plenty of perennials with seedheads that last into winter. They'll provide welcome food for your feathered friends and keep your flower beds looking attractive all year round. You have oodles of beautiful plants to choose from, but here are some of my favorites:

Astilbes *(Astilbe)*

'Autumn Joy' sedum *(Sedum 'Autumn Joy')*

Bee balms *(Monarda)*

Black-eyed Susans *(Rudbeckia)*

Joe Pye weeds *(Eupatorium)*

Purple coneflower *(Echinacea purpurea)*

Sea hollies *(Eryngium)*

Siberian iris *(Iris sibirica)*

Not Just for Show

Hummingbirds are famous as nectar sippers—and hovering showmen as well! But these jewel-

---

Quick Fix

Before you buy any plants for their berries, check to see whether they're dioecious types. This simply means that in order to get fruit, you need both a male (to send out pollen) and a female variety (to receive the pollen and produce the fruit). Bayberries, bittersweet, and hollies are just three examples of dioecious bird pleasers. You'll find a whole lot more in Chapter 14 (see "Take Comfort" on page 274).

toned acrobats also eat hordes of insects. In fact, quite often when they seem to be drinking nectar from a flower, they're really snatching up tiny bugs. Hummers are especially fond of tubular or trumpet-shaped flowers in bright shades of red, orange, yellow, and hot pink. Some of their all-time favorites are fuchsias, bee balms, daylilies, snapdragons, lilies, and trumpet vines.

Nest, Sweet Nest

Besides providing your feathered friends with food and sheltered nesting sites, the plants in your yard can supply building materials for the nests themselves. That's because nearly all songbirds make their maternity wards from just four basic materials: sticks, leaves, grass, and plant stems. Tiny hummingbirds build their equally tiny, eggcup-size hideaways from such things as moss, lichen, grasses, soft ferns, milkweed, and thistledown, all held together by strands of spiderweb.

Lessons Learned

I used to be a real stickler for keeping my yard tidy and free of all plant debris. Then one fine spring day, I spent a couple of hours watching a wren, a jay, and a cardinal searching for sticks to build their nests. Those birds worked so doggone hard to find just a few twigs in my tidied-up yard that I changed my ways, right then and there. Oh, I still sweep and rake the paving and the lawn, just to keep things looking good. But now I no longer clean up under my shrubs and hedges, which are the prime locations for stick-collecting songbirds.

Stick 'Em Up

Besides leaving twigs and small sticks on the ground where they fall from their parent plants, you can help the birds—and give yourself hours of viewing pleasure at the same time. Just collect handfuls of the little woody pieces that plants shed naturally, and pile them loosely in areas where you can watch the construction workers sorting through to find their favorites. Almost any tree or shrub in your yard will offer up a steady supply of droppings, but privet, willows, oaks, dogwoods, and lilacs are especially prolific. As for the shoppers you can expect to see in your mini lumberyard, here's a roster of the most common backyard stick builders:

- Cardinals
- Catbirds
- Doves
- Jays
- Mockingbirds
- Robins
- Thrashers
- Wrens

Size Does Matter

Some nest builders gather slender, short twigs, while others seek out sturdier branches that can be more than a foot long. And many birds combine all sizes and lengths in their construction projects. The secret to attracting the greatest variety of takers is to supply sticks that are about $1/2$ inch in diameter, in an assortment of lengths from 3 to 10 inches.

Beware of setting out any branches that are $1/2$ inch or more in diameter. Why? Because you will attract nesting birds all right, but they'll be large hawks, ospreys, and eagles—and you don't want those big guys around if you have cats, tiny dogs, or other small pets that roam around in your yard.

The Thorn Birds

Don't be surprised if you offer up some rose or berry canes, or other thorny twigs and get a "meow" of appreciation in return: Catbirds and their cousins, the mockingbirds and brown thrashers, all make a beeline to prickly sticks when it's time to settle down and raise a family. After all, those sharp spines make any predator think twice before he reaches for an egg or a baby bird! (Of course, this inhospitable building material is used only in the outer part of the nest, not near the unfeathered infants.)

I hope this goes without saying, but don't *you* reach for those spiny sticks until you've pulled on a pair of thick leather gloves!

Leave the Leaves

Here's another reason that birds flock to less than perfect yards: dead leaves. Now, don't get me wrong—I'm not suggesting that you quit raking them altogether. Just don't bother to collect every last little leaf. The strays that wind up in the corners of the yard or under hedges are in high demand during nesting season. That's because when dead leaves are worked into a twiggy foundation, they help keep the nest insulated on chilly nights, and they don't hinder air circulation on hot, stuffy days.

HOME REMEDY

When you cut back your perennials after blooming season is over, pile the plants where you can see them. You may spot orioles or other birds tugging at the stems to strip off the usable fibers. Asters and butterfly weed (Asclepias tuberosa) are just two plants with fibrous stems that make perfect nest-building material.

The Non-Green Grass of Home

Nesting birds go gaga for long blades of dead, dried grasses—ornamental types, that is, not turf grass. To attract the widest array of birds, set out clippings that are at least 6 inches long (so they can be easily woven into the nest) in a variety of widths. Popular choices include maiden grass (*Miscanthus* 'Gracillimus'), fountain grass (*Pennisetum*), and blue fescue (*Festuca*). You'll also find lots of takers for weedy grasses, such as orchard grass or timothy, which may be growing along your fence or in an overlooked corner. But skip the crabgrass and lawn clippings; few nest builders bother to collect them.

To present the grassy goods, just set aside the clippings whenever you cut back any of your ornamental grasses. Coil the blades into a loose circle, and store your treasure in a cool, dry place. Then offer up small amounts of it to your feathered friends throughout the spring-to-early-summer nesting season.

Here's Mud in Your Eye!

Remember how much fun you had making mud pies when you were a kid? Well, helping your avian pals can give you a great excuse to get out there and slop it up again! That's because many birds use mud in their nests—and you'll be a hero in their eyes if you make them a nice puddle. Just be sure to maintain it throughout the spring and summer because robins, swallows, and other "plasterers" often build more than one nest a season.

Your Building-Supply "Store"

Some birds are fearless and will instantly investigate your material offerings, no matter where you put them, or what you put them in. Other shoppers, however, feel more comfortable when you present the goods in a way that's close to natural. Here's a rundown of your supply options:

On the level. The simplest way to offer supplies is to put them right on the ground. This is just the ticket for robins, thrushes, towhees, native sparrows, and other birds that prefer to forage at low levels. There's only one disadvantage to this method: On a windy day, your whole stash is liable to blow away. You can counter that problem by putting out only a small amount of stuff at a time, and put it on the leeward side of a bush or fence.

A cagey cache. A clean wire suet cage makes a dandy "boutique" for hummingbirds, chickadees, titmice, nuthatches, and other clinging birds. If you fasten the cage to a solid support, so that it doesn't swing freely, chances are it will also attract orioles, tanagers, and other larger birds.

A tisket, a tasket. A shallow wicker basket makes a handsome holder for your collection of twigs, grasses, or soft specialty items, such as mosses and ferns. Set it directly on the ground, either in the open or tucked under a shrub, for robins, thrushes, sparrows, and other low-level roamers to discover. Or get a basket that has a handle, and hang it from a tree branch, or the kind of metal hook used for hanging plants and bird feeders. You'll be sending an advertising flyer to those that shop on the wing, like chickadees and jays.

Of course, this holder won't last more than a season or two out in the weather, so don't use one of your favorite handwoven treasures. Instead, pay a visit to your local thrift store, where you can find sturdy, good-looking baskets for next to nothing.

FINE FOOD AND WONDERFUL WATER

Even if you have a great big yard filled to the brim with bird-pleasing plants, a few well-stocked feeders will help you attract a whole lot more of the fine-feathered crowd, and keep them around longer. And that in turn means they'll be Johnnies-on-the-spot to solve your peskiest pest problems. In this section, I'll tell you how to provide a fine-dining experience without turning bird feeding into a second career—or spending a fortune on your "restaurant." We'll also take a look at the kind of birdbaths that will draw avian drinkers and bathers from near and far to your backyard.

Simply, Simplify

If you really want to simplify your bird-feeding life—especially if you're new to the pastime—just get yourself a high-quality, hopper-style feeder, and fill it up with black oil sunflower seeds. (You can find both seeds and feeders at most garden centers and hardware stores, as well as shops that specialize in birding supplies.) When birds find a feeder that's filled with this stuff, they think they've reached the mother lode, and for good reason. Make that four good reasons:

High meat-to-shell ratio. That's the fancy name for it, but all birds care about is that there's a plump, supersized kernel waiting for them under that thin shell.

Higher oil content. Fat is the fuel for birds' daily fast-action lives, and all those calories keep their little motors running. Black seed is higher in oil than the striped kind, so it's more beneficial to the hard-charging fliers—especially in cold weather.

Smaller size. Black seed is smaller than striped, so more kinds of birds can get it into their beaks. When you serve up striped seed, you'll attract plenty of big guys, such as jays and cardinals. But with black oil seeds, finches, song sparrows, and even tiny chipping sparrows can join in the fun.

Thinner shells. Because black seed has thinner shells than striped, more kinds of birds can crack it. In the old days, before this superfood hit the market, little gray juncos (which I grew up calling "snowbirds") had to pick through the leavings to find bits of overlooked kernels. Now they can eat right beside their big-beaked pals.

Believe it or not, this miracle seed is a budget saver, because pound for pound, it costs less than the striped variety. So stock up on it!

Roll Call!

Just about every kind of bird flocks to black oil sunflower seed. The only ones that usually pass it up are those that naturally chow down on soft foods: purple martins, which are insect eaters; robins, which like worms; and catbirds and orioles, which prefer fruit. But even these birds can decide to try a new taste treat every now and then. Why, I've watched a scarlet tanager enjoying the stuff, after "experts" tried to tell me they wouldn't touch it! But even without those adventuresome types, the list of regulars is a long one. Keep your eyes open, and you're sure to see some of these diners:

- Blackbirds
- Buntings
- Cardinals
- Chickadees
- Dickcissels (Yep, there really is a bird with this name!)
- Finches
- Goldfinches
- Grackles
- Jays
- Juncos
- Native sparrows
- Nuthatches
- Pine siskins
- Titmice
- Towhees
- Varied thrushes
- Woodpeckers

FAST FORMULA

Winter Warm-Up

When the weather turns cold, birds need extra calories to keep their little bodies warm. So do your feeder guests a favor by serving up big helpings of this power-packed snack.

1 cup of black oil sunflower seeds
1 cup of cornmeal
1 cup of peanut butter
$1/4$ cup of cracked corn

Combine all the ingredients in a bowl, and mix thoroughly. Pack the mixture into a wire suet cage, then sit back and enjoy the show!

Simple Serving

Even basic hopper-style "dining rooms" vary greatly in quality and price. So to make sure you get a model that will perform well for you and your resident diners, here's a list of questions to take with you on shopping day:

1. Is the feeder sturdy and well made with a good, strong hook or hangers?

2. Is there room for at least a dozen birds to perch at one time without running out of elbow room?

3. Will they be able to reach the seed easily while perched in a normal position?

4. Does the feeder hold enough seed so that you don't have to refill it more than once a day? (A quart of seed capacity is usually a good starting point.)

5. Can you refill it without taking it off its mount? You'll find this feature a big blessing on ice-cold mornings, or when you're running late for work.

6. Is it easy to fill with one hand? Remember, you'll probably be holding a scoop full of seeds in the other.

7. Does the design allow you a good view of your guests, or will they be hidden by the roof or other parts of the feeder?

Fundamental Fats

In late fall, natural foods start getting scarce, so from then on through winter, birds range far and wide to fill their bellies. This is the time to serve up two high-calorie, body-warming favorites: suet and peanut butter. Besides being a kind gesture to your avian guests, adding these goodies to the menu can offer a big benefit to you. First, you'll attract (and therefore get to watch and photograph) birds that don't normally visit your seed feeders. Second, some of those visitors may well remember your hospitality and return in the spring to build their nests—and eat your garden pests.

The quickest way to offer up this dynamic dietary duo is to mix equal parts of chopped suet scraps and peanut butter, and stuff the mixture into a wire-basket-style suet feeder (available anywhere you can find wild birdseed). If you want to stretch out the supply, simply add a cup or two of coarse-ground cornmeal to the mix.

Humming a Different Tune

Hummingbirds don't give a hoot about all the seeds in your feeder. It's nectar they need—that is, along with the protein they get from gobbling up the bugs in your yard. In the Deep South and Far West, the hummers stay around all year long, but in most parts of the country, they're on the job from midspring through early fall. If you want a fail-safe cue for setting out your nectar feeders, just watch for the first daffodils. When those pretty golden blooms burst forth, you know that hummingbirds won't be far behind.

As for what to put in your feeder, you can buy mixes to make hummingbird nectar, but there's no reason to spend the money. Just make your own, using 4 parts water to 1 part granulated sugar. Heat the water in a pan until it's almost boiling, then remove the pan from the heat, and stir in the sugar. Continue stirring until the sugar is completely dissolved. Cool, and fill your freshly cleaned feeder. Store any extra solution in the refrigerator in a tightly capped bottle or jar. It will keep for about three days. To speed up the mixing process, use superfine white sugar (the kind bartenders use). It dissolves almost instantly when stirred into water of any temperature, allowing you to skip the heating step. *Note:* Whatever you do, don't use honey in your feeder. It can infect hummingbirds with a fatal fungus.

Sweets for the Tweets

For all you budget-watching bird-watchers, this will be music to your ears: Some of the best, most user-friendly nectar feeders are the inexpensive models available at birding-supply stores, garden centers, or even your local supermarket—not the fancy "designer" creations you see in catalogs and upscale garden shops.

FAST FORMULA

Procrastinator's Protein Punch

Even hummingbirds can run a little behind schedule every now and then—or maybe some of them just like to avoid rush-hour traffic. No matter the reason, you may find yourself with a straggler that didn't catch the fall migration express. If the weather turns nippy for your stay-behind, add a protein boost to your nectar feeder. This recipe makes a little over 1 cup of solution, which should be plenty to nourish a lone bird until it, too, gets packing!

1 cup of water
Pinch of low-sodium beef bouillon
 granules
¼ cup of granulated sugar

Heat the water to or almost to the boiling point. Sprinkle the bouillon granules into the hot water, and stir to dissolve. Add the sugar, continuing to stir until completely dissolved. Cool, then pour the solution into a clean feeder.

But wherever you shop for your hummingbird diner, keep these tips in mind:

Consider the shape. There are two versions. One consists of a vertical tube reservoir with drinking holes at the bottom; the other features a wide, flattened disc that holds the nectar, with seats around the rim for the diners. Each type has its admirers, but I prefer the "flying saucer" model, simply because it can accommodate more birds and they can perch while they sip—giving me a chance to take long, admiring looks at these miniature marvels.

See the light. Or, rather, the sugar water. When you're shopping for a feeder, you'll see everything from elegant ceramic jars to big, red plastic apples. But you'll do yourself and the hummers a favor if you opt for a feeder with a transparent reservoir. That way, you can see at a glance when you need to refill it—you won't have to traipse outdoors and open the cap for a look-see, and you won't risk letting it run dry by mistake.

Try before you buy. Don't just buy a feeder based on looks. Take it apart and put it together again while you're still in the store. Make sure it's sturdy, the parts fit tightly, and the drinking ports are easy to reach for cleaning. I know this routine sounds a little tiresome, but if you have any doubts about the time you're spending, just remember that when you have to work with this gadget at home it will be full of sloshy, sticky sugar water!

Sip and Splash

Birds will drink from just about anything when they're thirsty, which may be why most birdbaths are made to look pretty to humans, rather than suit the needs of their real clientele. But that trend is changing. These days, you can buy birdbaths (usually made of fiberglass or molded plastic) that mimic the natural places, such as ponds, puddles, and streams, where birds prefer to refresh themselves. A model that has these features will make you a superhero to the avian crowd:

Ground-level construction. Water that's on the ground, where birds find it in the wild, is far more enticing to them than a bowl sitting on a pedestal, or a pretty saucer hanging from a chain.

Places to perch. The best birdbaths have faux rocks along the edges of the water and also protruding from the center, just like stones in a stream.

More than one pool. This is important because smaller birds, such as finches and titmice, need shallower water than their larger cousins, such as jays and robins. A bath that has areas of different depths will attract more kinds of birds. Just make sure that none of your compartments has water that's deeper than

---

HOME REMEDY

Filling nectar feeders outside is dang inconvenient, but carrying a freshly filled feeder from the kitchen to the yard can leave you with a sticky trail of drips to clean up. Fortunately, the solution is as close as your kitchen counter: Just hold a dishcloth under the feeder as you make your trek, and you'll leave no sloppy souvenirs along the way. When you return, give your cloth a quick rinse, and it'll be all set to resume its normal duties.

---

2 inches. Anything beyond that can make birds feel vulnerable and therefore, less likely to come calling.

A rough surface. When birds visit a water source, they like to have good traction underfoot—just as you and I do in a swimming pool or shower stall.

Sound effects. You'll get more winged visitors faster if they can hear your watering hole as well as see it. So look for a birdbath that comes equipped with an arched tube or other device that you can hook up to your hose, thereby allowing water to dribble gently into the pool. (You can also buy drip tubes separately to add the sound of moving water to your current birdbath.)

Tiny Toe Dabblers

Even the shallowest pool is too deep for hummingbirds. But here are a couple of ways you can say "Everybody into the pool!":

- Plant a few leafy "swimming holes." After a heavy rain, hummers love to bathe their cares away on foliage that's covered with a thin film of water. They're especially attracted to leaves that are large and horizontal (or close to it) with smooth, slightly concave surfaces that hold moisture for a while after the rain stops. Many beautiful trees and shrubs fill the bill nicely, including dogwoods (*Cornus*), sugar maples (*Acer saccharum*), spicebushes (*Lindera benzoin*), and eastern redbuds (*Cercis canadensis*).

- Set up a device that delivers water in a fine mist or small droplets. Bird-supply stores sell special, timer-activated systems that spew out misty clouds on a schedule of your choosing. You can also accomplish the same result with a nonoscillating lawn sprinkler, or even a hose nozzle that's set to a very gentle spray. (Just loop the hose over the crotch of a tree, so the water goes either outward or downward.) Whichever delivery method you choose, the key to building a loyal clientele lies in one word: regularity. Turn on your shower at roughly the same time every day, let it run for half an hour or so, and before you know it, hosts of hummers will appear at bath time.

GUARDING YOUR FLOCK

When you set out your feeders, songbirds and hummingbirds won't be the only diners you'll attract. Plenty of bigger birds and four-legged critters will flock to the scene, too. Sometimes, they'll simply want to get their share of the seeds and other goodies. Other times, though, they'll be gunnin' for your feathered friends. Here are some of my best tips for keeping furry *and* fearsome flying diners away.

Raiders in the Night

Except for squirrels, which grab their goodies in the daytime, furry feeder raiders mainly do their dastardly deeds under cover of darkness. And this habit gives you the perfect focus for the start of your antivarmint campaign. If you dish up the seed sparingly, and limit the offerings in open feeders to the amount that birds can clean up during daylight hours, there won't be many edibles left over to tempt nighttime raiders. You won't eliminate their visits, but you will save your wallet from being emptied!

Outfox Their Appetites

Feeder makers do a brisk business in styles that guard against animal use. Check your bird-supply store, or shop online, and you'll find a variety of anti-this and anti-that feeders. Look for these features:

Weight-sensitive. When a heavy customer steps onto the feeding platform, the door drops down, cutting off access to the seed supply.

Chew-proof metal. Gnawing teeth make short work of wood or plastic feeders, especially when real hunger (rather than mere curiosity) is the driving force. The best antipest styles are made with metal that can resist those munching molars.

Antitheft attachments. Dexterous paws often resort to carrying off feeders, hook, line, and suet! So look for feeders that attach with nails, screws, or other permanent moorings to prevent wholesale highway robbery.

Go the Extra Mile

I've tried just about every kind of "squirrel-proof" bird feeder on the market, and take it from me: A squirrel that's really determined can break into any of 'em! That is, unless you do a little remodeling. These two tactics have worked well in my backyard:

1. Mount your feeder on a 4- by 4-inch wooden post about 5 feet off of the ground. Then cover the post with strips of duct tape, run vertically. The squirrels' little feet will slip right off!

2. Hang your feeder from a rope or cable that's strung between two trees or posts. But before you attach it, cut the bottoms off some empty orange juice or soup cans, and thread them onto the rope. (Paint 'em green first if you

want them to blend into the scenery.) Three or four cans on either side of the feeder should do the trick. Then sit back and have fun watching the squirrels doing a jig right on down the line!

Whichever technique you use, just make sure you put the feeder out of leaping distance from tree limbs, garage roofs, or other handy launching platforms.

Make 'Em See Red

Unlikely as it may sound, squirrels often avoid the color red. Scientists speculate that the reason may be that in many places, squirrels and certain red-headed woodpeckers compete head-to-head for the same resources. And the woodpeckers' sharp beaks have taught the furry rascals not to be too pushy in claiming territory. I can't guarantee that the squirrels in your neighborhood are red-aphobic, but it can't hurt to test the theory. Try some of these simple measures to make them keep their distance from your feeders:

- Buy a red feeder or two, or paint your current ones red.

- Set out red lawn furniture.

- Plant beds of bright red flowers around your feeders, or set containers of them out on your deck.

Run, Raccoons!

These clever critters can clean out a bird feeder faster than you can say, "Who was that masked man?" But fortunately for you and your feathered friends, raccoons have ultra-sensitive feet that recoil from anything that's sticky, slippery, sharp, or just plain strange. So lay a 3-foot-wide strip of

any of these materials around your feeders, and those coons will clear out fast:

- Broken pot shards or jagged stones

- Nylon netting

- Plastic sheeting

- Smooth, round pebbles

- Thorny rose or bramble fruit canes

- Wire mesh

Not Here, Kitty!

Cats are some of the most wonderful pals you could ever hope to find—when they're inside the house, that is. Outdoors, they're the biggest threat to songbirds, bar none. Scientists estimate that each year, literally billions of birds fall prey to cats. You can take one big step for catkind simply by keeping your own felines indoors. On the other hand, controlling the kitties that roam your neighborhood is not that easy, but these tricks will help:

Think "location, location, location." Be sure to place your feeders and nesting boxes well out of leaping distance from trees, deck railings, or other pussycat perches.

Lay a prickly carpet. Cut thorny canes from rosebushes or bramble fruits, and lay them thickly on the soil at the base of feeders and nesting boxes.

Give 'em a hot foot. Sprinkle a wide band of ground hot pepper around your feeder area. When cats cross it to stalk the birds, they'll feel it, but good! It won't do permanent harm, but it may be unpleasant enough to discourage a return engagement. (For a more permanent variation on the foot-discomfort theme, build the flat fence described on page 266.)

Grow protection. Plant a climbing rose (the thornier, the better) below your feeder, and train the prickly canes to grow up the pole. The ornery felines will get their kicks elsewhere. This same protective device will keep cats from climbing into trees to rob nests—or leaping from them onto nearby feeders.

Quick Fix

Squirrels, possums, and raccoons are small potatoes when you live in bear country. If that happens to be your home, sweet home, here's good news: You can actually buy feeders that will allow you to entertain 2-ounce birds and keep 300-pound bruins at bay! Look for these surprisingly attractive, jaw- and claw-proof marvels in stores and on Web sites that specialize in birding supplies. The cost? Considerably more than you'd pay for a basic, bargain-basement feeder, but not much more than you'd pay for a sturdy, good-looking model that's resistant to smaller critters—and definitely a whole lot less than you could shell out for a fancy designer creation!

Do Fence Me In

A high, solid board fence will keep out all but the most determined cats—and just about every other critter, too. But if you can't, or don't want to, barricade your whole yard, just corral your bird feeder. All you need is some 4-foot-high wire fencing and a few wood or metal stakes. Pound the stakes a few inches into the ground, about 4 feet out from the feeder pole, and wrap the fencing around them (this will be a snap,

because the stuff will naturally coil in a circle when you remove it from the roll). To close your corral, simply overlap the ends of the fencing. That way, you can easily get in or out. Oh, one more thing: For the sake of your skin, be sure to snip off any sharp ends of the wire!

Soak It to 'Em

What do most cats hate more than anything in the world? Getting wet—that's what! (If you've ever tried to give your own cat a bath, you've probably learned that the hard way.) So take advantage of that antiaquatic feeling by adding a squirt gun to your antikitty arsenal. Then when you see Fluffy approaching your feeder, take aim and give her a shower. There's just one drawback to this method: It only works when you're riding herd on your feeding friends. Once you've blasted a kitty once or twice, she'll realize that you're the source of the dreaded shower, and anytime you're not around, she'll mosey on up to the bird buffet.

Soak It to 'Em, Take II

Even water-loving animals don't like it one bit when the wet stuff comes at them in a sudden blast. That's the secret behind a newfangled device that uses a motion detector to aim water at any varmints that are gunnin' for your birds or their mess hall. It's not a cheap solution, but it *is* easy and effective. All you do is push a plastic stake into the ground, hook up a hose to the outlet, and attach the battery-powered sensor. When any invader wanders into its sights (so to speak), the gadget lets loose with a short burst of water. Then it turns itself off, and resets to wait for the next invasion. A range of sensitivity settings lets you adjust the "fire" power to the size of the animal—so you can say "*sayonara*" to every size trespasser from chipmunks to deer.

Fan-Tastic!

Next to a blast of water, the thing that makes most feeder-robbing animals flee fastest is a sudden whoosh of air. So, just gather up all the fans you can beg, borrow, or buy, and set them in place around your feeders. (Be sure to use outdoor-grade extension cords.) Then just before you go to bed, turn 'em all on. The critters will hightail it for calmer pastures. Repeat this trick every night for a week or two. Your pest problems will be history—at least until a new bunch of foragers moves into the neighborhood!

Give Hawks the Heave-Ho

These majestic birds may be awe-inspiring to watch in the wild, but you sure don't want them gobbling up the invited guests in your yard. If you live where hawks only wander by every now and then, plant hemlocks, spruces, or other dense evergreens close to your feeder. That way, your little pals can make a fast dive for shelter when the need arises. But if a hawk begins a daily patrol, or perches frequently near your feeders, do your birds a favor and remove temptation—for both parties. Take down your feeders so that the songbirds disperse, and the predator will go a-hunting elsewhere. Once you're sure the coast is clear, you can reopen your restaurant, and before you know it, you'll have a capacity crowd again.

FAST FORMULA

Hot-Pepper Spray

This fiery condiment couldn't be simpler to make, but it's one of the most effective ways I know of to make seed stealers scurry in a hurry. (Don't worry—it won't harm the birds. They have no receptors in their brains for spicy flavors, so they can't even taste the pepper!)

$1/2$ cup of dried cayenne peppers
$1/2$ cup of jalapeño peppers
1 gal. of water

Add the peppers to the water, bring it to a boil, and let it simmer for half an hour. (Make sure you keep the pan covered, or the peppery steam will make you cry a river of tears!) Let the mixture cool, then strain out the solids, and pour the liquid into a handheld sprayer. Pour a shallow layer of seeds into an open tray feeder, and spray them lightly, but thoroughly. When they're dry, set them out. The pests will take one nibble—and rush off for cooler dining options.

Index

A

Acid rain, 91
Acne and blemishes, 217–219
Acrylic, 47
Acupressure, 172
Acupuncture, 131, 181, 184
Addresses, travel and, 109–110
Adrenal glands, 153, 172, 173
Aeration, 261, 265
Aftershave, alternative, 220
After Warranty Assistance
   (AWA), 88
Age-related macular
   degeneration (AMD), 120,
   146, 197–199
Age spots, 221
Aging. *See* Eye health; Hair
   loss; Hearing loss; Memory
   and mental acuity; Oral
   hygiene
Air bags, 94
Air conditioners, 42, 59–62
Air fresheners, 92, 184
Air leaks, in home, 50–53
Air travel, 101–104
Alaskan cruises, 106
Alcohol (distilled), 175,
   185–186
Alcohol (rubbing), 212, 270,
   310, 311
Alfalfa, 211–212
Allergies
   in pets, 15–16
   rashes from, 223, 224
   superfoods for, 147–148,
     151
   trees and shrubs and, 274
Alliums, ornamental, 290
Allowances, for children, 9–10
All-Purpose Pest-Prevention
   Potion, 289
All-Season Clean-Up Tonic, 265
All-Season Green-Up Tonic, 256

Allspice, 210
Aloe vera, 224, 225, 228, 242, 252
Alterations, 30
Aluminum foil, 91
American Automobile
   Association (AAA), 117
American Automobile Touring
   Alliance (AATA), 117
American Kennel Club, 103
American Medical Association
   (AMA), 191
Ammonia
   for cleaning, 63
   in cleaning formulas, 37,
     40
   in compost formula, 325
   in fertilizer formulas, 254,
     256, 262, 267, 283, 308,
     316, 337
   for insect bites, 239
   for lawns, 254, 255
   for pest control, 268, 311
   in pest-control formula,
     289
   in planting formula, 304
Analgesics, 134, 252
Anemia, 140, 144
Angina, 149
Animal pests. *See* Pest control
Annual flowers, 299, 300–301,
   307
Annual weeds, 269–270
Antibiotic ointment, 244
Antidepressants, 183
Antihistamines, 227, 246
Antioxidants, 196, 218, 242–243,
   251. *See also specific*
   vitamins
Ants, 238–239, 285, 332
Anxiety, 125–126
Aphids, 285, 332
Apple juice, 255
Apples
   for bad breath, 210

buying, 24
   recipes using, 159, 164, 168
   in skin-care formula, 219
   as superfood, 150–152
Applesauce, 151, 164
Appliances. *See also specific*
   appliances
   buying, 36–42
   cleaning, 40
   moving, 39
   owner's manuals for, 43
   vacations and, 67
Arginine, 153
Armyworms, 263
Arnica, 124, 130
Aromatherapy, 123, 174, 184
Arthritis, 122, 129–133, 151
Articulation agreements, 10
Asparagus beetles, 332
Aspirin, 134, 190, 223, 224, 252
Asthma, 122, 140, 145
ATM cards, 115
Avocados
   for hair care, 215, 220–221
   recipes using, 161, 166
   for skin care, 221
   as superfood, 152
Azaleas, 281

B

Baby gates, 71
Baby oil, 219
Baby powder, 288
Baby shampoo
   in garden formulas, 254,
     278, 299, 304, 325
   for lawns, 255, 267
Baby wipe containers, 74, 81
Baby wipes, 91, 92
Bacillus thuringiensis, 263, 264,
   330
Back pain, 132–134, 153

F